PRAISE FOR *WHAT'S*

"As a proponent of a holistic, personalized and preventative approach to medical care for over 30 years, it is clear to me that good health and disease prevention comes down to essentially living a balanced life and eating healthily. This well-thought-out book is an excellent guide to using diet and lifestyle choices to improve health outcomes. Every reader will benefit from the natural health principles, practical tips, and nutritious recipes presented here."
– **Jan Rydfors, MD, physician, author, and Assistant Clinical Professor at Stanford Medical Center**

"This book is a wonderful introduction to Chinese medicine and using natural healing principles to nourish the mind, body, and spirit. By following the seasonal principles and nutritious recipes, readers will be able to connect to nature's rhythms, align with the seasons, and learn how to truly thrive."
– **Jill Blakeway, LAc, DACM, Founder and Director of The YinOva Center, author, and host of CBS Radio's "Grow. Cook. Heal."**

"*What's Your Season?* is a well-thought-out presentation of the seasonal aspect of ancient Chinese healing wisdom combined with a plethora of new and refreshing food and lifestyle strategies. This highly useful and unique text has its theory grounded with delectable recipes and wholesome ingredients to match virtually every shade of appetite and health requirement."
– **Paul Pitchford, author of *Healing with Whole Foods: Asian Traditions and Modern Nutrition***

"I believe that all healing starts with Optimum Health and I start with a holistic approach to treating infertility in my IVF practice. *What's Your Season?* contains exactly the kind of information that will yield both short-term and long-term success. Although this book's unique approach to diet and lifestyle draws from the oldest medicine in the world, it is totally relevant today and will leave you feeling newly inspired."
– **Christo Zouves, MD, physician and author**

"A wonderful introduction to the principles of Traditional Chinese medicine, nutrition and vibrant living. Simple recipes that are easy to include in your life while being aware and conscious of current environmental concerns. An excellent addition to any conscious cook's collection."
– April Crowell, CHN, Dipl ABT, holistic nutritionist and Asian medicine therapist

"In this helpful and easy-to-understand guide, readers will find a holistic outlook that combines natural healing traditions with modern research. I will be recommending this book to my patients, colleagues, and anyone interested in alternative medicine therapies."
– Richard Antosek, DO, FACOS, physician

"Optimal health is dependent upon the balance of *yin* and *yang*. By merging timeless traditions from the East with scientifically proven ideas from the West, this book teaches you how to live in the balance and find the foods and activities that are right for your individual body and health condition."
– Philip Yang, OMD, acupuncturist, *qi gong* master, president of Nine Star University acupuncture college

"*What's Your Season?* is a fascinating and comprehensive guide to living seasonally for better health. The authors make it easy to understand the basics of Chinese medicine, offering specific exercises, health recommendations, and nutritious recipes for the different seasons. I would recommend this book to my patients and anyone interested in a natural lifestyle and a holistic approach that is attuned to nature."
– Brittany Petrick, LAc, MSOM, BSN, acupuncturist and nutritional consultant

"A new fusion of ancient and modern wisdom, *What's Your Season?* teaches an intuitive way to balance your health with the seasons as a guide. The approachable, multicultural recipes in this beautiful volume are sure to inspire!"
– Nishanga Bliss, DSc, LAc, professor, Acupuncture and Integrative Medicine College, and author of *Real Food All Year: Eating Seasonal Whole Foods for Optimal Health and All-Day Energy*

WHAT'S YOUR
SEASON?

Healing Principles and Recipes for Your Body Type

Brielle Kelly, Cherisse Godwin, and Kristy Hsiao

KELSIN ☘ PRESS

San Carlos, California

Kelsin Press
San Carlos, CA
www.kelsinpress.com

Cover design, book design, and art direction by
Gary Tooth / Empire Design Studio

Edited by Tom Pold

Illustrations by Narda Lebo

Photographs by Cherisse Godwin and Kristy Hsiao except as noted below

Shutterstock: Cover logoboom, Natasha Breen, yspbqh14, karelnoppe; page 118 Pinkyone

Creative Market: page vi Antonina Vlasova; page viii A_B_C; pages x, 60, 116 Foxys; page 1 Candid Hams Creatives; page 108 Ffforn studio; page 113 Smith Chetanachan; page 114 Zia Shusha; page 121 Zhekos; page 126 Boulevard de la Photo; page 131 Alexander62; page 133 etorres69; page 134 villorejo; page 140 Hello Goodbye Studio; page 142 EkaterinaPlanina; page 143 Phots; page 208 Zigzag Mountain Art; page 240 Kawizen

iStockphoto: page 182 maxsol7

Publisher's Cataloging-In-Publication Data

Names: Kelly, Brielle. | Godwin, Cherisse. | Hsiao, Kristy.

Title: What's your season? : healing principles and
    recipes for your body type / Brielle Kelly, L.Ac., Dipl.O.M.,
    Cherisse Godwin, and Kristy Hsiao.

Description: San Carlos, California : Kelsin Press, [2018] |
    Includes bibliographical references and index.

Identifiers: ISBN 9780999311417 (hardcover) | ISBN
    9780999311424 (paperback) | ISBN 9780999311431 (ebook)

Subjects: LCSH: Holistic medicine. | Seasons--Health aspects.
    | Somatotypes--Health aspects. | Medicine, Chinese.
    | Seasonal cooking. | Biological rhythms. | LCGFT:
    Cookbooks.

Classification: LCC R733 .K45 2018 (print) | LCC R733 (ebook)
    | DDC 615.5--dc23

Library of Congress Control Number: 2017959854

Printed in the United States of America

10 9 8 7 6 5 4 3 2 1

*To all those in search of vitality and wellness,
through all the seasons of life.*

Contents

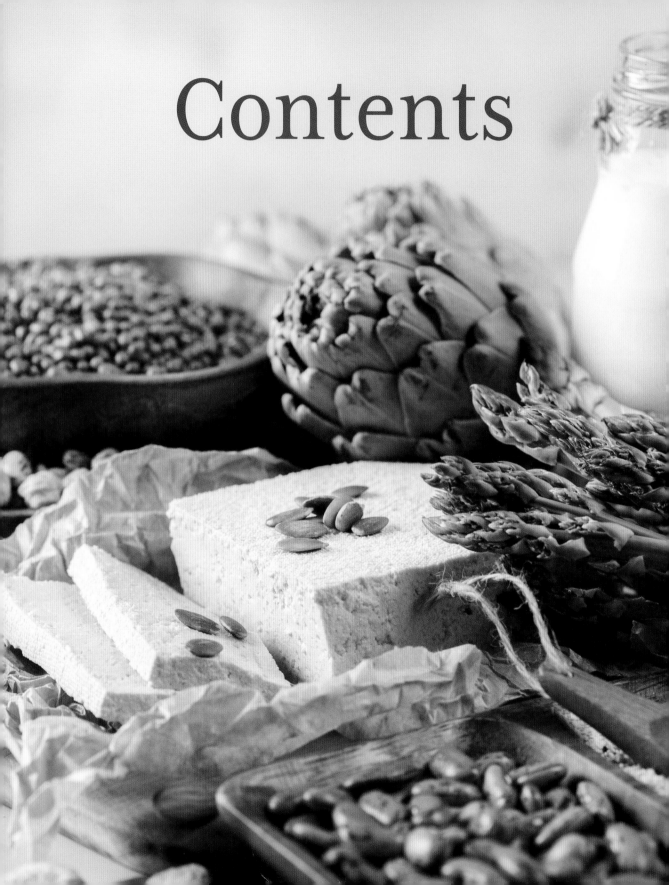

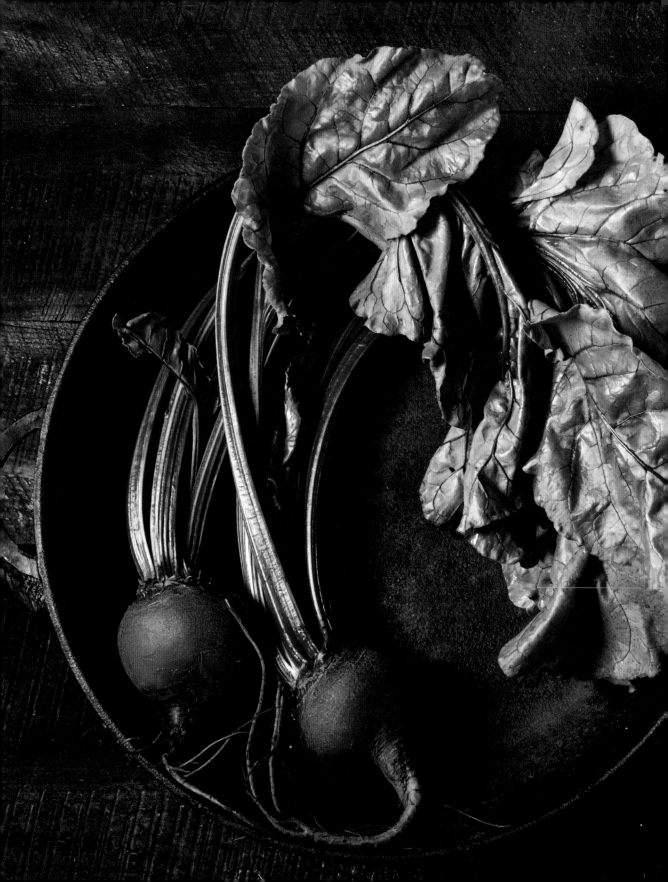

Introduction

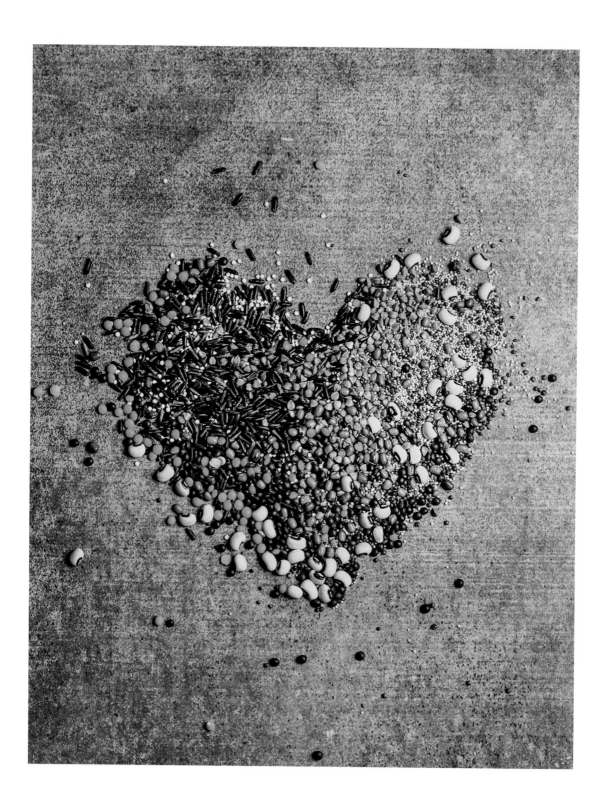

Introduction

The goal of this book is to present an individualized approach to eating and living for optimal health. It disabuses the notion that one diet fits all, and instead recognizes that each of us has a unique body type and our own specific requirements for good health. Using nature as a model for the ideal life, this book compares our body types to the seasons and prescribes a natural solution for restoring health and preventing disease. It helps us to identify our seasonal body types, understand our individual tendencies and needs, and discover the dietary practices, activities, and lifestyle choices that best support our well-being.

The longing for good health is universal. Each of our lives has been touched in some way by illness or pain; even if we have not experienced ill health personally, we know of someone who has suffered from chronic disease, such as diabetes, heart disease, or cancer. But what does living in good health mean exactly? For us, it means living our best lives and feeling our best, within our own individual potential, body types, and circumstances. Regardless of what our life paths entail, it is possible to find a way to feel good and live with joy, vitality, and energetic connection.

This book was born out of our desire to re-conceptualize what it means to live in good health and empower ourselves to create our own paths to wellness. As an alternative medicine practitioner and two culinary professionals, we are intimately familiar with the relationship between diet, exercise, and mental and physical health. Brielle is a licensed acupuncturist with a private practice in the San Francisco Bay Area. She applies an integrative approach to treating her patients, one which combines her scientific background in biomedicine and clinical nutrition with holistic therapies drawn from Traditional Chinese Medicine (TCM). Brielle believes that the best way to promote health is to use gentle, non-invasive treatments to support the body's inherent ability to heal itself. Cherisse is a culinary school graduate with professional cooking experience in both corporate and fine dining settings. She has worked with Hawaiian community organizations on outreach programs that address healthy eating and disease prevention. Having studied both whole foods nutrition and sports medicine, Cherisse takes a multi-disciplinary approach to health and wellness. Kristy has an educational background in science and the culinary arts, and has worked in the restaurant and food retail industries. She emphasizes high-quality, seasonal ingredients in her cooking, believing that foods are more flavorful when they are prepared simply and not masked by additional ingredients. Her interest in using food as medicine has led her to focus on ancient healing traditions and dietary therapies from the East.

Our approach is an alternative to quick fixes and silver bullets. It does not provide the cure for cancer or a miraculous weight loss solution. Instead, it offers perspectives on diet, health, and wellness, which are rooted in tradition, experience, intuition, and ultimately, our natural environment. In a time of rapid growth, technological advancement, and a relentless drive toward increased productivity, this book suggests a return to basics, a slowing down, and a restoration of balance. It suggests taking the long view: focusing on moderation over extremes, proactively preventing disease rather than reacting to it, nourishing the body instead of depriving it, and finding sustainable lifestyle choices that promote long-term health. What this book proposes is a return to a mindful and present life, one which is informed by nature's rhythms and lived in full awareness and accordance with its never-ending cycles.

Nature is our most ubiquitous teacher. It offers us a view of life as a constant process of renewal, from birth and growth to decline and death, and to rebirth once more. It is a study in contrasts, fluidly moving between light and dark, warm and cool, dry and wet, and expansion and contraction. Within nature's cycles, the only enduring constant is change. With each rising and setting of the sun, each ocean tide that rolls in and out, and each tectonic plate shift deep within the Earth's core, nature is continuously transforming and adjusting, balancing and re-balancing. Nature's lessons illustrate how we ourselves are meant to thrive: by navigating and embracing the change that is intrinsic to all life, and finding balance through it all.

The idea that nature should serve as a model for the ideal life is fundamental to Taoist philosophy and by extension, Traditional Chinese Medicine (TCM). Originating thousands of years ago, TCM is a medical system that views health in terms of natural elements and phenomena, the harmony of *yin* and *yang**, and the cyclical flow of energy known as *qi*. It is a holistic medicine that recognizes our fundamental connection to the universe which surrounds us and is embodied within us. And it is a form of

---

*Yin and *yang* are complementary and opposing forces, commonly represented by darkness and light. In TCM theory, the balance of *yin* and *yang* is necessary for good health, while the imbalance of the two leads to disease.

medicine that focuses on an individual's unique constitution and overall health, rather than just treating a disease alone. The goal of this book is to introduce an Eastern sensibility to modern lifestyles and to offer a complementary perspective for health and healing in the West. If the West is characterized by tangibility, a rapid pace, and a fiery hot *yang*, then the ideal counterpoint and complement lies within the ethereal, cool, and peaceful *yin* of the East. Both styles have their advantages and disadvantages. The most comprehensive approach to healthy living lies in the integration of the two, the merging of timeless traditions with modern science, and the balance of *yin* and *yang*.

When we adopt a truly holistic view of our lives and our health, it becomes clear that we as individuals are not only connected to each other, but to all living beings, to the energies that surround us, and to the greater collective whole. We are an extension and a product of our environment; as nature goes, so do we. Our bodies display the same qualities and variable phases that are observed in our natural environment. At times we may be hot, dry, or prone to feverish activity; at others, we can feel cold, damp, sluggish, or withdrawn. This book introduces the concept of a seasonal body type, relating our constitutions, health symptoms, physical characteristics, and personality traits to five different seasons: Spring, Summer, Indian Summer*, Fall, and Winter. It offers an approach for categorizing and understanding our health patterns in terms of universal phenomena and the fundamental laws that govern their balance.

The seasonal body type represents an imbalanced health pattern, one in which the body displays the same symptoms and characteristics throughout the year, rather than changing as the seasons do. The Summer body type, for instance, chronically embodies the characteristics of the summer season; he or she is often warm, red-faced, energetic, and talkative, regardless of the situation or circumstance. Physiologically, the Summer body type may also have health conditions like high blood pressure or diabetes. The Winter body type, on the other hand, always feels cold, even when others do not; he or she may have a pale complexion and a slow, quiet demeanor, and may experience infertility or low thyroid function. Most of us live with some kind of pathology or health pattern that defines what our seasonal body type is. We are figuratively "stuck" in one characteristic seasonal pattern throughout the year, continuously displaying the warmth or cold, the wetness or dryness, or the *yin* or *yang* found in one of nature's seasons.

This book suggests that when we live in optimal health, our bodies should move effortlessly along with nature and exhibit the characteristics of each of the five seasons throughout the year. Our ideal bodies are not chronically warm or cool, excessively damp or dry, nor are they imbalanced in *yin* or *yang*. Instead of being identifiable as a singular seasonal body type, ideally we should all experience, embody, and live along with each of nature's seasons. When our bodies are balanced and functioning efficiently, we possess a natural inclination to live and eat seasonally. In the warmer months, we tend to be more active and energetic, and our bodies inherently crave a lighter, more cleansing diet. In the cooler seasons of the year, we begin to slow down and retract, and we desire more warming and hearty

---

*Although Indian summer is not one of the four main seasons, for some regions it marks the period of time in which the climate fluctuates between long, warm summer days and the cool chill of fall.

foods, which build and store energy. The ideal body is neutral and adaptable to its surroundings. It follows nature's lead, aligns with its seasons, and fluidly transitions with its phases.

In order to restore the body to its natural state of health, we look to our environment to provide the cues, foods, and examples for how best to live within each season and heal each seasonal body type. For example, those with Spring body types benefit most from eating the leafy greens and tender shoots that nature offers in the spring and that symbolize the renewal of the season. For people with Summer body types, who have a tendency toward chronic heartburn, heat-related symptoms, and excess activity, the juicy fruits and vegetables available in the summer season help to cool, calm, and refresh the body. Indian Summer body types are characterized by a need for grounding energy which comes in the form of seasonal squashes and naturally sweet foods. Fall body types, who often feel sluggish and cold, benefit from the fall season's drying grains and pungent spices, which help to warm and invigorate the body. And finally, for the cold and reserved Winter body types, the winter season's root vegetables and rich, warming foods are most beneficial.

The Seasonal Body Type System presents a time-honored paradigm for health, one that encourages us to live seasonally and align ourselves with nature. The first section of this book begins by laying down a foundation for holistic health, providing background information on TCM, diet, exercise, the mind-body connection, and environmental influences. Readers who are already familiar with the general components of health may want to skip ahead to Part II, which focuses on a more individualized approach to health and the seasonal body type system. Through the use of a diagnostic checklist and seasonal profiles, the second section of the book helps us to identify what our "season" or seasonal body type is. It allows us to determine the season in which we are characteristically stuck, and provides a comprehensive set of dietary recommendations, recipes, activities, and suggested therapies for healing and re-balancing our body type.

For readers who are looking for information on healthy foods and seasonal eating, Part III describes the healing properties of a variety of whole foods and offers recipes which highlight the foods and themes of each of the five seasons. The recipes are designed to balance the seasonal body types, as well as support our individual progression through the seasons. Readers should begin by eating the foods and utilizing the recipes recommended for their individual body type; for example, Summer body types should eat from the Summer recipes and Winter body types should eat from the Winter recipes. After our bodies become more balanced and neutral, and we no longer exhibit the characteristics of one singular body type, we should cycle through the recipes and eat along with each of the five seasons, in accordance with nature's offerings throughout the year.

By identifying our seasonal body types and understanding our individual health patterns within the Seasonal Body Type framework, we can begin to embrace lifestyle choices that best serve our needs and gently guide ourselves back toward alignment with nature. In Brielle's health-care practice, her patients often ask her what kind of food they should eat in order to supplement their treatment. Although diet is an integral part of our lives and many of us take enjoyment and pleasure from the foods that we eat, a holistic approach to health must go beyond diet alone. Well-being relies on a multitude of factors, from our genetic makeup and constitution, to the foods that we eat, the physical activities that we perform, our environmental influences, and perhaps most importantly, the thoughts that we hold within our minds. Our mental perspectives, attitudes, intentions, and beliefs regarding ourselves and our health define our individual experiences on a daily basis. Making the commitment and choice to nourish our bodies and help ourselves succeed requires clarity of thought and mind. It requires us to quiet the judgment that comes with our ever-present attention to self and to honor what our bodies intrinsically know: how to be well.

As we deepen our self-awareness and develop a broader perspective of the world and our place within it, we recognize that the answers to good health are all around us. They are embodied in nature's cycles and universal rhythms, in its flexibility and resilience, and in its infinite and ever-lasting existence. Nature provides the insight, inspiration, and wisdom that we long for. This book proposes that one's best life is a seasonal life; optimal health lies in the fundamental ability to adapt to the seasons of change. When we are able to take the path of least resistance, to flow and yield like water, and to let nature run its full and variable course, that is when we know a life of ease, well-being, and balance. Regardless of our circumstances or the challenges that we may encounter, each one of our lives holds the promise of energy and vitality, and each one of us can learn to flourish and thrive in any season.

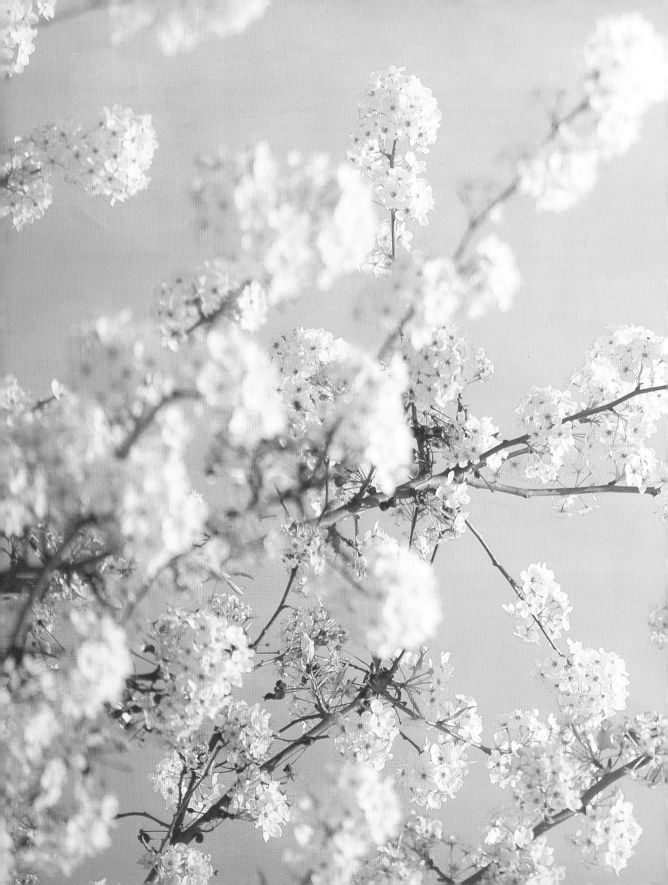

Part I

To Your Health

Chapter 1
East and West: tradition meets science

EAST MEETS WEST

The technological advances of the Information Age have dis-integrated the boundaries between the world's countries and cultures. The advent of the Internet and the rise of social media have made it easier than ever to exchange knowledge, search for information, and increase awareness of cultural ideas ranging from foods and spirituality to technology and health. Even the most seemingly disparate ideologies, like traditional Eastern philosophy and modern Western science, have begun to blend together. The integration of Eastern and Western medicine is a perfect example of how today's world merges information and in so doing improves our knowledge base.

Western medicine has begun to move eastward; for over fifty years, the health-care system in China has utilized a combination of both Western medicine and Traditional Chinese Medicine (TCM).[1] With roots over two thousand years old, TCM is a collective system of therapies that includes acupuncture, herbal medicine, acupressure, massage, and moxibustion (burning the dried mugwort herb known as moxa). In China, the majority of physicians are trained in Western medicine; however all medical students also receive some training in TCM and most hospitals offer both Western and TCM treatment options.[1,2]

At the same time, the West has begun to embrace the medicine of the East, as evidenced by the growing number of medical schools that teach curricula on acupuncture and holistic therapies. This push toward inclusion is in response to the surge of alternative medicine users in the United States.[3] With TCM at the forefront of this development, it seems that contemporary medicine is returning to a healing tradition that was established in the ancient texts and philosophies of the East. An Eastern approach to health may be the ideal choice to complement the strengths of Western medicine, while filling in the gaps and pitfalls of modern science.

Western medicine takes a molecular and mechanistic view of health. The body is divided into organs, tissues, and cells, and its functions are defined in a structured, quantitative manner. Utilizing a linear approach, the Western scientific method looks for a direct one-to-one relationship between cause and effect. Eastern medicine, on the other hand, employs a holistic view of the body, with no separation between mind, body, and spirit. Its qualitative perspective seeks to balance the body's energy systems and recognizes the complex interaction of multiple variables affecting health.

In the Western view, disease is a direct result of pathogenic factors. Its linear, causative model looks at present physical symptoms, their direct causes, and their subsequent remedies. Illness is only acknowledged in its final stage of manifestation; its symptoms are treated in a systematic, generalized way, largely irrespective of the patient. Within the macrocosmic view of TCM, however, disease is a process instead of an endpoint. TCM treats the whole individual as opposed to just the disease, acknowledging the subtle differences that exist between each patient. Consequently, TCM may attribute different causes to the same symptoms in different individuals. For example, five different patients with migraine headaches may require five different approaches to treatment. Each treatment is unique because TCM insists that the symptom (pounding headache) is the result of the disease, not the disease itself. Whether the migraine is due to hormonal changes, sensory stimuli, psychological stressors, consumption of monosodium glutamate (MSG), or dehydration, the symptom is addressed with a thoughtful consideration of all concomitant variables.

TCM focuses on the individual patient and treats the disease's underlying cause rather than its superficial symptoms. It suggests that instead of only treating the pain of a migraine headache, there may be a precursor in the disease process that deserves attention first. Treating disease is similar to weeding a garden; unless the roots are pulled and discarded, the weeds will survive and are likely to return stronger than ever. To achieve full disease prevention, TCM addresses the subtle, energetic precursors of disease and considers the non-physical influence of mind and spirit. Without this holistic view, there is little foreknowledge as to where the body is headed until it is too late.

This is not to say that modern Western medicine should go unheralded. Emergency treatment in the West is unparalleled, offering successful options for life-threatening injuries, illnesses, and other trauma. A mechanical perspective of the body lends itself well to surgical procedures like removing diseased organs or tumors. In addition, when the scientific advances made by Western medicine do work, they tend to work quickly; the drug penicillin saves hundreds of people from life-threatening bacterial infections every day. The powerful, fast-acting nature of Western medicine makes it ideal for acute conditions, but can also lead to unwanted side effects. The search for a singular cause of disease leads to a prescription for a singular intervention, or a magic pill. While an objective, scientific approach makes medicine for the masses, it also neglects the differences that distinguish us as individuals. As a result, iatrogenic disease (disease that is induced by medical treatment) is common, and medications come with warnings about side effects that have been observed, the causes of which are not well-understood.

*The part can never be well unless
the whole is well.*

–Plato

TCM treatments, in contrast, work slowly and are considered gentle on the body. Like other complementary and alternative therapies, TCM encourages the body to overcome illness on its own, through the application of minimally invasive techniques. It acknowledges the body's intrinsic capacity to heal itself and return to a state of homeostasis.[4] In addition, its medicinal herbs are used in their whole, natural forms, a contrast to pharmaceutical components and chemicals that are purified or synthesized in a laboratory. Because they use whole herbs, TCM formulas contain their own natural checks and balances, thereby minimizing side effects.[5] In their traditional application, herbal formulas are steeped for hours and ingested as a tea over a period of months; their effects tend to be more gradual than conventional pharmaceuticals. While TCM's mild nature may render it ineffective in emergency situations, it can be an ideal choice for the treatment of chronic illness and the long-term prevention of disease.

Because TCM utilizes slow-acting and long-term treatments, its efficacy as a medical system is difficult to study. Recovery times may take months or years, complicating the design and accuracy of clinical trials. Although TCM has been developed through thousands of years of empirical evidence, scientific validation is required before complete acceptance is achieved in the West. So, how does one prove the effectiveness and accuracy of TCM? In recent years, double-blind studies have validated the use of several herbal medicines. However, for acupuncture and other TCM treatments which do not have a suitable placebo, the double-blind standard is more difficult to establish.[6] Although the specific mechanisms behind TCM are not yet understood, the number of research studies demonstrating its efficacy in treating certain conditions suggests that it could play a complementary role to modern Western medicine.[7,8,9]

With their unique perspectives and methodologies, both Western and Eastern medicine bring value to health care. Both systems have their own drawbacks and merits, and they serve us best when combined together. An example of a medical treatment which integrates the practices of both East and West can be seen in a cancer patient who receives radiation and chemotherapy, while also being given herbal formulas to manage side effects and boost his or her immune system. As the nation's population grows older and the rate of chronic disease rises, a health-care system that emphasizes prevention and ensures longevity is essential.

THE ABC'S OF TCM

Before the written dissemination of information was widespread, knowledge was transmitted and verified through verbal claims and anecdotes. Given that TCM began some two thousand years ago, much of what we know today is based on oral traditions. With the arrival of written documentation around 200 BC came the publication of *Huang Di Nei Jing*, often translated as *Yellow Emperor's Classic of Internal Medicine* or *Yellow Emperor's Inner Canon*, the earliest extant record of one of the oldest forms of medicine in the world. Written as a series of questions and answers between the Yellow Emperor, *Huang Di*, and his teacher, *Qi Bo*, the book outlines the foundations and principles of TCM as we know them today. It also debunks the belief that supernatural forces control health and disease and instead cites the natural effects of diet, lifestyle, emotions, environment, and age as the reasons that diseases develop. Health, it suggests, depends on the preservation of harmony within the body, as well as harmony between the body and its environment.

The influence of nature is evident throughout the teachings of TCM. The human life cycle of birth and death echoes the flourishing and decline seen in nature: floods follow drought, cloudy skies clear for the sun, and wind-blown seeds offer a chance for new growth in once-barren soil. The *Inner Canon* postulates that the body is a microcosmic version of what we see in nature and spoke simply of aligning the body with nature in order to achieve optimal health. As the Earth cycles through the seasons, our bodies must follow suit.

With its strong emphasis on the natural world, the *Inner Canon* can also be considered a book about Taoism. The word "*tao*" is translated as "path" or "doctrine," and the theology that carries its name is more a philosophy about the ideal way of life than an organized religion. The way of the *tao* promotes naturalness, vitality, peace, receptiveness, and most of all, spontaneity. Being open to the influence of all points of view, the Taoist view is not rigid in its consideration of one perspective over another. This peaceful flexibility is infused throughout TCM and is perhaps the idea that most clearly distinguishes Eastern medicine from its Western counterpart's fixed and linear theories. Essentially, Taoism is what helps to make TCM a holistic medicine.

Classical Taoist texts emphasize the importance of harmonizing one's spiritual nature with one's physical body and surroundings. When we are aligned with our environment, there is no separation between ourselves and the cosmic whole. TCM's Taoist roots suggest that we reconnect with the natural world by spending time outdoors, climbing a majestic mountain, exercising under a shady tree, or simply taking a walk. Being in nature allows us to strengthen our connection to a power that is greater than our own and restore our connection to our true selves. When we are able to silence the stimuli of an artificial world, we can more easily attune to our deepest spiritual instincts and inner knowing.

The natural world also highlights the importance of using checks and balances. For example, when forest growth becomes too dense, wildfires clear out dead or decaying vegetation from the forest floor. When excess pressure builds up in the Earth's tectonic plates, the energy is released through earthquakes and tremors. TCM suggests that as human beings, we must also be careful to balance our lives by avoiding extremes and their often severe consequences. Just as a ship that is evenly weighted from bow to stern does not tip in rocky seas, a body that is balanced can adapt easily in the midst of chaos and live in great health and fortitude.

> *Humans model themselves on earth,*
> *Earth on heaven, Heaven on the Way,*
> *And the way on that which is naturally so.*
>
> – Lao Zi

WHAT IS *QI*?

Qi (pronounced chee) has been called the breath of life, the universal life force, or most simply, energy. One of the fundamental concepts of TCM philosophy, it is similar to the *ki, prana, pneuma,* and *mana* found in other cultures. Intangible and ethereal, *qi* is not only the energy that creates matter, but matter itself. This paradoxical statement highlights the powerful, yet elusive nature of this infinite force. A hint to its true meaning comes from the etymology of its Chinese character; originally, the word *qi* was represented with the pictogram symbol for vapor or air, symbolizing the fundamental connection between breath and life. Both physical and non-physical, *qi* is the air that we breathe and the spirit that breathes through us. It is the cosmos; we are made from it and we live within it. The concept of *qi* is a non-dualistic one. It implies that there is no separation between body and mind, or between man and universe. This theme of unification is found throughout TCM and serves as the foundation for a holistic view toward health.

    Qi is thought to travel within twenty different energetic channels or meridians throughout the body. Just as rivers carry water, these channels carry *qi*, bringing nourishment and support for all of the body's functioning. However, just like nature's rivers, these meridians can run dry or they can rage and overflow their banks. Similar to a fallen tree lying across a river, energetic channels can also become blocked, leading to an imbalance of *qi*. TCM suggests that a disruption or blockage of *qi* within the body results in illness or disease. Over time, an imbalance of *qi* that remains unresolved will result in more severe problems and chronic disease. The goal of TCM treatment, then, is to restore health by reordering and focusing *qi* within the body, allowing it to flow smoothly through the body's meridians at all times.

    With its patient-specific approach, TCM seeks to tailor its diagnosis and treatment to the individual. Recognizing the variability between patients is important when discussing the two basic types of *qi*: congenital *qi* and acquired *qi*. Congenital *qi* refers to a *qi* that is present from birth and inherited directly from our parents. Acquired *qi* is gathered daily from our surrounding environment, including the air we breathe and the food and water we consume. One's *qi*, and therefore one's health, is individualized and specific to one's ancestry and lifestyle. TCM philosophy states that if *qi* can be properly cultivated and balanced, vitality and longevity will be ensured.

WHAT ARE YIN AND YANG?

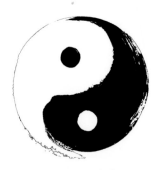

Taijitu symbol

The concept of non-duality also pervades TCM's ideas of *yin* and *yang*. In the *taijitu*, the familiar symbol shown here, *yin* is represented by the color black, and *yang* by the color white. Within each distinct area of black and white also lies a small circle of the opposite color; this suggests that within *yin* there is *yang*, as there is *yang* within *yin*. Each color is defined by a fluid region that transitions and blends into the other. Although black and white are distinct opposites, the *taijitu* symbol illustrates that *yin* and *yang* are both interdependent and coexistent, essentially representing a unified whole. Consequently, nothing is entirely *yin* or entirely *yang*.

The Chinese characters for *yin* and *yang* further demonstrate the relationship between the two. The symbol for *yin* depicts a hill covered by shadows, while the symbol for *yang* depicts a hill covered by sunlight. Although the sun sets on one side of a hill, it rises again to illuminate the other side; one event always occurs with the other. Like all opposites, *yin* and *yang* are defined by their relationship to each other and the contrast that lies between them. Without white there can be no black, and vice versa. The concepts of *yin* and *yang* are extensive and all-inclusive; every pair of opposites can be described in terms of *yin* or *yang*. Cold is *yin*, while hot is *yang*. Female is *yin*, while male is *yang*. The following table lists common associations used to describe the characteristics of *yin* and *yang*.

YIN	YANG
Black	*White*
Dark	*Light*
Moon	*Sun*
Female	*Male*
Cold	*Hot*
Decay	*Growth*
Winter	*Summer*
Soft	*Hard*
Slow	*Fast*
Earth	*Heaven*
Thought	*Action*
Internal	*External*

The characteristics of *yin* and *yang* can be seen throughout the natural world. First, *yin* and *yang* are direct opposites: the cool, tranquil evening (*yin*) provides respite from the hot, blazing sun (*yang*). Second, *yin* and *yang* coexist within each other: within the dormant seeds of winter (*yin*) lies the potential for the growth of summer (*yang*). Furthermore, *yin* and *yang* are interdependent: darkness (*yin*) is defined by the absence of light (*yang*), its opposing counterpart. As these examples illustrate, the concepts of *yin* and *yang* can be used to represent the unity, harmony, and constant change that are ever-present within nature.

Our modern lifestyles often lack this balance of *yin* and *yang*. New York City's Times Square on a Saturday night, for example, shows that some aspects of modern Western society exist in a severe *yang* state. With its flashing neon lights, stimulation as far as the eye can see, a cacophony of noise, and a myriad of wafting smells, *yang* is in full swing in the "city that never sleeps." *Yang* is everything that defines our overscheduled, over-achieving, over-fed, and under-rested lives. Without moments of silence or time for rest (*yin*), the intrinsic balance of *yin* and *yang* is absent; they do not coexist, nor do they interchange. Introducing Eastern philosophies into the Western lifestyle suggests that we slow down, embracing some *yin* activities while backing off from some *yang* ones. This can be accomplished simply by being still and making time to reflect, or by balancing the *yin* and *yang* aspects of the food we eat and the activities we perform. When *yin* and *yang* exist in complete harmony, the body and mind become more at ease, a state of being that inherently allows for the prevention of dis-ease.

A HOLISTIC FRAMEWORK FOR HEALTH

An integration of Eastern and Western thought represents a merging of experience and innovation, of tradition and science, and of *yin* and *yang*. Individually, each is distinct and valuable; unified together, they embody an even greater strength. To incorporate the *yin* style of the East in the *yang*-like West, we must recognize that we are part of a larger whole. Harmony within ourselves requires harmony with our surrounding environment. As nature cycles through its seasons, our lives also move through their own natural ebbs and flows. By following this external, macrocosmic design, we preserve the internal, microcosmic landscape of our own health and well-being.

A holistic approach to health involves the balance and fusion of mind, body, and spirit. In the chapters that follow, the quiet sensibility of the East will be introduced into all aspects of health, from diet and exercise to emotional awareness and environmental factors. With its unique ideas on Taoism, *yin*, *yang*, and *qi*, TCM offers a deeper understanding of the components of disease prevention. By incorporating these philosophies into our modern lifestyles, a prescription for optimal health can finally be written.

Chapter 2
You Are What You Eat

OUR DIET, OUR HEALTH

As the foundation of health, food supports and sustains life, fulfilling one of our most basic needs. At the same time, it is directly linked to the leading cause of death in the world, heart disease.[1] On one hand, it provides energy and nourishes the body; on the other, it can contribute to chronic illness and premature death. The contrasting nature of food can be seen in the wide array of food choices that are available to us. Our food can be as simple as a leaf of lettuce sprouting from the ground, or as complex as a stew that has been simmering on the stove for hours. It is a $2 cheeseburger eaten in a speeding car, or a $100 five-course meal savored in an extravagant restaurant. Food can be found in vast fields of wheat stretching as far as the eye can see, or concentrated in a box of fortified, sweetened breakfast cereal.

Food's dualistic nature is also exemplified in the relationship between nutrition and health. The concept of malnutrition was once the sole domain of undernutrition, hunger, and nutrient deficiency. Now it has also come to include overnutrition, excess consumption, and increasing rates of obesity, type 2 diabetes, and other diet-related diseases. Recently, the number of overweight people in the world has surpassed the number of underweight people.[2] Long considered to be a problem for only industrialized nations, overnutrition and obesity have quickly become prevalent in developing countries as well. According to the World Health Organization, over half of the world's diseases are attributable to the problems of undernutrition, overnutrition, and diet.[3]

> *Every time you eat or drink, you are either*
> *feeding disease or fighting it.*
> – Heather Morgan

One of the primary factors driving the worldwide rise in obesity has been the adoption of a Western diet and lifestyle.[4,5] As developing countries become more urbanized, traditional grain-based diets are abandoned for more cheaply manufactured and energy-dense foods rich in fats and sugars. An increased consumption of processed foods, inexpensive calories, refined oils, and animal-source foods is often accompanied by a decrease in physical activity and labor-intensive work; the resulting energy imbalance directly contributes to the problems of obesity and chronic disease.[6] Although modernization has led to great progress in food availability and diversity, it has also led to serious global health concerns. In terms of nutrition and health, packaged convenience foods are simply no substitute for fresh, whole, and unprocessed foods.

With the highest rates of obesity in the world, the United States has an estimated 64% of adults who are overweight and 30% who are obese.[7] Excess weight has been linked to an increased risk of chronic disease, disability, and death. In the U.S., diet plays a role in four of the top ten causes of death: cardiovascular disease, stroke, type 2 diabetes, and cancer.[1] Eating a Western diet that is high in fat, sugar, and salt also weighs on our economy. The U.S. Department of Agriculture (USDA) estimates the economic costs of health conditions attributed to diet to be at least $87 billion each year; this figure includes medical costs, lost productivity, and premature deaths related to diet.[8,9]

The effects of our dietary choices are not limited to our physical health. Several research studies have also demonstrated that certain foods can influence brain function and alter our emotional states, providing evidence that what we eat has an effect on how we feel.[10] Consumption of fish and omega-3 fatty acids, for example, has been associated with lower incidence of depression and bipolar disorder.[11] Many of us have firsthand experience with using foods to alter our mood states. We often crave comfort foods and sweet desserts when we are feeling down or low in energy. In fact, some research studies suggest that eating carbohydrates to elevate mood is a form of self-medication. Others propose that eliminating sugar and caffeine from the diet can reduce depression and emotional distress.[12] Although the mechanisms behind these food-mood interactions are not yet understood, it is clear that what we eat can impact our psychological well-being.

*The doctor of the future will no longer treat
the human frame with drugs, but rather will cure
and prevent disease with nutrition.*

– Thomas Edison

FOOD JOURNAL

*One way to increase awareness of the effects of different foods on your physical and emotional health is
to keep a food journal:*

» Record the details of your diet for one to two weeks. Include all meals, snacks, and drinks that
you consume.

» Take note of any physical or emotional symptoms that you experience, i.e. changes in energy
level, emotional moodiness, sleep quality, ability to focus, digestion, etc.

» What kinds of patterns do you notice? Do you feel tired after eating certain foods? Do you have
any headaches? What foods do you crave when you are feeling stressed?

» If you suspect that you have a food allergy or sensitivity, try eliminating that food from your diet
for two weeks. Then, gradually reintroduce it; do you notice any changes? Food intolerances are
commonly associated with refined sugars, wheat, caffeine, and dairy products.

IS THERE AN OPTIMAL DIET?

In our food-obsessed nation, there are countless magazines, websites, and 24-hour television channels
dedicated solely to food. Each year, Americans spend billions of dollars on diet books and weight-loss
products. We look to the latest nutrition studies to discover the health benefits of various foods and
nutrients, only to find out that the most recent research contradicts results that were published the year
before. Although there is an abundance of information on what we should eat, much of that information
is conflicting and confusing. For all of the nutrition research and scientific studies that have been
published over the last century, we have yet to discover the optimal, flawless diet.

Many of the problems with diet and nutrition research lie in the inherent nature of food and eating.
Because food generally has a long-term effect on health, there can be a significant lag time between the
consumption of a food and any measurable effects. While a drug like acetaminophen (commonly sold
as Tylenol) will have a noticeable effect on relieving a headache within a few hours, the same cannot
be said about a meal of lean protein, whole grains, and fresh vegetables, which may take weeks and
repeated consumption to show significant benefits. Additionally, different samples of the same food
may have different nutritional values, depending on where the food was grown or how it was prepared.

Subjectivity can also play a role in experimental outcomes; mental expectations and attitudes can influence how people perceive a food's taste and health benefits. Generally speaking, scientific studies tend to take a reductionist view of nutrition, attempting to single out the effects of specific vitamins and nutrients on health. By doing so, they ignore the fact that foods represent more than just the sum of their molecular components.

Establishing a single, linear cause and effect between diet and health has proven to be difficult, if not impossible. In an attempt to determine what foods are optimal for health and longevity, researchers have studied regional diets like the Mediterranean and Okinawan diets. While these studies have yielded useful information, their single population samples make them inadequate to be applied universally. One diet does not fit all. From genetic ancestry and environment to cultural customs and attitudes, the variations between how different people assimilate nutrients are just as important as what foods they choose to eat. Diet remains only one component in the myriad of factors that influence health.

The complex role of food in our lives extends beyond health alone; food and diet represent more than just basic nutrition and survival. Food unites us in cultural and social contexts, including daily family meals and festive celebrations. What we eat can define who we are; we may label ourselves "vegetarian," or "carnivore," or "foodie," or even a "chocoholic." Our attitudes toward food are important. Food can provide comfort and familiarity for some of us, while being a source of guilt and shame for others. The foods that we consume can also represent a connection to our Earth, community, and local resources. Each component of our food supply chain, from the land, plants, and animals to the people who harvest and produce our food, can have a direct effect on our lives. In order to fully understand the link between diet and health, we must recognize the variety of dietary influences that surround us and acknowledge our multi-faceted relationship with food.

A SENSIBLE APPROACH TO EATING

To many of us, the word "diet" implies a restriction of foods and calories to attain the often elusive goal of weight loss. From its original Latin and Greek roots though, the word originally meant one's "way of life," or "customary course of food." Diet should not be a daunting prospect or an exercise in self-deprivation; it merely represents what we choose to eat on a daily basis. As nourishment for the body, our diet should be a source of enjoyment and pleasure, instead of one of obsession and agony. It is the foundation of health, but it represents only one part of a holistic framework. By integrating dietary principles from both the East and West, a realistic and sensible approach to food and health can be developed. The following guidelines highlight this approach and reinforce food's ability to promote health.

TAKING A MACROCOSMIC VIEW

Diet represents a long-term investment in the prevention of disease. Through a slow and gradual process, the food choices that we make each day affect our future health and ultimately, our longevity. Because the effects of chronic diseases can take years to manifest, a focus on prevention remains the

YOU ARE WHAT YOU INGEST

While the foods you eat play an important role in your health, anything that you ingest can have an effect on your body.

» How do the things that you drink influence your health? Coffee, milk, juice, soft drinks, and water are all liquid forms of nourishment.

» Do you take any vitamins or herbal supplements on a regular basis? What are the ingredients in those supplements? How do you feel when you take them compared with when you don't take them?

» What kind of prescription or over-the-counter medications do you take? Do you notice any side effects? While medicine is used to support health, it can also have unintended consequences. For example, taking antibiotics not only destroys harmful bacteria, but also other microorganisms that benefit the digestive system.

key to enduring health. Taking a long-range and proactive perspective toward our diet suggests that foods should be eaten to nourish and sustain. The foods that we eat represent more than simple nutrients like carbohydrates, proteins, and fats; when combined with other health factors like exercise and the mind-body connection, they have the potential to enhance vitality and transform life.

LOOKING TO NATURE AS A GUIDE

Before a box of tube pasta and chalky orange powder masqueraded as food, our ancestors walked through aisles of farm crops and consumed fresh, natural, and healthful fruits and vegetables directly from the earth. In contrast, the convenience foods that are commonly found in the American diet today have been highly processed and are missing much of their original nutritional value, including micro-nutrients, dietary fiber, and protective phytochemicals.[13] The Industrial Revolution led to the creation of the modern food processing industry; food manufacturers began refining grains and processing foods in order to increase shelf life and prevent spoilage. Hardy brown grains like wheat and rice lost their nutrient-rich outer bran and germ layers, and were replaced with whiter, softer, and more palatable versions. Consumer preference for quick, tasty, convenient, and shelf-stable products has influenced dietary trends in the West. For example, instead of slowly cooking a pot of whole-grain oats over the stove, many of us would rather reach for a convenient box of breakfast cereal made from refined grains and sugars.

Ironically, most processed foods have also been enriched or fortified, in order to restore the original nutrients that were lost during processing. Other refined foods found on supermarket shelves contain long lists of unrecognizable ingredients, from preservatives and stabilizers to artificial colors and flavor additives. Many of these products tend to be high in fat or sugar, appealing to an innate human prefer-ence for energy-dense foods. While foods that are high in energy once represented a survival advantage in times of scarcity, today's increasingly sedentary lifestyles render them superfluous and they are now linked with rising rates of obesity and a decline in health.[14]

The ideal diet lies within nature and its seasonal variety of fruits, vegetables, and grains. A return to the traditional, plant-based diets of our ancestors allows us to enjoy nature's bounty and recall a simpler way of eating. Traditional food systems like the Mediterranean and Okinawan diets have evolved over generations. They are indigenous to a specific region and culture, emphasizing local, natural resources and time-honored methods of cultivating and producing food. Traditional diets also offer potential health benefits. While the adoption of a Western diet and lifestyle has been associated with chronic diseases like type 2 diabetes, hypertension, and stroke, traditional diets and lifestyle patterns have been shown to be protective against these health conditions.[15] Key components of indigenous diets include fresh, local, and seasonal foods, whole and unprocessed foods, small quantities of naturally raised meat and dairy products, fats from plant sources, minimally processed oils, fermented and pickled foods, and healing spices.[16]

Generally speaking, traditional diets emphasize whole and unprocessed plant-source foods that are rich in fiber and nutrients, while minimizing foods that are high in salt, fat, and refined sugars. In other words, these diets tend to be nutrient-rich and calorie-limited, whereas modern diets can be described as nutrient-poor and calorie-dense.[15] Adopting a whole foods diet encourages us to eat a single orange, fiber and all, instead of drinking from a carton of concentrated, pulp-free orange juice that has been manufactured from dozens of oranges. By eating foods in their whole, unadulterated, and natural forms, we respect the gifts that nature offers us and also show an appreciation for where they come from.

Tell me what you eat and I'll tell you what you are.

– Jean Anthelme Brillat-Savarin

OPTIMIZING *QI*

From an Eastern perspective, a food's *qi* is representative of its energy and vitality. Just as foods gather *qi* from the sun, water, air, and soil in which they are grown, our bodies directly absorb *qi* from the foods and drinks that we consume. The essence of a food's *qi* can be sensed simply by tasting, feeling, or looking at the food. For example, the vibrant green color of crisp, freshly steamed broccoli offers a sharp contrast to a limp, gray version that has been sitting on a cafeteria line for hours. Consisting of more than just minerals and vitamins, foods represent the essence and life force of their origin and environment.

Since a food's *qi* is directly related to its freshness, fruits and vegetables that have been picked and consumed at their peak offer the highest quality of *qi*. As foods are transported between the earth and the table, they begin to spoil and lose their vibrancy. Consequently, seasonal and locally grown produce provides a fresher, more vital alternative to processed foods that have indefinite shelf lives. Genetic modification and the use of pesticides, antibiotics, and hormones may also have intangible effects on a food's quality.[17,18] Similarly, the living conditions of animals being raised for food are important.

FROM THE EARTH TO THE TABLE – CEREAL PRODUCTION

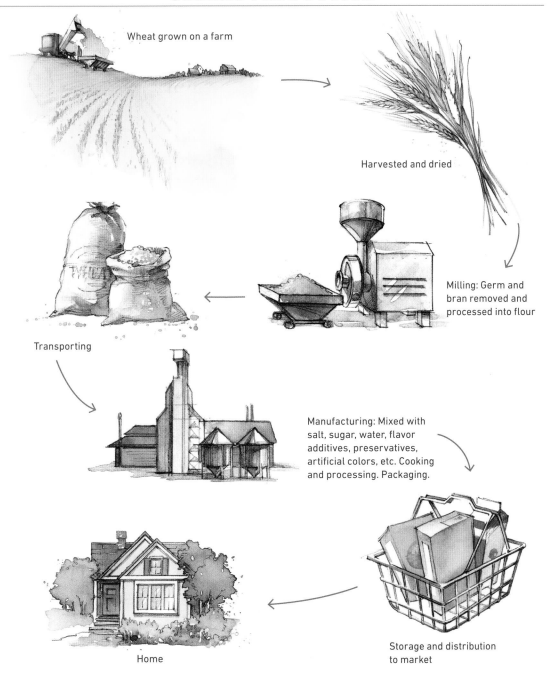

Wheat grown on a farm

Harvested and dried

Milling: Germ and bran removed and processed into flour

Transporting

Manufacturing: Mixed with salt, sugar, water, flavor additives, preservatives, artificial colors, etc. Cooking and processing. Packaging.

Home

Storage and distribution to market

Treating animals humanely may increase an animal's *qi* and consequently, its quality as food.

In addition to eating foods with high-quality *qi*, we must also enhance our bodies' ability to absorb that *qi*. This means minimizing the work required to break down and assimilate nutrients. Foods should be chewed well to encourage the action of salivary enzymes and to begin the process of digestion. Traditional Chinese Medicine (TCM) suggests that we limit our consumption of raw, cold, and frozen foods, since they counter our core body temperature and require more energy to digest. These principles may be especially important for people who show signs of weakened digestion, such as bloating, gas, constipation, or loose stool. The timing of our meals can also influence nutrient absorption. By eating larger meals during the daytime, we can take advantage of our bodies' increased digestive capacity during that time; likewise, smaller meals should be eaten in the evening when our digestive capacity is slower.[19,20]

EMPLOYING BALANCE AND MODERATION

A Western diet is often characterized by excess, from high-sodium snacks to rich, sugary desserts. Our meals typically include some type of animal protein as the centerpiece, with starches or vegetables served on the side as an afterthought. Once considered a luxury item and used in small amounts, meat now figures prominently in our diet. America's steakhouses are notorious for embracing the idea that "bigger is better," regularly serving up sixteen-ounce fillets that are four times the recommended portion size for meat.[21] A Western diet which emphasizes energy-dense foods is optimal for those who are looking to build strength or gain weight. It encourages rapid muscle growth and development. However, when taken to the extreme, a dietary emphasis on energy-dense foods can negatively impact our waistlines and our health. Practicing moderation suggests that we transition away from dietary extremes and consume a balanced diet filled with a variety of fruits, vegetables, nuts, legumes, and whole grains. Recent research has shown that high consumption of plant-based foods is associated with a reduced risk of cardiovascular disease and stroke.[22,23] By incorporating more of these foods into our diet, we can prevent chronic disease and shift the balance of health in our favor.

Moderating the amount of food that we eat may also be important to our long-term health. Studies of the diet in Okinawa, Japan, have shown that a mild restriction in calories may contribute to longer life expectancies and lower disease rates.[24] Okinawan dietary habits are represented by a common saying, "*hara hachi bu*," or "eat until you are 80% full." A balanced approach to eating is one in which we regulate not only the types of foods we eat, but also the amount.

USING THE POWER OF INTENTION

Our mental expectations and attitudes toward food can be just as important as the foods themselves. As a nation of habitual dieters, many of our thoughts about food revolve around anxiety and guilt. We worry about how many calories or grams of fat a food contains, or if a food is "good" or "bad" for us. In contrast, the French culture adopts a more relaxed approach that savors food, takes pleasure in eating, and emphasizes quality over quantity. Consequently, the French enjoy their bread, cheese, and wine, while also experiencing lower rates of heart disease and obesity than Americans.[25] By adopting a more positive attitude toward food, we may be able to have our cake and eat it too.

As we refrain from judgment and self-punishment, we begin to appreciate our food as a source of nourishment. By eating more slowly and mindfully, we can more fully engage in our meals and savor the foods that we eat. The practice of mindful eating entails placing one's attention and awareness completely on the process of eating. When we remove the distractions of television or reading materials, we can shift our focus to our food and increase our enjoyment of it, one bite at a time. Eating slowly has been shown to both increase satiety and help to moderate the amount that we eat.[26] By increasing our awareness of when we become full, the practice of mindful eating can help us to refrain from overeating and aid in any weight loss goals we may have.

Our intentions not only play a role in how we eat, but also in how we prepare our food. Cooking can be an expression of love and care for others, e.g. Grandma's home-made apple pie or a bowl of chicken noodle soup offered to a sick friend. Similarly, if a meal is prepared in a negative state of mind like anger or anxiety, that energy may be imparted to the food as well.[27] Cooking offers us an opportunity for sharing and communion, where intention and *qi* is both given and received.

MINDFUL EATING

For many of us, meals are mindlessly wolfed down in front of the television or in our automobiles on the way to our next appointment. What happens when instead we savor our food and engage in the practice of mindful eating?

» Begin with a peaceful environment: turn off the television and refrain from reading so that you can have full awareness of your surroundings and your meal.

» Show gratitude for the meal before you. Think of all the resources and lives that helped to bring this food to your table.

» Eat slowly, chewing each bite thirty to forty times before swallowing. Pay attention to the smells, flavors, and textures of each mouthful.

» Stay conscious and present in the experience of eating. Are the foods satisfying? Are you enjoying the meal? When do you become full?

» Do you notice a difference between mindless and mindful eating?

DISCOVERING YOUR INDIVIDUAL PATH

While the preceding principles offer general guidelines on eating for better health, it is important to remember that each person's health is unique and specific to that individual. There is no single diet that is optimal for everyone. Research studies have shown that there is considerable variability in how people respond to different diets; for example, some individuals may benefit from a low-fat diet, while others benefit from diets that are high in monounsaturated or polyunsaturated fats.[28,29] These differences are attributed in part to individual genotypes and the interaction between genes and diet.

Genetic and dietary factors can not only influence weight-loss outcomes, but also the body's metabolic response to certain diets.[30,31] With variability in ancestry, genetic makeup, body shape, and food preferences, different people have the potential to respond differently to the same foods. TCM philosophy suggests that the focus should be placed on the individual; each person therefore requires a health solution specific to his or her own body. This individualized approach is represented in the concept of seasonal body types, which will be described in more detail in Part II.

FACTORS OF INDIVIDUAL HEALTH

Take a moment to reflect on the unique nature of your diet, body, and health.

» What are the foods of your ancestors? How do the foods that you currently eat differ from those in a traditional diet?

» Are there any health problems that are common in your family? If so, what kind of preventive measures can you take in terms of your diet?

» What types of foods are native to or locally grown in your area? How often do you buy from farms raising food within a 100 mile radius of your home?

» Do you notice a difference between the foods available at your local farmers' market and those from the grocery store?

» Does the local climate influence your food choices (e.g. tropical fruit smoothies in Florida or hearty New England clam chowder)?

The dietary choices that we make each day are complex and have the potential to impact both our physical and emotional health. From a proactive health perspective, the foods that we eat represent an opportunity to nourish our bodies and transform our lives, and they should be enjoyed without guilt or self-criticism. With nature as our guide, we can choose a variety of fresh, whole, and unprocessed foods to provide the highest-quality *qi* and vitality to our bodies. Eating more vegetables, fruits, nuts, and grains brings balance to a Western diet often filled with animal products and refined and high-calorie foods. Using a mindful and holistic approach, we can discover the most optimal foods for benefiting individual health and ensuring longevity.

MUSCLE TESTING

*Muscle testing is a method for discovering how your individual body intuitively responds
to different foods or supplements.*

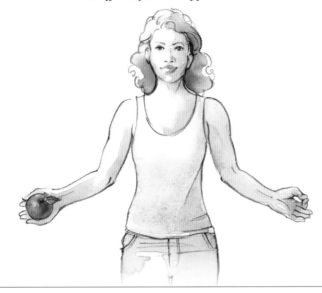

1.

Hold the item that you want to test in one hand. With your other hand, form a circle with
your thumb and your index finger. Hold it as tightly as possible. In your mind, ask yourself
if your body will benefit from this item.

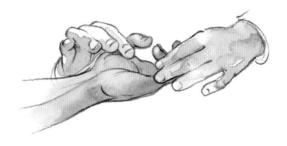

2.

At the same time, have someone pull your thumb and index finger apart, taking note of the
strength of your muscle response. How much effort did it take for that person to separate
your fingers? If your muscles remained strong during the test, your body may be respond-
ing positively to the item. If your muscles felt weak and put up little resistance, the item
may not be beneficial to your body.

*Try this muscle testing technique on various foods and supplements, even ones that
you think are "healthy." You may be surprised at the results.*

Chapter 3
You Are What You Think: the mind-body connection

MIND OVER MATTER

In the second century AD, the Greek physician Galen suggested that melancholy individuals were more susceptible to cancer than sanguine individuals.[1,2] In so doing, he became perhaps the first person to hypothesize that our minds have tremendous influence over our behavior. In this chapter, we will explore the link between mind and body, and offer examples of how to best utilize the power of intention to promote better health.

The mind-body connection is well-documented; evidence of its existence has been demonstrated in scientific journals for decades.[3,4] This large body of research falls under the heading of psychoneuroimmunology (PNI), or the study of the relationship between the central nervous system and the immune system. PNI explains how our conscious and unconscious thoughts affect both our voluntary and involuntary routines. For example, an anxious, busy mind is often accompanied by fast-paced breathing, whereas a relaxed, focused mind corresponds with slow, meditative breaths. A similar correlation can be seen in voluntary behaviors like eating. Our minds' arousal directly affects the speed at which we consume our food; the more stimulation or stress that our brains are experiencing, the faster, and therefore, the more, we eat.[5]

Where there is laughter there is always
more health than sickness.

– Phyllis Bottome

The findings of PNI suggest that our minds hold great influence over our bodies' functioning and health. By directing our thoughts, we can improve the way we feel. For instance, through mind-body techniques such as meditation, guided imagery, and biofeedback, we can learn to cope more effectively with chronic back pain or reduce the debilitating effects of a migraine headache.[6,7] While Eastern medicine has long understood that the mind and body cannot be separated, modern science is beginning to explore the reasons why.

HOW THE MIND AFFECTS THE BODY

Before we can unravel the mysteries of PNI and understand the effects of stress on the body, we must first understand the body at its ideal baseline: homeostasis. Homeostasis is a unique state in which complex, microscopic interactions come together to yield a finely tuned life form. When the body is in its natural homeostatic state, its biological systems function flawlessly as intended. The immune system attacks infections and heals wounds, the digestive system extracts energy from food and eliminates waste, and the respiratory system filters the air we breathe and infuses our blood with oxygen. However, once stress is introduced into the body, the whole system begins to falter.

Dr. Hans Selye, a forerunner in research on biological stress, showed that stressors can have a profound effect on our physiology and the development of disease.[8] PNI research suggests that stressors may compromise homeostasis by decreasing natural healing, weakening immunity, and lowering resistance to disease. Possible evidence of this decreased immune response has been observed in populations of stressed individuals, who were found to have fewer circulating immune cells and a higher susceptibility to viruses and common infections.[9,10]

Some research has even suggested that there is a direct link between the stress-induced reduction of immune cells (specifically natural killer (NK) white blood cells) and the initiation and progression of some types of cancer.[2] In fact, behavioral scientists have attempted to conceptualize a "Type C" personality that is inherently more at risk for developing cancer.[11] This personality type is characterized by the suppression and denial of emotions, the avoidance of confrontation, and an inability to express anger. Other research suggests that psychological factors like anger and hostility are associated with coronary heart disease.[12] In recent studies, depression has been linked to an increased mortality in cardiac disease patients; in contrast, men with high levels of optimism tend to have a reduced risk of cardiovascular death.[13,14]

The individual systems of the body do not function in isolation. The immune system is one part of a larger super-system that also includes brain centers that process emotion, glands that secrete hormones, and a vast network of neurons that comprise the nervous system. Whatever happens in one component of the system also affects the others.

HARNESSING THE POWER OF THE MIND

As with every realm of scientific study, there are critics who dispute mind-body research as faulty in both its methodology and accuracy. Some warn that psychosomatic explanations for disease etiology place blame on patients for their illnesses and are used to explain the things that medical science cannot. However, the mind's influence over the body should represent a tool of empowerment, rather than a burden of responsibility. Managing our minds to our advantage is an obvious, actionable remedy. Just as we make choices about the food we put into our bodies, we can make choices about the way we think and feel, within our own individual circumstances and states of health. By doing so, we can wield direct influence over our bodies' functioning. This understanding is the greatest gift of PNI.

The following section offers specific examples on how to reduce stress, increase awareness, and enhance the mind-body connection. As with any activity, these techniques will become more effective with practice. Daily practice, even for five or ten minutes per day, can yield both immediate and long-term results in mental and physical health.

REDUCING THE EFFECTS OF STRESS

The body's natural reaction to stress has been hard-wired since prehistoric times. In the presence of perceived danger, the fight-or-flight response puts the body on alert and prepares it for action; heart rate, respiratory rate, and blood pressure increase, while stress hormones like cortisol and adrenaline are released. Although our modern stressors are typically social or psychological in nature (e.g. job strain, interpersonal conflicts, and financial concerns) rather than physical threats to our survival, the body's physiological response remains the same.

Over time, constant and chronic stress can lead to elevated levels of stress hormones and a long-term activation of the stress response system. The physiological consequences of constantly elevated cortisol levels not only include hypertension and heart disease, but also impaired cognitive ability and lowered immunity.[4,15] Chronic stress can also lead to an increase and accumulation of abdominal fat, through the repeated activation of the hypothalamic-pituitary-adrenal (HPA) axis and an elevated secretion of cortisol. Additionally, it is linked to overeating and the consumption of foods that are high in fat and sugar, which in turn, contribute to overall weight gain.[16]

Diet, exercise, sleep, and relaxation are all important factors that can reduce the physiological effects of stress and enhance mood. A healthy diet lowers the risk of disease and boosts the immune system, helping the body to mitigate the effects of stress. Regular physical exercise has been shown to reduce levels of stress hormones like adrenaline and cortisol, while also reducing the body's reactivity to stressors.[17,18] Practicing relaxation techniques and getting adequate sleep are also helpful for stress reduction. By consciously commanding our minds and bodies to relax, we hold the ability to induce positive effects on our physiology.

DEEP BREATHING

As our bodies become burdened by stress, we replace our instinctive abdominal breathing with shallow chest breathing.[19] This type of constrained breathing is associated with high blood pressure and decreased oxygenation of the blood.[19,20] By practicing conscious and controlled breathing on a regular basis, we can restore optimal respiration. This simple technique can be used daily or whenever you feel stress creeping into your body.

1. To begin, breathe in slowly and deeply through your nose, counting to six. Focus on expanding your diaphragm.

2. Hold your breath while slowly counting to three.

3. Exhale slowly through your mouth, counting to eight.

4. Continue taking deep breaths while counting. You may want to keep your hand on your stomach to feel it rise and fall with each breath.

5. As you breathe slowly and deeply, feel your body becoming more relaxed and know that it is working efficiently.

Feelings come and go like clouds in a windy sky.
Conscious breathing is my anchor.

– Thich Nhat Hanh

PROGRESSIVE RELAXATION

Progressive relaxation is a two-step process of sequentially tensing and relaxing different muscle groups in your body, through a systematic progression from your feet to your head. Although you may think you are relaxed while watching television or even sleeping at night, your muscles are often still holding the day's stress; teeth clenching is one example of subconscious muscular tension. Progressive relaxation encourages the mind to become more aware of the body, where it is holding tension, and what it feels like to release that tension.

1. Practice this exercise while lying down or reclining in a comfortable position.

2. To begin, focus your attention on one muscle group, e.g. the muscles in your left foot.

3. Inhale and activate these muscles as hard as you can for eight seconds; in this example, curl your toes and flex your arch.

4. Be careful to tense the intended muscle group only; in this example, make sure that your calf and thigh muscles stay relaxed. With practice, you will learn to make very fine distinctions between your muscles.

5. After eight seconds, release the tension gradually. Notice the difference between contraction and relaxation.

6. Repeat with your right foot, then move to your calf muscles. Continue this process for the remaining muscle groups, from your legs to the top of your head. The entire process may take twenty to thirty minutes.

IMAGINING A POSITIVE OUTCOME

When our minds drift to sandy beaches or pleasant memories, we can catapult ourselves out of the tedium of a corporate meeting or the frustration of a grueling airport layover. Daydreaming allows us to engage in escapism and it can be just as effective at helping us escape from illness. Recent research has shown that when it comes to seeking relief from pain, a combination of guided imagery and medical care is superior to standard medical care alone.[21,22] Encouraging the mind to create images that conjure positive feelings of power, control, hope, or relief can alleviate stress, depression, and anxiety.[23]

The power of guided imagery can be demonstrated when we imagine eating a sour lemon. When we engage our senses in vivid detail, we picture the lemon's bright yellow color, feel the tiny bumps of the fruit's skin, and smell its zesty fragrance. As we imagine ourselves biting into the fruit's tart, juicy pulp, we may discover that our mouths actually begin to pucker. From this illustration, it is clear that genuine manifestation and physiological response can occur through simple imagery and visualization.

GUIDED IMAGERY

Guided imagery is a program of directed thoughts and suggestions; it activates all of your senses and leads you to believe that what you are imagining is real. One goal of guided imagery is to attain a focused state of relaxation that ultimately helps to enhance creativity, performance, healing, and learning.

1. Find a comfortable position and begin by breathing deeply and slowly.

2. Choose a relaxing scene for your visualization, e.g. a snow-capped mountaintop or a warm, tropical beach.

3. Imagine yourself in your new, peaceful surroundings. Using all of your senses, create the scene in your mind with as much detail as possible.

4. What do you see? Describe the colors and sights around you. What sounds do you hear? How does the air feel on your skin? Take a deep breath. What do you smell?

5. Allow yourself to unwind and enjoy the scene you've created. Remember this feeling of relaxation within your body. When you feel ready to depart, carry the feeling with you as you leave. With practice, you will be able to enter this relaxed state more quickly and easily.

FORMING INTENTIONS AND EXPECTATIONS

Intention has been described as directing thought in order to perform a determined action.[24] It can also be conceptualized as the conscious application of one's *qi*, or energy, to positively affect oneself and others. The idea that one person's intentions can influence the health of another person falls under the concept of distant healing intention (DHI). Prayer is one example of DHI; other forms include practices like energy healing, spiritual healing, and remote mental healing.[25] While the mechanism of distant intentionality is not yet understood, research has shown that sending healing thoughts from a distance may actually influence the activation of certain brain functions in its recipients.[26]

Expectation works similarly to intention, and serves as the foundation for the placebo effect, the safeguard of the scientific method. The placebo effect explains why a group of patients who are told they are receiving an expensive medication feel greater relief than those in a different group who receive the same medication, but are told it is cheaper.[27] Similarly, patients who expect a treatment to alleviate pain will often experience activity in parts of the brain responsible for analgesia and report a reduction in their pain levels, even before the treatment is administered.[28] Research involving cancer patients demonstrates that both real and false expectations can affect the way that patients respond to their illnesses. When cancer patients expect that their treatments will cure them, they tend to experience a better quality of life compared to patients who believe their treatments will only control pain or manage their symptoms, without the expectation of curative healing.[29] It seems that we hold the potential to realize an outcome just by believing in it.

AFFIRMATIONS

Affirmations are specific personal statements made in the present tense that create feelings of support and confidence. Positive affirmations have the power to affect positive change; they should be repeated or written down frequently until they are as much belief as they are encouragement.

1. Begin by finding a comfortable position; you may want to do this exercise while lying in bed before falling sleep, or in front of the mirror upon waking.

2. Choose a target word or phrase that you wish to reinforce as a goal. For example, at times when you are feeling frustrated or angry, you may want to choose one of the following phrases: "Peace," "I am calm and relaxed," or "There is nothing I cannot handle."

3. Repeatedly recite the affirmation to yourself, speaking aloud if desired. Feel the intention and power in your words and declarations.

This process can be repeated daily or whenever you would like to reinforce positive thoughts and attitudes.

EXPERIENCING GRATITUDE

The concept of gratitude has been described as an emotion and state of appreciation, as well as a dispositional trait and life orientation toward noticing and appreciating the positive in the world. Research demonstrates that gratitude is strongly related to well-being and may be causal to it, leading to physical, psychological, and interpersonal benefits.[30] Grateful people tend to be more optimistic, experience positive emotions more frequently, have lower levels of stress, and have less anxiety and depression. Experiencing gratitude is not only associated with enhanced mood, life satisfaction, and psychological resilience, but also with positive relationships and prosocial behavior.[30]

Studies show that simple interventions can be used therapeutically to increase gratitude.[30] One method involves making lists of things for which one is grateful; these "gratitude lists" can be recorded on a regular basis. Another method involves writing a thank-you letter and reading it aloud to the recipient. By reflecting on blessings rather than shortcomings, we can foster gratitude and create a better quality of life for ourselves. In research studies involving university students, regular gratitude exercises were associated with fewer reported physical ailments, better sleep quality, and higher levels of positive affect.[31] Although gratitude exercises are considered temporary interventions and may not lead to a deep sense of gratitude or alter one's fundamental life orientation, researchers suggest that applying an intentional and regular focus toward gratitude may have a beneficial effect on long-term levels of well-being.[31]

INCREASING AWARENESS AND MINDFULNESS

Perhaps the most essential way to enhance the mind-body connection is by becoming aware of one's whole self (mind, body, and spirit). Mindfulness is commonly defined as "paying attention in a particular way: on purpose, in the present moment, and non-judgmentally."[32] With roots in Buddhist and Eastern traditions, it is a practice that cultivates attention and awareness of what is presently taking place. Living consciously and being fully aware allows us to utilize the power of the mind to maximum effect. For instance, to truly reduce the effects of stress, it is helpful if we can first identify that we are feeling stressed, while also trying to understand the origins of that stress. Only through recognition and understanding can we use the mind to influence change.

Scientific research has shown that mindfulness training is associated with less emotional distress, more positive states of mind, and a better overall quality of life. It not only contributes to a state of relaxation, but also beneficially influences the mind, the brain, the body, and our behavior.[33] Mental training, in the form of meditation, has been shown to affect brain function and actually induce long-term neural changes; during electroencephalogram-monitored meditation, highly experienced Buddhist monks were observed to have higher gamma brain wave activity than people with little meditation experience.[34]

MEDITATION

Meditation is an ancient technique that can be used to calm and focus the mind. There are many different types of meditation practices, including emptying your mind, reciting a mantra, practicing awareness, or focusing on an object. One of the simplest techniques involves focusing on your breath:

1. Begin by clearing a quiet space, free from distraction or stimulation.

2. Sit in a chair or cross-legged on the floor with your spine erect. You may keep your eyes closed or partially open.

3. Breathe naturally through your nose. Become aware of the sensation of your breath as it enters and leaves your body. Notice your abdomen moving in and out with each breath.

4. If your mind begins to wander, accept the thoughts without judgment, release them, and return your attention to your breath.

5. Allow yourself to remain in a relaxed state for a minute or two before gradually coming out of your meditation.

If you are new to meditation, you may want to start with just five minutes of daily practice, gradually increasing your practice in five-minute increments each week.

BIOFEEDBACK

Biofeedback uses an external measuring device to help you increase awareness of and gain conscious control over specific biological processes. By using therapeutic biofeedback machines, bodily functions like heart rate, blood pressure, muscle tension, and skin temperature can be monitored in real time. With the help of a qualified practitioner, you can train your thoughts and control your body's physical response. Biofeedback has been shown to be effective for treating tension and migraine headaches, chronic low back pain, and urinary incontinence.[6]

Life can be found only in the present moment.
The past is gone, the future is not yet here, and if we do not
go back to ourselves in the present moment,
we cannot be in touch with life.

– Thich Nhat Hanh

THE MIND-BODY CONNECTION IN DAILY LIFE

With growing evidence of the link between mind and body, the benefits of incorporating mind-body techniques into daily practice are obvious. When our minds are strong, our bodies respond accordingly. From simple thoughts and expectations to visualization and awareness practices, there are a variety of ways that we can mentally influence our physiology and health. To maximize the effect of these practices, it is also important that our minds be clear and completely engaged with our bodies and their surrounding environment. The more attuned we are with our bodies and ourselves, the greater control we have over our health.

Enhancing the mind-body connection includes living mindfully and making a conscious decision to be aware and present in our daily activities. For many of us, this can mean turning off the auto-pilot switch on our morning commute, or listening actively during our next business meeting. Perhaps we will practice mindfulness by choosing to eat our meals away from distractions such as televisions, computers, and newspapers; in addition to being able to actually taste and appreciate our food, we may also experience better digestion and more weight loss. Exercise also becomes more effective when it is performed more consciously. Research shows that when athletes focus internally on bodily sensations like muscle tension and breathing, their physical performance improves.[35] Mindfulness practice can be used to enhance performance by promoting greater awareness of thoughts, emotions, and physiological states.[36] Instead of focusing on external stimuli or tuning out the sensations of physical exertion, we can actually feel our bodies' systems working together and sense the energy flowing through us.

Each time that we engage the mind, we strengthen the mind-body connection and provide ourselves with one more tool to use in the prevention of disease. It is estimated that we have an average of 70,000 thoughts each day.[37] In effect, this also means that we potentially have 70,000 opportunities a day to command good health. We know that our thoughts impact our emotions and our emotions impact our physiology, therefore the incentive for positive and conscious thinking is abundantly clear. Regardless of what is happening around us, the mind offers us control of our internal environment; we alone hold the power to choose our thoughts and influence the way we feel.

We are what we think.
All that we are arises with our thoughts.
With our thoughts, we make our world.
– Buddha

Chapter 4
You Are What You Do: activity and exercise

THE HEALTHY APPEAL OF EXERCISE

Thirty years ago, it would have been hard to imagine that we could buy groceries, communicate with business colleagues around the world, or send someone a birthday present without ever picking up a telephone or moving from the recliner. We owe this victory of convenience to the technological revolution and the innovative engineers and entrepreneurs from Silicon Valley and beyond. However, for every winner there is a loser, and the loser in this revolution is the human body. No longer required to toil on farms, engage in hard manual labor, or even walk to the corner store, our bodies have become soft, both literally and figuratively. Although we enjoy greater efficiency and ease in our lives, our bodies bear the burden of our increasingly sedentary lifestyles.

As a recurring factor in the top ten causes of death in the United States, physical inactivity places a heavy economic burden on the U.S. health-care system.[1,2] Heart disease, type 2 diabetes, obesity, and cancer are just a few of the health conditions that can be improved or prevented with regular physical activity. With both physiological and psychological benefits, exercise can increase longevity and promote health for people of all ages. Although the Centers for Disease Control and Prevention (CDC) report that U.S. adults have become more physically active in recent years, more than half of us still do not meet the recommended levels of physical activity (at least thirty minutes of moderate-intensity activity, five times a week).[3] In addition, about one in four adults report that they do not engage in any leisure-time physical activity at all.[4]

For some of us, retiring to the couch at the end of the day to watch television seems more appealing than finding the time and energy to get up and exercise. When instant gratification is as rewarding as it is, it is hard to sell prevention. However, disease prevention is where exercise shows its best effects.[5] Perhaps one of the most visible benefits of exercise is weight loss.[6,7] With rates of overweight and obesity reaching epidemic proportions, diet and exercise remain the most essential ways to regulate caloric intake and expenditure. Maintaining a healthy body weight is also important in the prevention and treatment of type 2 diabetes, a condition commonly linked to obesity.[8,9] Researchers suggest that physical activity benefits those with diabetes by improving both the body's glucose control and its sensitivity to insulin.[10]

Aerobic exercise has a major impact on cardiovascular health, not only lowering blood pressure and improving blood flow, but also reducing levels of triglycerides and cholesterol. By improving vascular function and the body's ability to take in and use oxygen, exercise can increase physical capacity and decrease levels of fatigue.[11,12] Regular physical activity has also been seen to reduce the incidence of breast and colon cancers. It may increase survival rates in cancer patients, improving both longevity and quality of life.[13,14] To prevent osteoporosis and bone loss, weight-bearing exercises (ones that place compressive forces on the bone) are particularly helpful.[12] When performed regularly, activities like brisk walking, jumping, running, and resistance training have been shown to increase bone mineral density.[15,16] Even simple balance exercises can offer important health benefits, like counteracting the deterioration of muscular strength, physical function, and postural control that occur with aging.[17,18] Balance training and exercises like *tai chi* (sometimes known as *tai ji* or *tai ji quan*) can improve coordination and reduce the likelihood of falls or injuries among the elderly.[19,20] Being physically fit not only prevents injuries from occurring, but also lessens the severity of an injury and helps to speed up recovery.[21,22]

> *Those who think they have no time for exercise will sooner*
> *or later have to find time for illness.*
> – Edward Stanley

In addition to strengthening our bodies, physical activity also benefits our minds, improving cognition, learning, and brain function. Using neuroimaging scans, scientists have discovered that exercise can actually change the structure and volume of the brain.[23] Not only does exercise boost our brain power, but it also makes us smarter. In older adults, exercise training has been shown to improve performance of cognitive tasks and control processes like planning, scheduling, multi-tasking, and working memory; this suggests that exercise can protect against cognitive decline.[24] There is also evidence that physical activity can benefit academic performance in school-age children, based on evaluations of perceptual skills, achievement in standardized tests, and academic grades.[23]

By improving mood states, quality of sleep, and self-perception, regular physical activity can also affect how we feel. Research studies show that exercise helps to enhance mood and reduce feelings of both anxiety and stress.[25] Exercise enhances the circulation of the brain's "feel-good" chemicals, including serotonin, norepinephrine, and endorphins. In experiments on rats, scientists have discovered that running can induce biochemical changes in the brain and increase the ability to handle stress.[26,27] Numerous studies also demonstrate that exercise is effective in the prevention of depression; it not only benefits mental well-being but also improves quality of life.[25] In the U.S., the prevalence of depression and mental illness has increased to the point that antidepressants have become the most commonly prescribed class of drugs.[28] Regular exercise may offer a natural, low-cost alternative or supplement to the use of these pharmaceuticals.

EXERCISE IN THE EAST AND WEST

Given the myriad of health benefits that physical activity can offer, one might ask what kind of exercise is the best? In the West, we celebrate athletic feats of superhuman strength, speed, and endurance. Our heroes compete in grueling triathlons and military-style obstacle courses, crossing the finish line in glory and sometimes exhaustion to the point that they can no longer stand; they are iron men and women, bodies chiseled and minds focused. As a nation, we honor hard work and achievement. Mantras like "no pain, no gain" and "go big or go home" provide inspiration to weekend warriors and encourage us to push ourselves to the extreme. For an additional dose of motivation, we rely on personal trainers to bark at us like drill sergeants and light our competitive fire. Typically, our workout routines parallel our energetic, fast-paced lifestyles; high-intensity, sweat-yielding, heart-pounding exercise is part of the American way. However, this is not the only approach to exercise.

In most Eastern cultures, the goal of exercise is not to burn calories, but to move and enhance *qi*, the energy force found in all living things. Slow, meditative styles of exercise that incorporate deliberate movements and stretches are common; these practices encourage the smooth flow and circulation of *qi* throughout the body. Eastern philosophy suggests that energy should be preserved and cultivated, instead of expended or burned away through intense effort.[29] In the West, a typical workout may include running at maximum speed while sweating profusely; in the East however, common exercises include yoga, *tai chi*, and *qi gong*, which are slower and more deliberate forms of activity. With an emphasis on spiritual connection and mindfulness, these Eastern-style exercises use the breath to focus the mind, engage the body, and develop *qi* from within. Many of their forms and poses also highlight a connection to the natural environment, drawing inspiration from elements of nature and mimicking the graceful movements of animals. Although the gentle movements of Eastern modes of exercise lack the physical intensity of those typically found in the West, they still offer a wide variety of health benefits. Recent research suggests that meditative forms of exercise like yoga, *tai chi*, and *qi gong* can not only reduce stress and alleviate depression, but also decrease hypertension and boost immune function.[30,31,32]

With their contrasting styles of exercise, the East and West offer fundamentally different, yet complementary approaches to health. If the West represents an intense and fiery *yang*, then the East symbolizes a cool and fluid *yin*. One perspective inspires us to take action to energize our bodies; the other encourages us to conserve and cultivate our energy from within. Each approach provides unique benefits to the body, but the greatest contribution to health occurs when the two are combined together. In the ideal case, both *yin* and *yang* are equally nurtured; one is not emphasized more than the other. As with any study in extremes, moderation is the key to longevity. Only when *yin* and *yang* are in harmony can the body thrive to its fullest.

> *When genuine energy is stored within, diseases cannot invade the body.*
>
> – Li Dong-Yuan

FINDING BALANCE

Traditional Chinese Medicine (TCM) teaches the value of an individualized approach, suggesting that we all have different requirements for staying fit. In general, we tend to gravitate toward activities that are most like us, because they are the most comfortable. While *yang* individuals may enjoy the exhilaration of speeding down ski slopes as fast as possible, *yin* individuals may prefer to engage their minds through slow Pilates movements and stretches. However, balance is essential, and one way to promote it is by choosing activities that contrast with our natural tendencies.

If we find that our days are mostly *yang*-dominant, i.e. we are rushing to and fro, fueled by caffeine, and constantly dealing with heart-pounding stressors, then we might consider choosing exercises that focus on nourishing our *yin*. Low-intensity activities with slow, fluid movements like yoga, golf, and swimming help to calm the fire generated by an excess *yang*, while meditative, internally focused exercises like *tai chi* and *qi gong* emphasize the connection between breath and body. For those of us with *yang* tendencies and lifestyles, *yin*-style exercises can seem boring and excruciatingly slow; however, gentle movements and soothing activities are precisely what our overworked bodies and minds crave. Constantly pushing the body's physical limits actually does us a disservice if it leads to fatigue and repeated injury. When the body breaks down from excessive *yang* exercise and work, stretching, massage, and bodywork therapies are beneficial ways to cultivate *yin* and restore balance. Rest and renewal are essential for those who are accustomed to burning the proverbial candle at both ends.

For people on the *yin* side of the spectrum, *yang* activities can counterbalance slower-paced and sedentary lifestyles. Those of us who work in solitude or sit in front of a computer all day long can benefit from revving up our internal *yang* with invigorating, endorphin-boosting workouts. Exercises that elevate the heart rate, such as kick-boxing or cycling, will help to combat lethargy by moving *qi* and circulating blood throughout the body. If getting started is the hardest part, group exercise classes or playing league sports like tennis, basketball, and soccer can offer some external motivation. Since the natural tendency of *yin* is to withdraw, those of us with *yin*-dominant lives must focus on developing *yang*. Outdoor activities such as hiking and mountain biking allow us not only to connect with nature, but also to rejuvenate our bodies with fresh air and energy from a bright, *yang* sun.

Finding our individual *yin-yang* balance does not mean that we must give up activities that we enjoy. While many physical activities can be classified as *yin*-dominant (e.g. yoga and golf) or *yang*-dominant (e.g. boxing and sprinting), nothing is entirely *yin* or *yang*. Elements of both can be found in all forms of exercise and emphasized according to our individual needs. For example, although yoga is primarily considered to be a spiritual practice, those who want to build *yang* may choose a more strenuous form, like Ashtanga, or opt for sweat-inducing Bikram yoga. Similarly, competitive athletes who typically embody an intense *yang* can nourish their *yin* by enhancing fluidity in their movements or focusing on the mental aspects of their sport. Balancing *yin* and *yang* can mean switching between heart-pounding kickboxing routines and *tai chi* in the park at sunrise, or simply incorporating a mindful stretching routine into daily running workouts. As our lifestyles and health conditions cycle naturally between *yin* and *yang*, we can choose different activities to provide restorative balance to our individual bodies. Regular physical exercise and movement, both *yin* and *yang*, can help to promote health throughout the course of our lives.

> *Be kind to your body –*
> *it's the only place you have to live.*
> – Jim Rohn

INTEGRATING BODY AND MIND

The previous chapter explored the relationship between mind and body, showing that mindfulness is an essential component of good health. With any activity, whether it be eating or exercising, we receive the most benefit when we are fully engaged and present. Most of us are familiar with mindless exercise; when we run on a treadmill, headphones in and music blaring, all while watching the news headlines scroll by on television, we are purposely disconnecting ourselves from our bodies. In comparison, when we look at an Olympic diver executing an intricate combination of twists and somersaults before slicing into the water with barely a splash, we see an example of a mind and body that are merged and working in perfect unison.

Physical feats are best executed when the mind is actively participating. When mindfulness is applied to physical activity, it enhances performance through the increased awareness of inner psychological and physiological states. Researchers suggest that sustained attention and awareness may give athletes a more accurate perception of their levels of physical exertion and fatigue.[33] Exercising mindfully allows us to receive constant feedback on how our bodies feel and ensure that they are working efficiently and without pain. It also encourages us to enjoy the process of exercise and experience the flow of energy throughout the body, from the heart and lungs to the muscles and bones. Mindfulness can be incorporated into any exercise program if we eliminate distractions, focus our attention in the present moment, and release our judgments about outcome or results.[34] When the mind and body are in complete unity, we can begin to achieve a state of consciousness that can be described as a "runner's high," "being in the zone," or "flow." In this state of optimal performance, the mind is totally absorbed in the moment and physical movements become fluid and effortless.

MINDFUL EXERCISE

Mindful exercise is the practice of being fully aware of your internal and external environment during physical activity.

» Begin with an intention to be mindful during your exercise session. Turn off electronic devices and distractions, such as audio players, televisions, or tablets.

» What do you notice about your surroundings? Are there any specific sounds, sights, or smells that enter your awareness?

» How does your body feel? Pay attention to your muscles as they contract and relax. Can you sense your heart rate elevating or slowing? Are you experiencing pain in any areas of your body? If you become aware of any tension, try to mentally release it and allow that part of your body to relax.

» Focus on your breath. Are you breathing through your nose or your mouth? Is your breath steady or labored? Try exhaling during the active phase of your movement and inhaling during the rest phase. Recognize that your body is fully capable of this physical effort.

» What are you thinking about? Are you trying to distract yourself from the discomfort of working out? Are you worrying about work or things that you have on your to-do list? Focus on form, rhythm, and flow. When your mind wanders, bring your awareness back to the experience of your body in motion.

Perhaps the best way to keep our minds engaged during exercise is to make fitness fun. If the idea of working out in the gym doesn't excite us, we should find an activity that we do enjoy, whether it is playing beach volleyball, dancing to our favorite music, or playing catch with our kids. Physical activity should be an expression of vitality and energy, not a chore to be dreaded. For those of us who are starting an exercise program for the first time, we can begin by choosing simple activities that get the body moving and encourage the flow of *qi*. Exercise does not have to mean competing in ultramarathons or bench-pressing two hundred pounds; it can simply mean taking long walks to rediscover our neighborhoods or riding our bicycles to work. By providing opportunities to create social ties, learn new skills, and connect with nature, regular physical activity can offer us a wide range of lifelong benefits that go beyond physical fitness alone. Being active both supports health and enhances life; it represents joy, vitality, and freedom, embodying the essence of what it means to be alive.

This is the real secret of life – to be completely
engaged with what you are doing in the here and now.
And instead of calling it work, realize it is play.

– Alan Watts

AN INTRODUCTION TO EASTERN-STYLE EXERCISES

The following activities highlight an Eastern approach to exercise that nourishes *yin* and emphasizes mindfulness. When practicing exercises like *qi gong*, yoga, and *tai chi*, the movements should be as slow and fluid as possible. Focusing on the breath will help to cultivate awareness and strengthen the connection between mind and body. Group classes and individualized instruction can also enhance the practice of these exercises.

QI GONG—DAN TIAN BREATHING

Qi gong is an energy practice used to enhance and strengthen qi, *the energetic life force. In Eastern medicine,* qi *is thought to travel in channels throughout the body. The storage center for this energy resides in the* dan tian, *which is located in the lower abdomen, a few centimeters below the navel and close to the body's physical center of gravity. The following exercise is designed to cultivate* qi *and focus it into the body's center.*

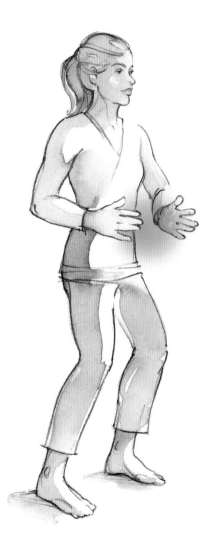

1.

To begin, stand with your legs shoulder-width apart and feet firmly rooted to the ground. Your posture should be upright but relaxed, with your knees slightly bent.

2.

With your elbows by your sides, hold your hands up in front of your abdomen, with palms facing each other and thumbs pointing upward. Your hands should be in a comfortable, relaxed position about six inches apart; imagine that they are loosely holding a small ball of energy between them.

3.

Breathe in deeply through your nose, expanding your diaphragm and lower abdomen. Exhale slowly and completely.

4.

Be aware of any physical sensation between your hands. Some people describe the feeling of *qi* energy as warmth, tingling, or pulses; others visualize it as light or color. You may find that closing your eyes makes it easier to increase your awareness of *qi*.

5.

Continue breathing slowly and deeply while you begin to focus your energy into the lower abdomen and *dan tian* area. Imagine that the *qi* in your body's center is gaining strength and intensity with each breath in and out.

Try this exercise for three to five minutes at a time, increasing to ten minutes as you gain more practice.

TAI CHI—WALKING CRANE

It is thought that a Taoist priest created the practice of tai chi *or* tai ji quan *after observing a fight between a snake and a crane. Originally developed as a martial art,* tai chi *emphasizes soft, circular maneuvers to counter hard, fast strikes. In recent years, it has become a popular health practice due to its use of slow, meditative movements and its ability to enhance the body's healing capacity. In this exercise, imagine that you are a crane or an eagle, stretching your powerful wings and preparing to fly.*

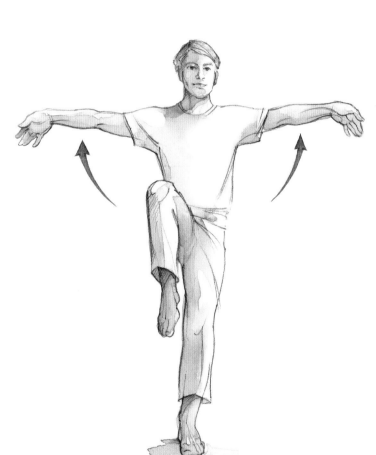

1.

Start by standing with your feet about shoulder-width apart from each other and your arms relaxed by your sides. Take slow, deep breaths in and out.

2.

While inhaling, shift your weight to your right leg and lift your arms straight out to your sides. As you lift your arms, let your hands drop down naturally from your wrists; with your fingers relaxed and pointing downward, draw your fingertips together in a slow, grasping motion. Continue raising your arms as you lift your left leg; bend your leg at the knee and raise it toward your chest.

3.

When your hands reach the height of your head, exhale and gradually begin to release your arms downward; relax your fingers, drop your wrists, and allow your arms to float down to your sides. At the same time, slowly lower your left leg one step in front of your original starting position.

4.

Gradually shift your weight to your left leg and repeat the crane movement by lifting your right leg and raising your arms to your sides again.

5.

Continue alternating your legs and walking forward with fluid, controlled motions. Repeat the exercise for five to ten steps per leg.

YOGA – HALF SUN SALUTATION
(*ARDHA SURYA NAMASKAR*)

Derived from the Sanskrit word meaning "union," yoga is a practice that emphasizes spiritual connection and transformation. It cultivates awareness by keeping the mind still through a series of meditative poses and breathing techniques.

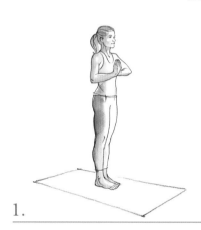

1.

Stand in a relaxed and upright position with your feet together or a few inches apart. Press your hands together, palms touching, and hold them in a prayer gesture in front of your chest.

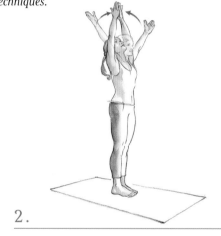

2.

With a deep breath inward, reach your arms out to either side, sweep them straight above your head and place your palms together. Slightly tilt your head back and look up toward your hands.

Hold each pose for five seconds. Coordinate your movements with each breath in and out.

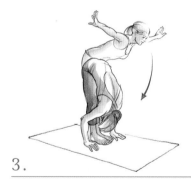

3.

Exhale, release your hands to your sides and bend forward at your waist with your legs straight. Let your arms hang down and your head drop toward your feet. Touch your hands to the floor, bending your knees slightly if needed. Notice any unnecessary tension being held in your body and completely release it.

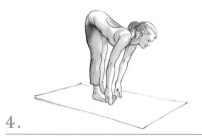

4.

As you inhale, lift your torso and head away from your legs with your back straight; keep your fingertips on the floor or bring your palms to your shins. Slowly lengthen your spine one vertebra at a time as you look directly in front of you.

The Sun Salutation is a sequence of poses designed to pay respect to the sun as a symbol of light and the giver of life; accordingly, it is often practiced at sunrise. For those new to yoga, this half sequence can serve as a good introduction to the practice.

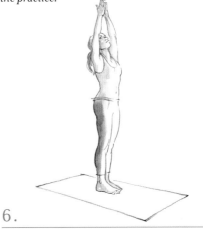

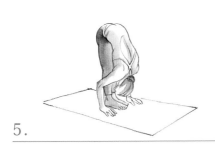

5.

Exhale and release your body into a forward bend once more. Press your forehead into your knees.

6.

Inhale, sweep your arms up, extend your body upright, and bring your palms together overhead. Reach up to the sky and direct your gaze upward.

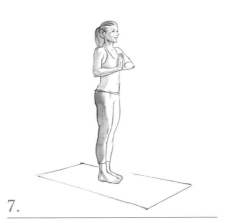

7.

Finish by exhaling and letting your hands drift down together to the initial prayer position at your heart.

Repeat this sequence five times; focus on receiving the power of the sun with each slow and rhythmic breath.

Chapter 5
You Are What You Absorb: environmental influences

THE NATURE OF OUR ENVIRONMENT

The debate over "nature vs. nurture" is a passionate one. Are we the susceptible consequence of our environment, or are our destinies mapped out by microscopic cartographers in utero? The answer is likely a bit of both. Evidence suggests that our health does not depend on our inherited genes alone, but rather on a complex interaction of genetic, behavioral, and environmental factors.[1,2] From the perspective of Traditional Chinese Medicine (TCM), the *qi* that we gather from our environment combines with the *qi* that we inherit from our parents to create a unique and dynamic picture of life. From the air, water, and food that we ingest, to the physical spaces in which we live and work, our environment helps to define who we are and how we behave. The quality of our health, therefore, is directly proportional to the quality of our environment. We are in part what we absorb.

As environmental awareness increases, so do concerns about the purity of our air, water, and land, and our potential exposure to toxic chemicals, heavy metals, and pesticides. Although we know that pollutants exist in the air we breathe, the water we drink, and the soil in which our food is grown, they are often invisible to the naked eye and seemingly out of our direct control. According to the Environmental Protection Agency (EPA), exposure to environmental contaminants may be a risk factor for a wide variety of diseases and health conditions, including low birth weight, respiratory disease, cardiovascular disease, and cancer.[3] Environmental contamination is particularly harmful early in life, its impact on the growth and development of children and fetuses different than its impact on adults.[4,5]

Within Taoist philosophy, breath is the foundation of our connection to nature, and it exemplifies one of the ways in which we embody our surroundings. TCM suggests that the air we breathe is directly transformed into *qi*, or energy, for use by the body. Air quality, therefore, is of utmost importance. It is not surprising that the toxic effects of air pollution are chiefly observed in diseases of the lungs and respiratory system. One of the more obvious examples of this relationship is the correlation between cigarette smoking and the incidence of lung cancer. The EPA and the U.S. Surgeon General confirm that even secondhand smoke can lead to lung cancer, respiratory disease, an increase in the frequency and severity of asthma attacks, as well as premature death.[6,7] On a larger scale, environmental air pollution results from activities that support our modern lifestyles, from the burning of fossil fuels for energy to industrial manufacturing and transportation. Breathing air pollutants on a daily basis can actually lead to an accumulation of black carbon deposits in our lungs over time. Air pollution is not only associated with decreased lung function and respiratory disease, but also with cardiovascular disease, genetic damage, and reproductive health problems.[8,9]

> *For breath is life, and if you breathe well you will live long on earth.*
>
> – Sanskrit Proverb

Our drinking water can also become polluted; contaminants in bottled and tap water can include bacteria and viruses, chemicals and solvents, and minerals like arsenic and lead. In developing countries, the lack of clean water and adequate sanitation results in millions of deaths every year; access to clean water is critical in the prevention of health problems like diarrheal diseases, parasitic infections, and arsenic poisoning. In the U.S. and other developed nations, the disinfection and treatment of drinking water with chlorine has significantly minimized the risk of water-borne disease. However, the process of chlorination also comes with its own hazards. Chlorination by-products have been associated with bladder and rectal cancers, as well as reproductive health problems.[10,11,12] It is important to retain the benefits of water chlorination and to control microbial disease, while also considering the risks of chlorinated water systems.

Like a porous, permeable sponge, our land readily absorbs contamination from industrial waste and heavy metals, agricultural pesticide and fertilizer runoff, and the leaching of waste from landfills. Since many of these toxic chemicals and compounds do not degrade easily or at all, the environmental impact of soil pollution can be extensive and long-lasting. Soil contamination is absorbed by plants and crops which are eaten by animals and humans, and its toxic effects are amplified along each step of the food chain. It also contributes to water pollution through runoff to lakes, rivers, and oceans, and to air pollution through the release of volatile compounds into the atmosphere. Heavy metal contamination in soil can be particularly hazardous to our health; chronic exposure to cadmium, mercury, lead, and arsenic has been associated with such health effects as kidney damage, neurological impairment, cardiovascular problems, and an increased risk for certain cancers.[13] One example of widespread soil pollution is in China, where rapid industrialization and the application of agricultural chemicals has led to increasing rates of heavy metal contamination. It is estimated that more than 10% of China's farmland is now polluted with heavy metals, impacting both food safety and public health.[14]

ENVIRONMENTAL INFLUENCES ON THE FOOD CHAIN

Not only do we absorb chemicals in the air, water, and soil that surround us, we multiply their effects by ingesting foods grown in those elements. Environmental contamination affects land, crops, and grazing animals, and eventually works its way up to the top of the food chain. As a direct representation of their surrounding environment, foods capture the essence and *qi* of their original source. Environmental contaminants and toxins compromise the quality of our foods and diminish their *qi*; consequently, polluted foods offer less vitality to the body. Emphasizing the quality of the foods we eat requires an awareness of how those foods are grown, including any use of pesticides, hormones, antibiotics, and genetic modification in the production process. It is not clear what the long-term health risks are of consuming foods that have pesticide and chemical residue. However, concerns over their potential effects have contributed to a revival in recent years of traditional farming practices, now known as organic farming. By excluding the use of synthetic herbicides and pesticides, organic and sustainable farming practices may enhance both soil fertility and the diversity of local birds, plants, and insects.[15,16] Reducing chemical contamination and preserving biodiversity benefits the health of the ecosystem, and indirectly benefits human health as a result.

SAFEGUARDING AGAINST ENVIRONMENTAL CONTAMINATION

Consider the following to minimize your exposure to environmental contamination:

Air

» Reduce air pollution and your carbon footprint by conserving energy, using public transportation or carpools, and recycling.

» Avoid outdoor activity when air pollutant levels are high.

» Use high-efficiency particulate air (HEPA) filters in indoor ventilation systems, portable air filtration units, and vacuum cleaners.

Water

» Learn where your drinking water comes from and how it is treated by your local water utility.

» Protect your water supply and local watershed by minimizing the use of pesticides, using biodegradable cleaning products, reducing waste, and conserving water.

» Use a supplemental water treatment system in your home (e.g. activated carbon filtration, reverse osmosis, or distillation).

Land

» Shop at farmers' markets. Get to know your local food suppliers and what agricultural practices they use.

» Buy organic fruits, vegetables, and meats when possible to minimize your exposure to pesticides, synthetic fertilizers, and toxic chemicals.

» Thoroughly wash and scrub fruits and vegetables before eating.

» Start your own garden so that you can control how your food is grown and what goes into it.

» Remove your shoes when entering your home to avoid tracking in polluted soil, dirt, and other contaminants.

RADIATION IN OUR ENVIRONMENT

Like chemicals, heavy metals, and other pollutants, radiation can be a source of environmental contamination. In addition to the natural electromagnetic fields (EMFs) created by the Earth and sun, we are also exposed to man-made sources of radiation that result from the use of electrical energy. Examples of high-frequency radiation include ultraviolet rays, x-rays, and radioactive material; low-frequency waves include those generated by power lines, household appliances, radio and television transmissions, and electronic devices.

High-frequency x-rays and gamma rays are known to cause DNA damage and cancer, and low-frequency radiation may be carcinogenic to humans as well.[17,18] Although the long-term effects of EMF exposure are not yet known, we can take precautionary measures to minimize our exposure to radiation. Just as we use sunscreen to protect ourselves from ultraviolet rays, we can limit our exposure to other sources of radiation by using a wired headset or speakerphone when talking on cellular phones, turning off wireless routers when they are not in use, and reducing our proximity to major sources of EMF.

THE INFLUENCE OF OUR SURROUNDINGS

In addition to the elements that we absorb and ingest from our environment, the physical spaces that surround us can also have an effect on our health, often in an intangible way. Studies of environmental and socioecological psychology suggest that how we relate to our physical surroundings and social environments can impact our health, well-being, mood states, and behavior.[19,20] For example, the experience of sitting in a noisy traffic jam on a hot summer day usually induces a distinctly different state of being than the experience of hiking a scenic ridge trail while breathing cool mountain air. Researchers have found that climate and weather can affect human behavior in both pro- and antisocial ways. Some studies have shown an association between heat and violence, with higher temperatures being linked to higher rates of violent crime. Other studies have shown that people tend to exhibit more helpful, altruistic behavior on days with pleasant weather than on days with unpleasant weather.[20] We are constantly being bombarded by a variety of sensory stimuli from our surroundings, each of which contributes to varying degrees of arousal and stress on our nervous systems and has the ability to influence our well-being.

Any space in which we choose to spend our time, whether it is for living, work, or play, holds influence over our health. In our built environments, like our homes and workplaces, interior design features like sound, lighting, air quality, physical layout, and color choice can all play an important role in our mental well-being and our levels of stress.[21,22] Anyone who has spent time working in a tiny, windowless cubicle under a buzzing fluorescent light is familiar with the impact of workplace conditions on productivity and job satisfaction. With a proven relationship between the physical, chemical, and social factors of a work environment and the incidence of mood disorders and suicide, evidence confirms that quality work demands a quality work environment.[23] Occupational stress not only affects mental health, but can also lead to physical health consequences. Job strain and psychosocial conditions in work environments have been shown to contribute to cardiovascular disease, hypertension, and atherosclerosis.[24]

Imposing a wide range of effects on our health, our surroundings can also influence the quality of our lives in positive ways. The Chinese practice of *feng shui* suggests that the optimal layout of our homes and work spaces can enhance our *qi* and create harmony for our personal finances, relationships, and health. Health-care facilities are also recognizing the significant role of our surroundings in health and healing. An increasing number of hospitals and cancer treatment centers are changing the design of their facilities to improve the quality of patient experience. Features like open spaces, natural lighting, soothing colors, music, and outdoor gardens are all being incorporated into hospital designs to positively influence patient outcomes.[25,26] Research studies suggest that allowing patients to view landscape scenes or natural elements like trees, plants, and water can also have a therapeutic effect, reducing stress, anxiety, and the need for strong pain medication during recovery.[27]

The innate bond between human beings and nature explains why contact with our natural environment is so beneficial to our health. Evidence demonstrates that exposure to animals, plants, landscapes, and wilderness can increase feelings of relaxation and improve mental well-being.[28] Furthermore, being outdoors in nature, or even the act of imagining oneself in nature, has been shown to increase levels of energy and feelings of vitality.[29] Fresh air and sunshine supply our bodies with more than just oxygen and vitamin D; these environmental sources of *qi* provide us with the opportunity to supplement and strengthen our own *qi*. Through our interactions with the natural world, we enhance our connection to the surrounding environment and the universal life force present in all living things.

THE HUMAN FOOTPRINT

Just as the environment holds influence over our lives and health, our actions and behavior have an effect on the environment in return. The "green" movement of the last several decades has brought awareness to the reciprocal relationship between man and Earth, recognizing the need for responsible environmental stewardship. One example of this can be seen in the 2010 Gulf of Mexico oil spill. As one of the largest examples of environmental contamination in U.S. history, the spill not only damaged the surrounding ecosystem and marine wildlife, but also highlighted the indirect consequences of depending on fossil fuels for energy. Each action that we engage in as humans has broader, global implications and contributes to our overall ecological footprint. When we conserve natural resources and engage in eco-friendly practices, we not only benefit the Earth, but also its inhabitants.

Protecting the environment begins with an awareness of our actions and their ability to affect our surroundings. Even small steps like carpooling or taking public transportation to work can contribute to an overall reduction in vehicle emissions, air pollution, ozone layer damage, and ultimately, global warming. Similarly, minimizing the use of pesticides and toxic chemicals in both home and commercial settings can help to ensure the safety of our land, water, crops, and food supply. With limited reserves of natural resources and a growing population worldwide, conservation is critical to the longevity of our planet for generations to come. As we invest in renewable and clean energy sources, we can begin to reduce our reliance on fossil fuels and benefit both environmental and personal health.

*What is the use of a house if you haven't got
a tolerable planet to put it on?*

– Henry David Thoreau

RESPECTING MOTHER EARTH

Environmentalism highlights our fundamental connection to our surroundings and echoes the Taoist philosophy that our bodies are microcosmic reflections of the macrocosmic universe. Taoism recognizes the interdependent relationship between man and nature, viewing the Earth as our mother, the heavens as our father, and all living things as our brothers and sisters. Its teachings emphasize the interconnectedness between heaven, Earth, and humanity. Man is not seen as separate from nature; rather, he is an integral part of the cosmic whole. Consequently, Taoism suggests that the natural world deserves the

EVERY DAY IS EARTH DAY

Here are a few steps that you can take at home, at work, and in your community to promote environmental health:

» Save energy – use renewable energy sources, cut back on electricity usage, and install energy-efficient appliances and light bulbs.

» Conserve water – repair faucet leaks, turn off the faucet while you wash dishes and brush your teeth, install low-flow showerheads and water-efficient toilets, plant native vegetation in your yard, and water your lawn during the coolest part of the day.

» Cut back on vehicle emissions – walk, bicycle, carpool, use public transportation, drive a hybrid, electric, or hydrogen vehicle, and buy local goods that have not been transported over long distances.

» Minimize your use of pesticides and fertilizers.

» Properly dispose of hazardous materials and electronic waste.

» Buy locally and sustainably grown foods.

» Reduce the amount of waste that will end up in landfills, buy products with fewer packaging materials, and minimize your use of natural resources.

» Reuse products and containers, use cloth bags for shopping, use cloth napkins and towels, and sell or donate used goods instead of throwing them away.

» Recycle metals, plastics, glass, cardboard, and paper, compost your food scraps and yard trimmings for use in your garden, and buy products made from recycled materials.

same level of respect and care that we grant ourselves. As we receive nature's bounty and gifts, we must also ensure that we protect and support the environment in return. The Earth's well-being can no longer be viewed as something separate from us; we are dependent on our planet and responsible for the consequences of our actions upon it.

The environmental ethic found in Taoist philosophy can be traced to its reverence for nature. Nature is upheld as the model for the ideal life and guides us to act accordingly. The Taoist concept of *wu wei*, or non-action, suggests that we should harmonize with natural processes and avoid interfering with nature's course. Our interactions with nature should be based on a spirit of cooperation and preservation, rather than exploitation. By taking our cues from Mother Earth, we can follow her ebbs and flows and live in accordance with her seasons. Taoism teaches us to align with nature, synchronizing with its dynamic patterns and adopting its vigor, instinct, and resilience. As we unite our minds, bodies, and spirits toward wellness, our silent but omniscient partner is the environment, alongside us all the while.

Chapter 6
A Holistic Picture
of Health

CONSTITUTIONS AND BODY TYPES

The recipe for humankind requires the perfect execution of
a myriad of chemical and biological processes. Although we
all share the same basic needs, each of us is born unique. The
differences between us are apparent from birth, from physical
traits like skin tone, body shape, and structural makeup to
psychological characteristics like temperament and the ways in
which we view and interact with our surroundings. Traditional
Chinese Medicine (TCM) philosophy suggests that an individual's
constitution is inherited from one's parents and influenced by
one's *yuan qi*, or the original *qi* with which each person is born.[1]
In some ways, our constitution represents our most fundamental nature, a symbol of our origins and an essential part
of our character.

Through the observation of body structures, physical characteristics, and personality traits, constitutionology attempts to
account for the differences that exist between individuals and
correlate those differences to specific patterns of health and
disease. Constitutions can be hardy and robust, weak and frail,
or something in between. Constitutional factors can influence

our current state of health and our future susceptibility to disease. Although some of us seem to catch a cold every time the weather changes, others are able to ride out the flu season without a single sniffle. Constitutional body types can also help to explain why one person responds well to a certain diet, while another does not lose weight when following the same guidelines.

Formed at birth, our constitution represents an intrinsic framework of health that is influenced by extrinsic and environmental factors. Although our genes may predispose us to certain health characteristics and conditions, our daily choices about what to eat, think, do, and absorb help to determine the final outcome. Conceptualized as a complement to the human genome, the term "exposome" encompasses all of the non-genetic exposures that we are subjected to throughout our lifetime.[2] Researchers suggest that these environmental factors play the principal role in human disease, comprising 70% to 90% of all disease risk.[3] Our diet, exercise, and environment affect the regulation of our genes on a molecular level.[4] Epigenetics is the study of how environmental signals lead to changes in gene expression and activity, switching genes "on" or "off" and influencing our susceptibility to disease or health. Studies by Dr. Dean Ornish and the Preventive Medicine Research Institute demonstrate that comprehensive changes in diet and lifestyle can modulate gene expression in the prostate and even reverse severe cases of coronary heart disease.[5,6] In order to obtain a comprehensive picture of health, we must interpret the human constitution within the full context of our lifestyle factors and environmental influences.

A PERSONALIZED AND MULTIFACTORIAL APPROACH

Each individual is metabolically, physiologically, and genetically different. We not only vary in our response to different foods and environmental stimuli, but also in our age, lifestyle, preferences, and health status. The science of nutrigenomics examines the complex interactions between our genetic constitution and our environment, highlighting the differences between individuals and the need for a personalized approach to nutrition and health.[7,8] Personalized medicine offers us the ability to maximize our individual health potential and prevent disease by tailoring our diet and lifestyle practices to our specific needs, genetic characteristics, and health requirements. It focuses on the individual, considering a broad range of factors from nutrition and physical activity to psychological influences and environmental exposures.[9]

When diet, exercise, the mind-body connection, and environmental influences are combined, together they weave a web that represents optimal wellness. Each strand of this web is equally important and mutually inclusive, offering its own contribution to the overall picture of health. With each addition to the intricate pattern, the web is strengthened and bolstered. Holism, one of the distinguishing tenets of TCM theory, considers how these separate pieces come together to form a fortified center that is rich with energy and endurance. It also suggests that when we consider the concept of health, we should ensure that our view is expansive in both scope and time.

At any given moment, our state of health represents a single point along a continuum between ease and disease. Our well-being is dynamic and variable, reflecting a myriad of inputs. Because

FACTORS INFLUENCING HEALTH

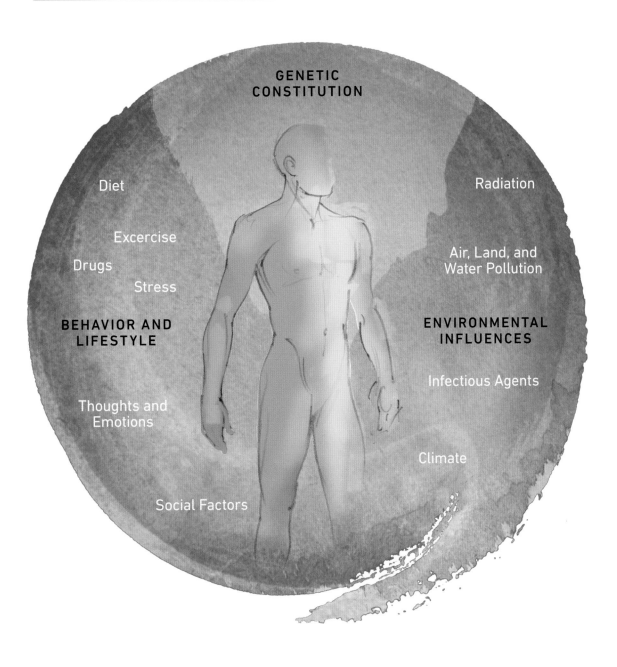

GENETIC
CONSTITUTION

Diet

Radiation

Excercise

Air, Land, and
Water Pollution

Drugs

Stress

BEHAVIOR AND
LIFESTYLE

ENVIRONMENTAL
INFLUENCES

Infectious Agents

Thoughts and
Emotions

Climate

Social Factors

each person's health is unique and constantly changing, there are no hard or fast rules that apply to everybody. By staying flexible and taking a long-term view, we can, however, bring all the strands together to build a foundation of good health.

ADOPTING A GOOD ATTITUDE

The idea of health is a subjective one; we all characterize our health differently based on our individual perceptions and beliefs. For some, being healthy can mean having a body that is in prime physical condition, energized and prepared for any adventure. For others, it can mean having mental clarity, a feeling of vitality, and freedom from emotional stress. Although the constant stream of images from the media might lead us to believe otherwise, a healthy body does not necessarily mean having a thin waistline or sculpted muscles. Health represents much more than just our appearance. The benefits of a healthier lifestyle go beyond weight loss; they also include resilience, the absence of pain, and the ability to meet life's challenges with readiness and grace. Our ideal state of health is ours to define. Consequently, we alone choose our individual attitudes toward health and determine if those beliefs are serving us well. Are our goals realistic? Have we confused health with body image? When we recognize that the process of health is a long-term prospect, we can adopt a sensible outlook toward it and discover its true meaning: feeling and living well.

The journey toward healthful living should include things that we enjoy and help us to feel good. The daily choices we make about what to eat, think, do, and absorb become opportunities to relish instead of burdens of responsibility. Envisioning the things that we want for ourselves and what it feels like to have them allows us to inspire change and propel ourselves to a new reality. Whether our goal is to fit into a new pair of jeans or have enough energy to play with our kids, our thoughts and intentions are what set the tone for our future behavior and actions.

> *He who can believe himself well, will be well.*
>
> – Ovid

ADAPTING TO CHANGE

Change is inherent for all living things. As a series of transformational processes, life challenges us to constantly move, grow, and evolve. The energy of nature continuously ebbs and flows; the bright sunlight of the day yields to the cool darkness of the evening, the heat of summer subsides into the cold of winter, and a white *yang* flows seamlessly into a black *yin*. Our bodies thrive on variety and contrast. When we engage in different activities and embrace new experiences and environments, we become stronger and more prepared to respond to any challenge. For example, by including both low-intensity yoga and high-intensity aerobics into our workout routines, we activate different muscle groups and ensure that our bodies are balanced as a whole. Doing so not only helps us to avoid injury, but also prepares us for spontaneous and variable activity. Similarly, exposure to different types of environments can be beneficial to our health and immune systems; the more contact we have with a variety of microbes in childhood, the greater defense we have against them as adults. As life offers up a variety of conditions and circumstances, we must change and adapt along with them. Flexibility is the key to navigating change, whether this includes our changing states of health, our changing environment, or external conditions which may be out of our control.

NOURISHING THE BODY AND MIND

In order to truly promote health, we must nourish our bodies with more than just the basic nutritional requirements necessary for survival. Optimal health demands that we choose that which "feeds" and sustains our whole selves. Although we take care of our families and friends, we often fail to take care of ourselves. Making personal health a priority means treating ourselves with the same care and compassion that we show to others. Health is best maintained when there is more appreciation than criticism, more indulgence than deprivation, and more forgiveness than punishment. When we treat ourselves well, our bodies respond accordingly.

> *Have patience with all things,*
> *but first of all, with yourself.*
> – St. Francis de Sales

By nourishing ourselves, we can influence every aspect of wellness. Home-cooked meals prepared for our families become expressions of love, representing more than just nutrients or calories. Exercise is an act of nourishment for the body; it strengthens our hearts and muscles, while circulating blood, oxygen, and *qi*. As we practice awareness and other mind-body techniques, we support our minds and enhance the connection to both our bodies and our surrounding environment. When we nurture ourselves with simple acts like practicing a hobby, curling up with a good book, or taking a walk after a long, busy day, we are able to reap immediate benefits. What is it that makes us happy? We should immerse ourselves in experiences that breed enjoyment, while feeling gratitude for the foods, activities, and surroundings that support our well-being. When we set forth with positive intention and take pleasure in the gifts that life offers us, optimal wellness is well within our reach.

TRUSTING OUR INDIVIDUAL WISDOM

There are a great many guides and a great many teachers, none more revered than the omniscient one sitting upon the highest mountain in the most foreign land. It seems that the more remote the source of information, the wiser the guidance appears to be. With thousands of books on diet and health being published every year, there is an abundance of information available to us. While many experts offer recommendations on how to achieve optimal health, we must rely on our own individual wisdom to determine what feels best for *our* bodies. As our greatest resource and earliest knowledge base, our inner guidance serves as an internal compass, helping us to navigate through life's choices along our unique paths to well-being.

Our intuition arises from a source deep within us. Motivational phrases like "trust your gut" and "follow your heart" exemplify this inner knowing. When we use our senses to describe something that "feels right" or "resonates" with us, it is as if we know that all of the individual cells in our bodies are vibrating in harmony and agreement. Our bodies express knowledge that is not necessarily learned or verbalized, but that is inherently understood. Physical cravings and feelings of discomfort or pain can all serve as examples of a body that is communicating with the mind, its partner in health.

In order to hear the messages that our bodies are sending, we must ensure that the mind-body connection is functioning smoothly and freely. Through the practice of meditation and awareness exercises, we can quiet the mind and re-train it to access our deeper intuition. As we filter through the cacophony of noise and conflicting messages that surround us, we become more attuned to our bodies and aligned to their present state. Our bodies hold the keys to wellness; to access them, we must listen, trust our individual wisdom, and place our faith in the process of health.

The only way to live is to accept each minute as an unrepeatable miracle, which is exactly what it is – a miracle and unrepeatable.

– Margaret Storm Jameson

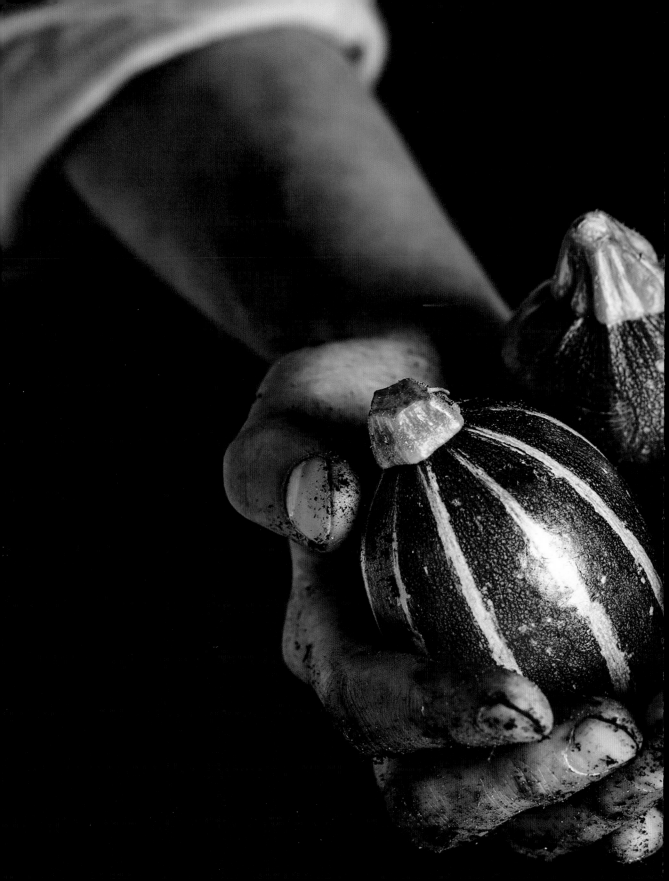

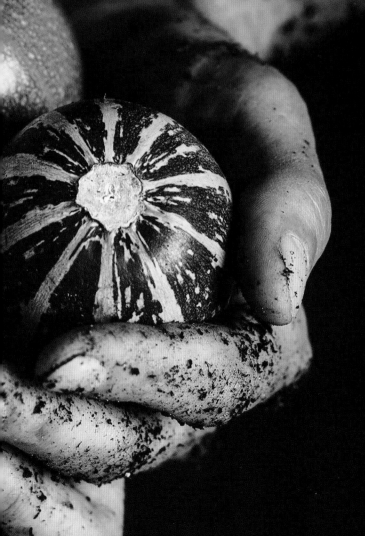

Part II
The Seasonal Body Type System

Chapter 7
Foundations
and Philosophy

HOT AND COLD: HUMORAL THEORY

The idea that individual health should be viewed in the context of one's environment is central to humoral medicine. Practiced in the ancient civilizations of Greece, China, India, and Latin America, humoral medicine is one of the oldest and most widely influential belief systems in the world.[1,2] Humoral traditions are still used today in many cultures as comprehensive principles for understanding everyday health and disease.[3] Taking a macrocosmic view of man in relation to his natural environment, humoral theory defines health as the balance of opposing elements. Hot and cold, wet and dry, light and dark, growth and decay: these terms can be used to describe elements in the natural world, as well as elements of our individual health. Humoral theory links our diet, lifestyle, and state of health to the natural phenomena that surround us. It emphasizes the fundamental connection between man and nature.

The basis of all forms of humoral medicine is the balance between opposing elements or humors. Ancient Greek medicine proposed that the body is governed by four humors or bodily fluids: blood, phlegm, yellow bile, and black bile.[4] The relative proportion of humors to each other or the dominance of one humor over another was thought to correlate with a certain set of physical traits, health conditions, and emotional temperaments. Similarly, the Ayurvedic medicine system from India suggests that individual constitutions are dependent on three elements: *vata, pitta,* and *kapha.* Balance of these elements, or *doshas,* is necessary for optimum health, while an imbalance contributes to the process of disease.[5] Furthermore, Traditional Chinese Medicine (TCM) describes the elemental forces that affect the process of health in terms of *yin* and *yang.* In all forms of humoral theory, it is the balance of opposing elements that defines optimal health, and the imbalance of those elements that leads to disease. Humoral medicine suggests that the excess or deficiency of any one element will present itself in the form of health symptoms or ailments. For example, excess *yang* or deficient *yin* may be experienced as a fever or a red skin rash, while excess *yin* or deficient *yang* may be characterized by a pale face or the physical sensation of being cold. Over time, these imbalances will lead to the manifestation of more severe symptoms and eventually illness.

Hot and cold are perhaps the most basic and primordial pair of opposites. In their simplest form, the terms "hot" and "cold" can be used to characterize the thermal nature of an object. If *qi* is defined as energy, then temperature is simply a measure of *qi* in motion. Consequently, when *qi* moves quickly, there is heat, and when *qi* moves slowly, there is cold. Similarly, heat signifies tension while cold represents withdrawal. The thermal quality of the body can be described by the degree of energy, or the amount of heat or cold, present at any given point in time. Hot and cold are also relative states. Just as *yin* and *yang* exist on a spectrum, varying thermal intensities (warm, neutral, or cool) can be found on a range from extreme heat to extreme cold.

Symbolically, the words "hot" and "cold" have meanings that go beyond temperature alone. Cultural and social information are often encoded into these terms, like descriptions of our emotional states (e.g. "hot-tempered" or "cool as a cucumber") or the ways in which we interact with each other (e.g. "he was warm and affectionate" or "she was cold and distant"). The TCM concepts of *yin* and *yang* can be used to express the relationship between hot and cold, as well as other opposing universal pairs: slow and fast, light and dark, and male and female. There are *yin* and *yang* people, *yin* and *yang* body types, and *yin* and *yang* seasons and stages of life. In nature, there is an inherent inclination for all living things to seek equilibrium; as such, the optimal state of existence is one that is defined by the balance of both hot and cold and *yin* and *yang.*

The key to balancing health is to balance our individual constitutions through the foods we eat, the activities we do, and the lifestyle choices we make. To apply humoral theory to our health, "hot" foods are used to treat cold conditions and "cold" foods soothe overheated states. *Yang* activities like mountain biking and jogging invigorate those with a placid *yin* constitution, while soothing *yin* activities like *tai chi* and yoga benefit those with excess *yang.* Throughout our lives, our individual needs change depending on age, gender, and overall condition. Our environment and climate also influence what our bodies require for balance. While a cold fruit smoothie may be the ideal refreshment when we are sitting on a beach in Hawaii, the same drink may not seem so appealing if we're standing in Alaska in the middle of winter. Using heat and cold to balance the body requires a holistic perspective of individual health within the full context of our environment.

The law of yin *and* yang *is the natural order
of the universe, the foundation of all things, mother
of all changes, the root of life and death.*

– The Yellow Emperor's Classic of Internal Medicine

CLASSIFICATIONS OF HOT AND COLD

In humoral medicine, classifications of hot and cold are based on observations of how the body responds to various stimuli. Historically, these characterizations have been applied to both diseases and foods. Humoral theory relates the etiology and incidence of disease to the external environment and the seasonal variations between hot and cold. Different illnesses are associated with different climates or changes in the weather; "hot" diseases are more common in the summertime, while "cold" diseases are observed more often in the winter.[6] For example, too much heat in the body is often characterized by symptoms like dry mouth, thirst, fever, skin rashes or irritations, dark-colored urine, high blood pressure, and many inflammatory conditions. In contrast, excess cold can manifest itself as chills, clammy skin, weakness, fatigue, arthritis, rheumatism, and respiratory problems. The same principles that govern heat and cold in natural phenomena can also be seen in their effects on the human body; heat causes expansion and expulsion, while cold can induce solidification and congestion. Generally, hot illnesses are thought to radiate from the center of the body outward to its surface, while cold illnesses manifest themselves internally, staying deep within.[6]

The characterization of a food as either hot or cold depends on an intrinsic, abstract quality; consequently, a food's thermal nature may not necessarily be the same as its actual, physical temperature. Eating heating foods like garlic or onions can cause the body to flush or experience warmth, while eating cooling foods like watermelons and coconut juice can refresh or cool down the body. TCM suggests that consuming too many heating foods can lead to excess heat in the body and eventually, to the manifestation of "hot" illnesses such as rashes and fevers; heating foods can also exacerbate health symptoms in individuals with a "hot" or *yang* body type. Correcting an imbalance between *yin* and *yang* involves using cooling foods to treat a hot, *yang* body and warming foods to treat a cold, *yin* one.

Using different foods to balance health is a fundamental component of disease prevention. The familiar quotation from Hippocrates, "Let food be thy medicine and medicine be thy food," still holds true today. As a daily source of *qi* and energy, the foods that we eat form the most basic building blocks of our health. Humoral theory emphasizes a natural inclination to use hot and cold foods for healing, a practice which has been built into generations of dietary traditions and habits. For example, when we catch a cold, we often crave a bowl of warming chicken soup to help us feel better. After a long day in the sun, a tall glass of iced lemonade refreshes our overheated bodies. Just as we balance a dish of hot buffalo wings with a side of celery sticks, we eat spicy Indian curries with a cooling yogurt raita.

Sometimes we even use hot and cold foods externally on the body; cooling cucumber slices are used at the spa to soothe puffy eyes, and muscle balms made with capsaicin (an ingredient found in hot peppers) activate a healing response in sore muscles. Even though we may not be aware of it, we are constantly applying the principles of humoral theory to balance the elements of hot and cold in our lives.

HOT AND COLD FOOD THERAPY

For the most part, humoral classifications of hot and cold foods are similar across different cultures throughout the world.[1] Foods that are higher in protein, fat, and calories are generally considered to be heating; they build, energize, and increase tension within the body. Examples of warming foods include animal products, meats, and other rich, fatty foods. They tend to create warmth in the body and help to sustain it in colder climates. For example, in extreme cold and Arctic regions, the traditional Inuit diet includes foods like whale blubber, which is extremely high in fat and energy and is very warming. Some plant-source foods also have a warming thermal nature. Typically, plants that grow deep within the earth or take longer to grow (e.g. carrots, potatoes, and cabbages) store more energy and tend to be more warming. Foods and drinks that have a stimulating effect when consumed (e.g. coffee, spices, and sugar) also tend to be warming. Alcohol is not only heating in the physiological sense, but it can also "heat" one's temper, intensifying emotions like anger and aggression.

On the other end of the spectrum, cooling foods generally have a lower caloric value and a higher water content. Cooling foods are beneficial for soothing, cleansing, and relieving irritation within the body. Most fruits and vegetables are considered to be cooling; this includes foods like watermelons and tomatoes, and citrus fruits, like lemons and grapefruits. Vegetables that grow quickly, like lettuce, cucumbers, and summer squash, also tend to be cooling. In contrast with root vegetables, leafy greens and other cooling vegetables typically sprout and grow above ground, with only a short growth time before harvest.

In most humoral classifications, neutral foods tend to be staples, like grains and starches. Most beans and legumes also tend to be neutral or slightly warming. Many cultures classify these staple foods as thermally neutral because they generally can be consumed without disrupting the body's humoral balance or causing illness.[3]

There are exceptions to the broad classifications of hot and cold foods. For instance, while most vegetables are cooling, certain crops like mustard greens, fennel, and horseradish have a spicy flavor and a more warming effect on the body. Similarly, while many fruits like melons and pears are cooling, there are some that are warming, like cherries and peaches. Most meats and seafood are neutral to warming, except for pork and crab which tend to be more cooling. TCM classifications of hot and cold foods have been developed over centuries of use and observation; the following chart shows the thermal nature of some common foods, ranging from most cooling to most heating.

THERMAL NATURE OF SAMPLE FOODS

	COLD	COOL	NEUTRAL	WARM	HOT
Fruits	Grapefruit	Apples	Grapes	Cherries	
	Watermelon	Pears	Pineapple	Peaches	
Vegetables	Seaweed	Broccoli	Asparagus	Bell peppers	Garlic
		Celery	Beets	Cabbage	Ginger
		Cucumbers	Carrots	Fennel	Onions
		Lettuce	Cauliflower	Mustard greens	
		Summer squash	Green beans	Parsnips	
		Swiss chard	Potatoes	Winter squash	
		Tomatoes			
Grains		Barley	Amaranth	Oats	
		Millet	Corn	Quinoa	
		Wheat	Rice	Rye	
Nuts and Legumes		Mung beans	Almonds	Black beans	
			Chickpeas	Chestnuts	
			Kidney beans	Walnuts	
			Lentils		
Meats and Seafood	Crab	Clams	Mackerel	Beef	Lamb
		Pork	Sardines	Chicken	
			Tuna	Salmon	
				Shrimp	
Spices		Peppermint		Basil	Black pepper
				Cloves	Chili pepper
				Cumin	Cinnamon
				Nutmeg	
				Rosemary	
				Thyme	
Beverages		Green tea	Water	Coffee	Alcohol
		Orange juice			

A food's inherent thermal nature (hot, cold, or neutral) can also be affected by how it is cooked or prepared. Generally, raw foods tend to be thermally cooler than foods that are cooked. Raw foods require more energy to digest and the resulting loss of internal energy has a cooling effect on the body. When foods are prepared with high-heat methods like frying, grilling, roasting, or baking, or using slow cooking techniques like stewing or braising, they tend to have a more warming effect on the body than if they are steamed, blanched, or boiled. Additionally, dried foods tend to be more warming than fresh ones. Both the cooking method used to prepare a dish and the temperature at which it is served can enhance a food's thermal nature. For example, chicken served hot off the grill has a more warming effect than the same grilled chicken served at room temperature.

THE EFFECTS OF DIFFERENT COOKING METHODS ON THE THERMAL NATURE OF FOODS

VERY COOLING	COOLING	NEUTRAL	WARMING	VERY WARMING
Chilled	Raw or uncooked	Steamed	Stir-fried	Deep-fried
Frozen		Blanched	Boiled/simmered	Roasted/broiled
		Poached	Braised	Grilled
			Baked	

In addition to a food's thermal nature, other properties are important in the application of dietary therapy. TCM theory suggests that the different flavors of sour, sweet, salty, bitter, and pungent* affect the body differently and provide distinct benefits for each body type. In TCM, flavor refers to a food's properties and effect on the body, and does not necessarily correspond to the taste of the food when eaten. Bitter flavors, for instance, have a drying effect on the body, while pungent flavors promote circulation, naturally sweet flavors build and nourish, sour flavors are cleansing, and salty flavors have a moistening effect. In general, foods with a mild taste, like grains and other staples, can be eaten in larger quantities. On the other hand, foods with stronger flavors, like certain spices and herbs, tend to have a correspondingly stronger effect on the body and are best consumed in smaller quantities, for more medicinal use. Using different foods to balance individual health requires consideration of thermal nature, flavor, and cooking method.

Dietary therapy has been a central component of TCM for thousands of years. Although humoral classifications of hot and cold have been developed primarily through experiential use and cultural observation, scientists are now beginning to understand the underlying mechanisms and biochemical properties that make different foods "hot" or "cold." Some research suggests that the *yin* or *yang* nature of certain fruits may be related to their copper, iron, and magnesium content.[7] In other studies, foods thought to have a heating effect have been associated with the production of prostaglandin E2 (PGE2), a hormone-like substance that promotes the inflammatory response in the body. In comparison, foods with a cooling effect have been found to inhibit the production of PGE2.[8] Lastly, research on the properties of traditional Chinese herbs shows that *yin*-tonifying herbs have higher antioxidant activity than *yang* herbs, suggesting that *yin* may relate to the process of antioxidation, whereas *yang* relates to oxidation.[9]

---

*In classical TCM texts, the fifth flavor is commonly translated as "pungent" or "acrid." Traditionally, umami is not recognized as one of the five therapeutic flavors in TCM philosophy.

TCM FLAVOR CLASSIFICATIONS OF SAMPLE FOODS

SOUR	BITTER	SWEET	PUNGENT	SALTY
Adzuki beans	Alfalfa sprouts	Almonds	Black pepper	Duck
Apples	Amaranth	Beef	Cayenne	Octopus
Cheese	Asparagus	Cabbage	Cinnamon	Oysters
Grapes	Celery	Carrots	Fennel	Pork
Kiwis	Coffee	Chicken	Garlic	Seaweed
Lemons/Limes	Dandelion	Coconuts	Ginger	Soy sauce
Mangoes	Lettuce	Corn	Kohlrabi	
Olives	Rye	Eggplants	Mustard seeds	
Pineapples	Tea	Figs	Onions	
Plums	Turnips	Milk	Peppers	
Tomatoes		Oats	Radishes	
Vinegar		Potatoes		
Yogurt		Rice		
		Spinach		
		Sweet potatoes		
		Walnuts		
		Wheat		

BODY TYPES AND THE SEASONS

The fundamental Taoist principles of TCM suggest that optimal health can only be achieved when we live in harmony with the universe around us. The body as a microcosm matches the Earth as a macrocosm, while its internal climate balances with its external surroundings. As the seasons change, our bodies and constitutions should follow. When summer rays shine down upon us, we become more energetic and *yang*-like, flourishing and reveling in the sun. When the frigid cold of winter arrives, we curl up and retreat into the introspective *yin* of the season. Transformation is necessary and intrinsic to all forms of life.

In TCM, each of the five seasons represents a unique stage of life and a distinct phase of *yin* or *yang*. Spring, with its delicate blossoms and hint of *yang*, is the harbinger of new beginnings and a season filled with hopeful optimism. It is followed by summer, a time of flourishing, bountiful growth that is fueled by a hot, *yang* energy at its peak. As the heat of summer transitions to the cool of fall, Indian summer represents the ideal balance between *yang* and *yin*. Its seemingly endless days of sunlight and its mild, temperate weather offer a fleeting glimpse of perfection. Fall arrives with a cool, brisk gust of air and the final harvest of the year; colorful leaves are shed as nature loses its vibrancy and begins its decline into *yin*. Finally, the cold of winter encourages retreat and withdrawal, marking the period of deepest *yin*. Time slows to a peaceful standstill as the world awaits the rebirth that comes with spring and the start of a new cycle.

A LIFE CYCLE THROUGH THE SEASONS

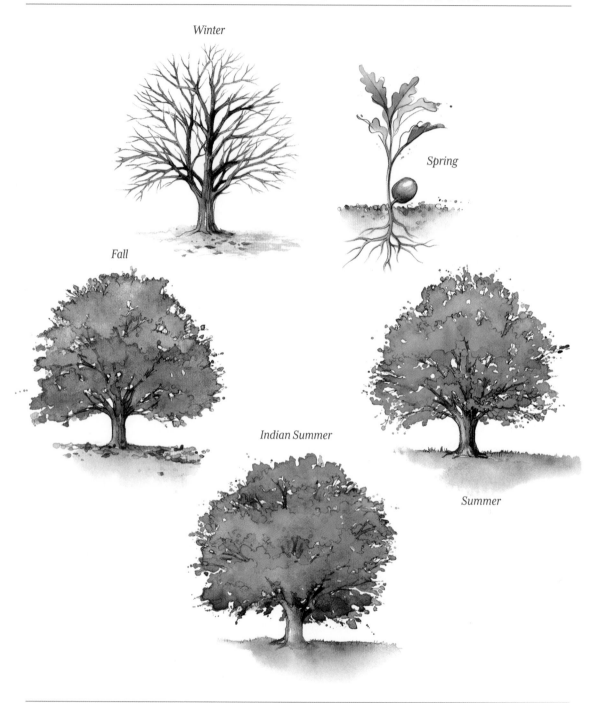

Winter

Spring

Fall

Indian Summer

Summer

There is an appointed time for everything,
and a time for every affair under the heavens.
A time to give birth, and a time to die;
a time to plant, and a time to uproot the plant.
– Ecclesiastes 3:1-2

A body that is in harmonious balance with its surrounding environment is one that directly reflects nature's seasonal changes; it experiences phases of hot and cold, wet and dry, expansion and withdrawal, and growth and decay synchronously along with the Earth. In most cases, our bodies exist in some state of imbalance, either due to our inherent constitutions, lifestyle choices, or natural preferences. An imbalanced body behaves as if it is perennially stuck in one season. Instead of adapting to nature's seasons, it remains stagnant; a "summer" body displays the hot, *yang* characteristics and blazing excitement of summer all year long, while a "winter" body is pale, cold, and withdrawn, regardless of the season or external environment.

The Seasonal Body Type System categorizes our individual constitutions and tendencies into five seasonal body types: Spring, Summer, Indian Summer, Fall, and Winter. Each body type relates to one of the five seasons of TCM and to that season's climate, theme, foods, and activities. Individuals with a more *yang*-like nature resemble the *yang* seasons of spring and summer. They often display characteristics of "heat," like a flushed complexion or a warm body temperature; they are marked by the same fast-paced energy and intense activity found in those seasons. In order to balance the *yang* in Spring and Summer body types, these individuals should eat more cooling foods and engage in slower, *yin*-like activities. On the other hand, Fall and Winter body types tend to be more dominant in *yin*, showing signs of coldness like cold hands and feet, and exemplifying the calmer, slower tempo of the later seasons of the year. Countering excess *yin* and restoring balance in these body types calls for more warming foods and *yang* activities. Indian Summer body types lie within the middle ground between *yin* and *yang*. Neutral and mild foods are appropriate for this type, as well as for the four other body types, as they help to sustain energy and build a general foundation of health.

Often, our natural tendencies actually aggravate our constitutional types and underlying health conditions. Hot Summer types, who thrive on blood-pumping excitement and intensity, enjoy eating spicy and fried foods that warm their overheated bodies even more. Although they prefer life on the fiery, *yang* edge, they may find it difficult to sustain that fire all year long. Meanwhile, Winter body types often consume cooling foods, like raw fruits, salads, and ice cream, which only exacerbate their feelings of cold and lethargy. Instead of eating warming foods and engaging in *yang* activities to balance themselves, they make choices that cause them to withdraw even further into a state of *yin*. In order to harmonize our bodies with the environment and achieve optimal health, we must choose the foods and activities that are appropriate for our seasonal types and constantly engage in a balancing act that matches hot to cold, and *yin* to *yang*.

A NATURAL SOLUTION

Look to the seasons when choosing your cures.
– Hippocrates

The keys to balancing health lie within nature itself. The Earth prescribes a natural solution by providing foods in each season that inherently support the body's activities within that season. The seasonal foods of summer include cooling tomatoes, cucumbers, and watermelons that are ideal for countering the long, hot days of the season. Corn and pumpkin highlight the Earth's seasonal offerings in Indian summer, and are appropriate in the diet during that time because they are thermally neutral and naturally sweet. In the colder months, warming root vegetables and winter squash become available, offering a way for the body to sustain itself through the cold. When we look to nature as our guide, we discover that the foods our bodies require in each season are the same ones that nature already offers. At the times we need to balance *yang*, the Earth gives us *yin* foods; when we need to protect against excess *yin*, the Earth offers us warming, *yang* foods.

A LIST OF SEASONAL PRODUCE IN NORTH AMERICA*

SPRING	SUMMER	INDIAN SUMMER	FALL	WINTER
Asparagus	Apricots	Apples	Broccoli	Brussels sprouts
Beets	Avocados	Avocados	Cauliflower	Cabbage
Carrots	Basil	Eggplants	Cranberries	Chestnuts
Fava beans	Bell peppers	Figs	Kale	Grapefruit
Leeks	Blueberries	Grapes	Pears	Kale
Lettuce	Cherries	Green beans	Persimmons	Kohlrabi
Onions	Corn	Melons	Pomegranates	Lemons
Peas	Cucumbers	Okra	Pumpkins	Oranges
Spinach	Eggplants	Onions	Quince	Tangerines
	Garlic	Potatoes	Sweet potatoes	Winter squash
	Green beans	Summer squash	Turnips	
	Melons	Swiss chard		
	Nectarines	Tomatoes		
	Onions			
	Peaches			
	Plums			
	Strawberries			
	Summer squash			*For more information on local foods in your specific area, see the Appendix.
	Swiss chard			
	Tomatoes			

Eating seasonally means eating foods that are grown within a specific season and geographical region. By consuming seasonal foods, we also promote the use of environmentally friendly and sustainable agriculture practices. Instead of eating bananas grown in tropical areas thousands of miles away, we eat the foods that nature offers us nearby. Buying locally grown produce allows us to enjoy freshly picked fruits and vegetables, save transportation costs and fuel, and also support our local farming community.

The following diagram illustrates how the five seasons and body types relate to the seasonal themes, climates, foods, and phases of *yin* and *yang* throughout the year.

SEASONAL PHASES OF *YIN* AND *YANG*

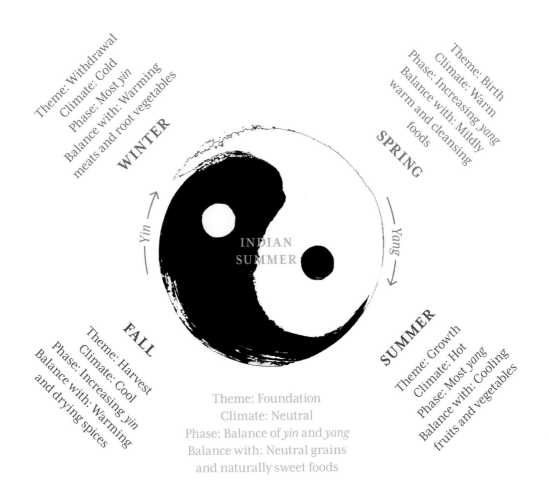

WINTER

Theme: Withdrawal
Climate: Cold
Phase: Most *yin*
Balance with: Warming meats and root vegetables

SPRING

Theme: Birth
Climate: Warm
Phase: Increasing *yang*
Balance with: Mildly warm and cleansing foods

— Yin —

— Yang —

INDIAN SUMMER

FALL

Theme: Harvest
Climate: Cool
Phase: Increasing *yin*
Balance with: Warming and drying spices

SUMMER

Theme: Growth
Climate: Hot
Phase: Most *yang*
Balance with: Cooling fruits and vegetables

Theme: Foundation
Climate: Neutral
Phase: Balance of *yin* and *yang*
Balance with: Neutral grains
and naturally sweet foods

THE SEASONAL BODY TYPE PHILOSOPHY

In the next few chapters, we will further explore the five seasonal body types, looking at their defining characteristics, related health symptoms, and specific principles for healing. Each of our bodies requires a personalized prescription for wellness, one that is governed by a unique set of factors: our constitutional body types, our diets and lifestyle choices, and our environment. The Seasonal Body Type approach allows us to understand all of the factors of individual health within one comprehensive system. It applies a holistic framework to the process of health, viewing the body within the full context of its surroundings and comparing it to elements found in nature. As we relate our bodies to the seasons, we can begin to recognize how the seasonal phases of hot and cold, wet and dry, and *yin* and *yang* influence our health. Instead of transitioning with nature's seasons, we often find that the characteristics of one season or seasonal body type dominate all year long. Our bodies exist in a perpetually "hot" state, like Summer, or a "cold" one, like Winter. When our bodies are in a state of imbalance, we can apply the principles of humoral theory to restore balance and harmony once again.

Living seasonally means that we must align with all aspects of nature, attune to its cycles, and embrace its every ebb and flow. As we follow nature's seasons, eat its foods, and synchronize with its phases, we pay respect to the Earth and honor the gifts that it offers us every day. To live seasonally is to live mindfully, with full awareness and reverence for our connection to the greater universe. When we are able to exist in complete harmony with the changing seasons and truly live as nature intended, our bodies will be free from disease and wellness will be all that we know.

Everything in the universe is within you.
Ask all from yourself.

– Rumi

Chapter 8
What's Your Season?

IDENTIFYING YOUR SEASONAL BODY TYPE

There are several ways to assess which seasonal type best represents you. For self-diagnosis, you can complete the body type checklist in this chapter, evaluate your physical features and character traits, and compare yourself to the five profiles. Another tool you can use to determine your body type is tongue analysis; according to Traditional Chinese Medicine (TCM), your tongue's appearance is an indicator of your state of health. For a more thorough, professional evaluation, you may also want to consider visiting an acupuncturist or a TCM practitioner.

WHAT YOUR TONGUE SAYS ABOUT YOU

As a representation of your internal bodily climate, your tongue's color, shape, and coating can offer invaluable information about your state of health.[1] By looking at your tongue, a trained eye can determine the general state of your digestive and circulatory systems, your body's thermal nature, and the patterns of imbalance that exist in your body. Tongue analysis can help you diagnose your body type, as well as monitor changes in your health condition.

Look at your tongue in the mirror and take note of its color and appearance. The way your tongue appears within the first five seconds will be the most accurate representation of your body type. After five seconds, your tongue's characteristics will begin to change due to exposure to the surrounding air. What color is the body of your tongue? Is it pink, red, pale, bluish purple, or purple in color? A healthy tongue will be pink or light red across its entire surface. A red tongue exemplifies the warmth of Summer body types and a bluish purple tongue is common to the colder Fall and Winter body types. A purple or lavender tongue is indicative of Spring types, while a pale tongue can be seen in both Indian Summer and Winter types. Does your tongue have any spots or small bumps on its surface? Similar to the color of your tongue, red-colored spots may be seen in Summer types and purple-colored spots in Spring types. If you notice that your tongue has spots on it and they are a different color than the body of your tongue, then your tongue is displaying signs from two different pathologies or body types. For example, if your tongue has purple spots and a red surface, you have characteristics of both Spring and Summer body types.

In addition to its color, the shape and surface of your tongue may also show characteristics of hot and cold, *yin* and *yang*, and wetness and dryness. Is your tongue skinny and narrow or large and puffy? Does its surface appear wet and smooth or is it dry and cracked? Is there any coating or fur on your tongue? Ideally, the size of your tongue should be proportionate to the interior of your mouth, neither too small nor too large. The perimeter of your tongue should barely touch the inside surface of your teeth. A large, swollen tongue is associated with an accumulation of fluids in the body, whereas a small, thin tongue relates to dryness. The tongue should have a slightly moist body and a thin white coating. A yellow coating is a sign of heat, which is associated with a Summer body type, while a thick white coating is a sign of cold found in Fall and Winter body types. If the coating is thick and resembles fur, there is a strong imbalance toward *yin* (cold) or *yang* (heat). If the coating is moist with a sticky or pasty consistency, then that indicates an internal climate that is wet or damp. For example, those with a Fall body type are generally prone to feelings of cold, edema, and sinus congestion, and their tongues may appear to be wet and swollen with a sticky white coating. In contrast, some Summer body types have a warmer, drier internal climate and tongues that are red and thin, with a dry, cracked surface and a yellow coating.

Your tongue might exhibit a combination of both *yin* and *yang*, hot and cold, or wet and dry characteristics within different areas. Generally, the more prominent characteristics will indicate your overall tendencies toward *yin* or *yang*. Your tongue's appearance can also vary depending on if you are sick, are taking any medication, have just eaten, or regularly scrape your tongue as part of your oral hygiene routine. Use tongue analysis in combination with other diagnostic techniques to gain a comprehensive picture of your health. The following illustrations include tongue characteristics that are commonly seen in each of the five seasonal body types, as well as a person in balanced health. Which illustration does your tongue most resemble?

TONGUE CHARACTERISTICS OF THE SEASONAL BODY TYPES

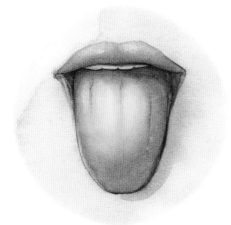

Balanced Body

Pink color, slightly moist surface,
thin white coating

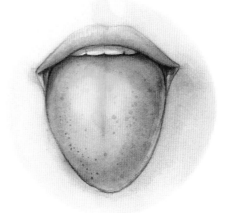

Spring Body Type

Purple color, purple spots

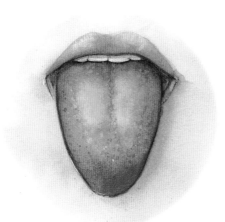

Summer Body Type

Red color, yellow coating, cracks, red spots

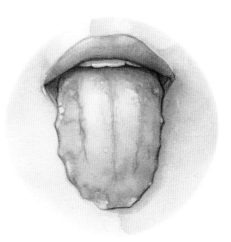

Indian Summer Body Type

Pale color, thin white coating, scalloped edges

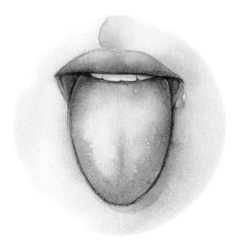

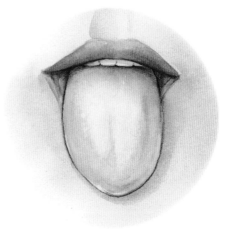

Fall Body Type	Winter Body Type
Light bluish purple color, swollen body, wet surface, sticky/pasty white coating	Pale or bluish purple color, white coating

SEASONAL BODY TYPE CHECKLIST

Because of the complexity of the human body and the constitutional, environmental, and lifestyle factors that influence health, you may find yourself identifying with more than one seasonal body type. Generally, our bodies tend to display characteristics from the cooler seasons (fall and winter), the warmer seasons (spring and summer), or the neutral center (Indian summer). For those with both warm and cool symptoms, usually one health pattern will be more predominant. If you have a pressing health concern or a chronic condition, use that as an indication of your primary seasonal body type. As you review the following lists of symptoms, check off the characteristics that regularly apply to you and add up your totals for each of the five seasons to determine your seasonal body type. Although your responses may be influenced by changing health conditions, illnesses, medications, or stress levels, try to provide answers that represent your general state of health most of the time.

Check below if any of the following regularly apply to you:

SPRING BODY TYPE

☐ I am prone to headaches.

☐ I sigh frequently.

☐ I have frequent bouts of hiccups.

☐ I am often irritable, moody, or easily frustrated.

☐ I often have chest discomfort or tightness.

☐ I have chronic pain in my muscles or joints.

☐ I experience pain or clotting with menstruation.

☐ I experience premenstrual symptoms like mood swings, food cravings, irritability, or trouble concentrating.

☐ I have eye conditions like twitching or blurry vision.

☐ I experience chronic muscle spasms, cramps, or tightness.

☐ I often have hard stools or hemorrhoids.

☐ My tongue has a purple, reddish-purple, or lavender color, and/or purple spots.

☐ I tend to be idealistic, tenacious, or impatient.

☐ I have a passive-aggressive approach to conflict.

___ **Total**

SUMMER BODY TYPE

☐ I run warmer than most people, my palms and soles are warm or hot, or I have an aversion to warm weather.

☐ My skin is easily flushed or prone to rashes.

☐ I am often thirsty or have night sweats.

☐ I have chronic heartburn.

☐ My urine is scanty and has a dark color.

☐ I have high blood pressure or diabetes.

☐ My gums bleed easily.

☐ I have bad breath.

☐ I have yellow or green sputum with post-nasal drip, sinus congestion, or cough.

☐ I have arthritis, edema, or swelling that feels worse in hot, humid weather.

☐ I have difficulty sitting still and often feel antsy.

☐ My tongue has one or more of the following: a red color, a pointy shape, a dry surface, a yellow coating, cracks, or red spots.

☐ I am an adventurer, extrovert, or natural leader.

☐ I have a quick temper, a talkative nature, or exaggerated gestures and emotional responses.

___ **Total**

INDIAN SUMMER BODY TYPE

- ☐ I get sick (e.g. a cold, flu, or sinus infection) three or more times a year.
- ☐ I often lack energy, feel tired, or feel listless.
- ☐ I bruise easily.
- ☐ I have asthma that gets worse with physical activity.
- ☐ I have environmental allergies.
- ☐ I often feel dizzy.
- ☐ I see spots or floaters in my eyes.
- ☐ I have dry eyes, skin, or hair.
- ☐ I experience digestive issues such as gas, bloating, constipation, loose stool, pain, or irritable bowel syndrome (IBS).
- ☐ My menstrual period begins or ends with spotting.
- ☐ I feel tired after a bowel movement.
- ☐ My tongue has scalloped edges or teeth marks.
- ☐ I tend to be nurturing, reliable, level-headed, or reserved in demeanor.
- ☐ I tend to worry a lot.

___ **Total**

FALL BODY TYPE

- ☐ I have cold and clammy hands or feet.
- ☐ My pain and moods are worse in cold, damp weather.
- ☐ I have white or clear sputum with post-nasal drip, sinus congestion, or cough.
- ☐ I often get a stuffy feeling in my head or a band-like headache, both of which are worse in cold, damp weather.
- ☐ I have arthritis that feels worse in cold, damp weather.
- ☐ I have edema or swelling in my body that feels worse in cold, damp weather.
- ☐ My urine is cloudy and pale in color.
- ☐ My stool is sticky or has mucus in it.
- ☐ I often have white vaginal discharge.
- ☐ My body feels heavy or sluggish in cold, damp weather.
- ☐ I am more than 15 pounds overweight.
- ☐ My tongue has a wet surface and a sticky/pasty white coating.
- ☐ I am self-reliant or deliberate in demeanor. I tend to be disorganized or have difficulty concentrating.
- ☐ I tend to linger in sadness or grief.

___ **Total**

WINTER BODY TYPE

- ☐ I run colder than most people or have cold hands and feet.
- ☐ I prefer warm drinks or have an aversion to cold weather.
- ☐ I have a pale complexion.
- ☐ I urinate frequently and my urine is pale in color.
- ☐ I have hypothyroidism or sluggish thyroid function.
- ☐ I have dark circles under my eyes.
- ☐ My appetite is weak.
- ☐ I have a low sex drive or I experience erectile dysfunction.
- ☐ I have alopecia or premature graying of my hair.
- ☐ I like to sleep for long periods of time (more than 8 to 9 hours).
- ☐ My physical movement tends to be slow.
- ☐ My tongue has a white coating that is not sticky/pasty.
- ☐ I tend to be quiet, introverted, sensitive, or intuitive.
- ☐ I tend to be insecure or fearful.

___ **Total**

PROFILES OF THE SEASONAL BODY TYPES

The following section includes sample profiles of the different seasonal body types, with descriptions of each type's common characteristics, personality traits, and physical symptoms. You may not relate to all of the traits described for each type; however, there should be one or two types with which you generally identify.

THE SPRING BODY TYPE

Connie is a successful businesswoman who works twelve-hour days and is a confident go-getter with a competitive edge. Her optimistic outlook and dedication to her work are inspiring to those who work under her lead. She is known to be tough, but fair. Connie makes decisions quickly and emphatically; however, because she tends to trust her own opinions and gut instinct over ideas presented by others, she can appear to be inflexible. Socially, she can be passive-aggressive, displaying an amiable exterior to cover up the frustration she feels when things don't go according to plan.

Connie's desire to achieve extends to her devotion to long-distance running. Her rigorous exercise routine and high training mileage has left her tendons and muscles dry and tight. Every year, she suffers from at least one musculoskeletal injury (e.g. a hamstring pull, crick in her neck, or ankle sprain). Connie also complains of an intermittent, irritating twitch in her eyelid that seems to go away only when she is on vacation. She takes a stool softener to treat her chronic constipation and hemorrhoids. Each month, her menstrual periods arrive with severe cramping, pain, and mood swings.

In general, Spring body types may exhibit one or more of the following symptoms: tension headaches, migratory pain, eye conditions (e.g. blurry or poor vision, or twitching), constipation, bloating, hiccups, and frequent sighing. Women with this seasonal body type may also have menstrual pain or irregularities, cysts, or soreness in their breasts. The characteristic body structure of Spring types is lean with taut musculature. They tend to be determined and ambitious, but easily frustrated, and rigid in both body and mind.

THE SUMMER BODY TYPE

Simon is gregarious and outgoing; he loves to socialize, but has never been good at setting boundaries. He is an engaging storyteller with pizzazz, using his powers of persuasion to great success as a sales manager. He enjoys meeting new people and networking with potential clients and contacts. Quick with a joke, Simon makes friends with ease, though his gestures of affection toward complete strangers display an unintentional disregard for personal space. His boundless enthusiasm is embodied not only in his loud voice and hearty laugh, but also in the explosive tirades that he goes on when he loses his temper.

Always on the move, Simon relies on caffeine to fuel his busy lifestyle. He gets warm easily and often dresses in short-sleeved shirts and shorts, even in cold weather. His face gets flushed easily and he complains of a thirst that he can never seem to quench. Simon takes antacids to calm his chronic heartburn and sleep medication to help him fall asleep. However, the medication never settles him as it should and his racing mind and restless legs keep him awake most nights.

Like Simon, most Summer types exhibit some form of sleep disturbance, such as night sweats, restlessness, insomnia, or profuse dreaming. They typically feel hot and thirsty, and their palms and soles are warm. A rosy complexion, dry skin, acne, and skin rashes are also common for this type. Summer body types often have chronic heart disease, high blood pressure, or diabetes. While their stools can be dry and hard, or loose and unformed, they tend to be very malodorous. Summer types are exuberant and boisterous, but can be quick to anger. They often exhibit inappropriate social behavior or laughter.

THE INDIAN SUMMER BODY TYPE

Helen is known both at work and among friends as a faithful and steadfast mediator. She likes to feel needed and works to make a difference, but does not demand any professional or financial recognition for her efforts. A social worker, Helen takes on the problems of her clients and sometimes returns home from work feeling overwhelmed. She is loyal and trustworthy, and has an affinity for keeping the peace. She is often seen resolving disputes, trying to save a marriage, or sitting by the bedside of an ill friend. Helen is the kind of person who constantly gives to others, but often neglects to look after herself. She frequently finds herself internalizing other people's problems, which can contribute to feelings of anxiety and personal worries of her own.

Helen is round at the waist and ankles and a few pounds heavier than her ideal weight. She feels low in energy all day long and complains of a poor appetite, but craves sweet foods to give her a boost. Alternating between having loose stool and constipation, she also suffers from irritable bowel syndrome. Helen bruises easily and has varicose veins, which are especially obvious on her pale skin. She has a history of miscarriages and menstrual periods that begin or end with spotting.

In general, Indian Summer types tend to lack energy and complain of fatigue. They often have a passive manner and a soft voice. Their immune systems are weak and they are frequently sick with colds or flu. Having a diminished appetite along with frequent cravings for sweet foods, these body types are also likely to have weak digestion; this often results in gas, bloating, gastrointestinal pain, constipation, or loose or watery stool. Indian Summer types often have a pale skin tone that easily shows their frequent bruising. They may also suffer from recurring bouts of dizziness. Indian Summer types tend to be mild-mannered and reliable, but they can also be prone to worry and anxiety.

THE FALL BODY TYPE

Roger can often be found nestled in his study, reading a textbook on applied mathematics. A respected professor by day and a creative inventor by night, Roger spends most of his time alone, lost in thought. He is deliberate and methodical with his work, ruminating over the problem at hand until he reaches the ideal solution. His slow, cautious nature helps him to avoid taking unnecessary risks, but it can also limit his ability to bring his projects to fruition. His mind often feels as though it is in a fog, making it difficult for him to concentrate on the task at hand; his body often feels heavy, making his physical movements appear slow and labored.

Roger is often congested from seasonal allergies and he suffers from band-like headaches. Through-out the day, he can be heard clearing his throat or blowing his nose, due to a constant post-nasal drip. His arthritis is aggravated by cold and damp weather, but even on sunny days he feels most comfortable sitting by the warmth of the fireplace in his study. Roger consumes the standard American diet (SAD); he craves processed foods that are high in fat, salt, and sugar. He is twenty pounds overweight and the extra weight on his frame contributes to his feelings of heaviness, laziness, and sluggishness.

Fall types generally exhibit the following signs and symptoms: water retention, edema, or swollen, arthritic joints which feel worse in cold, damp weather. They often have cold and clammy hands and feet. These body types tend to store weight more easily than others and may have a hard time losing it. They complain of a heavy sensation in the body or a congested, muzzy feeling in the head. Sinus congestion or post-nasal drip with white sputum is common in these types. In addition, they may have sticky stools, incomplete bowel movements, or yeast infections. Cautious and deliberate, Fall body types can have trouble making decisions. They may also have a gloomy outlook and a hard time recovering from loss.

THE WINTER BODY TYPE

Trish is a budget analyst at a software company. Preferring to work on her own, she rarely associates with her fellow co-workers outside of the office. Trish likes to spend her free time in the peaceful and quiet solitude of her home; on weekends, she can often be found on her living room couch, curled up under a wool afghan reading a book. Shy and introspective, Trish is admired by a few close friends for her empathy and thoughtfulness. She never forgets a birthday or anniversary.

Because she often feels cold, Trish wears sweaters and multiple layers of clothing, even in the summertime. Despite the multiple cups of hot tea she drinks, she can never seem to get warm. Trish has a weak bladder and makes multiple trips to the restroom throughout the day. She lacks the energy to sustain her daily activities; even the most routine tasks tend to tire her out. A sound sleeper, she enjoys sleeping as much as she can.

In general, Winter types can be quiet and withdrawn. Their complexions are often ashen and they have dark circles under their eyes. In addition, these types typically feel tired and move in a slow, measured way. Due to their lack of appetite, they often skip meals or eat only very small amounts of food. Winter body types feel cold and frigid, especially in their hands and feet. They may complain of sexual dysfunction or a low sex drive. They also tend to urinate frequently. People with this body type are intuitive and sensitive, but may be prone to feelings of fear and insecurity.

USING YOUR INTUITION

After you have completed the checklist, examined your tongue, and compared yourself to the different body type profiles, you can determine which seasonal body type or types you most resemble. Do you identify with the *yang* of Spring and Summer types, with the *yin* of Fall and Winter types, or with neutral Indian Summer type in between? As you read through the remaining chapters and the seasonal recipes found in Chapters 11-15, you can gain further insight into what your seasonal type is. Do you gravitate toward the information and recommendations listed for a certain body type? Are there recipes from one season that appeal to you more than from others? The most practical approach to determining your seasonal body type may involve replacing logic and reasoning with your natural instinct and intuition.

Trial and error can also help you discover which seasonal type and healing principles are most appropriate for you as an individual. As you follow the diet and activity guidelines recommended in the following chapters for the seasonal type you have identified, see how your body responds to these lifestyle changes. Do you feel more energetic? Have your symptoms improved? Do you feel better emotionally? If you have picked the correct seasonal representation of your body type, you should notice positive results within three to four weeks. However, if the season's foods and activities leave you feeling worse than before or if you do not see any change, you may need to adjust your self-diagnosis.

Every patient carries her or his own doctor inside.
– Albert Schweitzer

GETTING A PROFESSIONAL OPINION

If you have trouble determining your seasonal body type, you may want to consult an acupuncturist or TCM practitioner. These professionals will perform a holistic examination of your health, including your current physiological and psychological symptoms, as well as your prior medical history. During the initial evaluation, you may be asked about health conditions and lifestyle factors, from pain, chronic disease, and stress levels to your daily diet, exercise, and digestive function. In addition to using tongue analysis, TCM practitioners may also use pulse diagnosis to render a more complete picture of your body's state of health.

After a thorough review, TCM practitioners may diagnose your health condition using terms like "excess," "deficiency," and "stasis" in relation to your levels of *yin, yang, qi*, or blood. Alternatively, they may use the Five Element Theory. To correlate the common diagnoses used in TCM to your seasonal body type, see the summary chart of the five body types in the Appendix. Depending on your specific health condition, TCM practitioners may recommend acupuncture treatment, in which very thin needles are inserted into the skin at different points along energetic channels known as meridians. These needles may also be stimulated by hand, or inserted with the application of heat or electric current. During acupuncture, you may feel tingling sensations, pulsing, or feelings of heaviness. Typically, you will be asked to remain still after the needles are inserted; each acupuncture session generally lasts fifteen to thirty minutes.

Additional TCM treatment therapies can include *tui na* massage (a therapy that uses forceful kneading, rolling, pushing, and pulling to increase the flow of *qi*), cupping (the application of glass cups or vessels through suction), and moxibustion (burning the dried mugwort herb known as moxa). All of these treatments are used to tonify and stimulate the circulation of *qi* within the body. Some TCM practitioners may also suggest dietary changes or prescribe herbal remedies, which can be taken as pills, oil tinctures, or teas. See the Appendix for resources for finding a licensed acupuncturist or alternative health practitioner near you.

CONCLUSION

Once you have determined your seasonal body type or types, you can focus on the specific recommendations and lifestyle changes necessary to feel your very best. In the following chapters, you will find guidelines, healing principles, and recipes for each of the five body types. Although these lifestyle choices and activities may be potentially new and unusual to you, stay flexible and approach them with a positive attitude. As your life proceeds and stressors come and go, your body's needs may change, along with your body type. Stay mindful of those needs, listen to your body, and adjust your approach to eating and exercise as necessary. By doing so, you will find your individual path and harmonize with nature's seasons.

To find an open road, have an open mind.

– John Towne

Chapter 9
Healing Your Seasonal Body Type

In an ideal world, our bodies would cycle through the seasons along with nature. We would embody the spirit and characteristics of each season in turn, feeling warm and energetic during the summer and cool and peaceful during the winter. A body that exists in complete balance should not be recognizable as any one seasonal type; it is neutral and comfortable within all five seasons, showing strength and vitality within each. Our ideal bodies should directly reflect nature's cycle of seasons and experience the growth and renewal that comes with its ever-changing contrast.

Harmonizing our bodies to the Earth's seasons requires a balancing of *yin* and *yang*. For Summer body types, this means choosing *yin* foods and activities to cool down their frantic *yang* energy and provide them with much-needed rest. Winter body types can find balance by warming up their cold hands and feet and coming out of their *yin*-like shells. Each seasonal type benefits from an individualized and holistic approach to healing; this includes specific foods, physical activities, and awareness exercises which are appropriate for that particular body type.

Live in each season as it passes; breathe the air,
drink the drink, taste the fruit, and resign yourself
to the influences of each.

– Henry David Thoreau

SPRING

Spring is a time for new possibilities and reawakening after a long, cold dormancy. Leafy greens sprout from once-barren fields, animals emerge from their dens to birth their young, and the air becomes warm and energizing. Although the spring season is characterized by renewal and transformation, Spring body types do not embrace the change that is intrinsic to their season. Typically, these body types are rigid in every way, displaying an unyielding nature in both mind and body.

HEALING PRINCIPLES

Think

The overall focus of Spring body types should be the release of both mental and physical tension. From a Traditional Chinese Medicine (TCM) perspective, the physical pain and emotional frustration typically experienced by these types results when *qi* is stagnant or when the flow of energy becomes interrupted within the body. Like the season of spring, Spring body types thrive by way of movement, change, and growth: letting go of the old and welcoming the new. Instead of repressing their emotions, these types benefit from finding an effective outlet for their thoughts and feelings. Cognitive therapy can assist them in learning to express their emotions more freely, while also helping them to manage the stress and tension that they feel. Awareness exercises or support groups that focus on forgiveness may also help Spring types to let go of old thought patterns like resentment and judgment.

By adopting a more flexible and forgiving attitude toward themselves and others, Spring body types can encourage flow and movement in all areas of their lives. As they release their need to control and plan every outcome, they can learn to loosen their tight grip and rigid ways, live with more ease, and relax into their natural well-being. These types benefit from embracing risk and opportunity despite the initial discomfort they may feel. The spring season calls for the free flow of new ideas and energies, prompting us to look forward and be receptive to whatever changes life may bring.

Each morning we are born again.
What we do today is what matters most.

– Buddha

Do

When it comes to physical activity, Spring types should focus on activities that circulate blood and *qi*, encouraging energy to flow both through them and within them. *Qi gong*, an Eastern-style exercise that focuses on enhancing one's *qi* and promoting its circulation, can be helpful for these body types. (For a brief introduction to *qi gong*, see the activity box at the end of Chapter 4.) Finding ways to release tension in the musculoskeletal system is important. Activities like yoga and gentle stretching done in a warm setting can help to improve flexibility in the tight muscles, tendons, and ligaments that are common to Spring types. Regular massage therapy and bodywork are also beneficial for improving circulation and releasing tension.

Spring types should consider incorporating expressive and free-form activities into their often rigorous and unyielding routines. An emphasis on fun and play can provide balance to more structured and competitive forms of exercise. Enjoying physical activity for the simple pleasure of motion and movement, rather than for the achievement of concrete goals or specific results, can be very liberating. Spring types also benefit from expressing themselves creatively through activities like art and music. For example, modern dance or drumming classes can help them to express and release harbored emotions like anger and frustration, while loosening up their bodies and freeing their energy in a social, non-competitive way.

Eat

A Spring diet should be filled with the naturally abundant greens of the season. Chlorophyll-rich leafy greens are both ideal for the annual rite of spring cleaning and the everyday diet of these body types, because they allow for a gradual cleanse and detoxification of the body. For this seasonal type, it is best to consume foods that encourage the flow and circulation of *qi* throughout the body. Pungent foods like mustard greens, watercress, and members of the onion family help to promote movement, while fresh herbs and spices aid in digestion.

Light eating and simple meals are also important for Spring body types. Because dietary fats tend to weigh the body down and hamper liver function, they should be consumed in limited quantities. One way to counteract the effects of greasy foods is to consume sour foods like vinegar and lemons.

SPRING BODY TYPE DIETARY PRINCIPLES

Emphasize:
» Light meals
» Leafy greens and vegetables
» Sour flavors
» Lightly cooked foods prepared through steaming, stir-frying, or sautéing

Minimize:
» Fatty, greasy, and heavy foods
» Refined oils

Quick cooking methods like steaming and sautéing are recommended, since they only require minimal amounts of added oils. A lighter and more cleansing diet improves the body's circulation of *qi*, promoting the release of tension from the body and stuck emotions from the mind and heart.

SPRING BODY TYPE FOOD RECOMMENDATIONS

Grains
Buckwheat
Rye

Legumes
Black soybeans
Yellow soybeans

Vegetables
Bell peppers
Broccoli
Carrots
Eggplants
Fennel
Green onions
Kohlrabi
Leeks
Mustard greens
Onions
Radishes
Turnips
Watercress

Fruits
Cherries
Kumquats
Lemons
Limes
Lychees
Oranges
Peaches
Plums
Tangerines

Seaweeds
Arame
Hijiki
Kombu
Nori
Wakame

Meats and Seafood
Chicken
Crab
Eel
Sardines
Shrimp

Nuts and Seeds
Almonds

Herbs and Spices
Caraway
Cardamom
Cayenne pepper
Chili pepper
Cinnamon
Fennel seeds
Garlic
Turmeric

Other
Vinegar

SUMMER

Summer is a time for bright, bold crops and farmers' markets that are bursting with the season's fruitful bounty. Its long, hot days entice us to play outdoors and partake in cooling drinks, crisp salads, and refreshing fruits and vegetables. Summer is characterized by heat, energy, and growth. People of this body type generally feel warmer than most and have difficulty sitting still; they also tend to be enthusiastic, expressive, and hot-tempered.

HEALING PRINCIPLES

Think

For Summer body types, the inability to relax or settle down at night is similar to a never-setting sun. In order to be free of their heat-related symptoms, these types need to embrace the softer, quieter, and slower ways of winter. This means balancing an excess *yang* with a cool and calm *yin*. One option for Summer types is to employ mantra-style chanting, an activity that soothes the mind with a single, repetitive thought. Meditation practice, especially if done regularly, can help these body types to develop restraint, find peace within themselves, and learn to be comfortable with silence. In addition, progressive relaxation exercises can be beneficial since they train the mind to quiet and control the body. They are excellent for encouraging relaxation before going to bed, allowing for a gradual transition from the clamor of daytime to a restful night. Summer body types should also avoid using electronics such as televisions, computers, and cell phones at bedtime, since these devices are too stimulating for an already racing mind.

Typically, Summer types tend to express every thought that comes to mind, often times monopolizing the conversation. They may also become easily agitated or blow up at the slightest provocation. To balance their fiery tendencies, these body types should consider pausing before speaking and focusing on their breathing. By setting boundaries in both their personal and professional relationships, Summer body types can learn to rein in their flagrant, unrestrained *yang*. These types can preserve their *yin* by keeping to their own personal space and developing more patience and self-control.

Do

Ideal forms of exercise for Summer types may include yoga (but not Bikram-style yoga, as it is too hot) and other meditative practices like *tai chi* or *qi gong*. These slow-paced activities can provide balance to the high-speed careen through life common among Summer body types, teaching them both patience and restraint. Lap swimming is not only cooling for an overheated body, but its repetition can also be soothing for an overactive mind. Another alternative for these body types is golf; often played in a serene setting, golf has a slow pace and requires a calm, yet focused mind.

No matter what kind of activity Summer types choose, they should focus on nurturing *yin* and making their physical movements as smooth and fluid as possible. Instead of relying on brute strength or energetic intensity to achieve a physical result, these body types benefit from emphasizing breathing, control, and proper technique. Whether they are hitting a tennis ball, kicking a soccer ball, or carving s-turns on their downhill skis, Summer types' primary focus should be on flow, economy of motion, and the conservation of energy. Because Summer body types tend to push themselves to the extremes, one of the most important principles for them is to ensure that they allow adequate time for rest and recovery. Relaxation is essential for these body types to balance the strung-out energy that motivates them to excessive activity.

Eat

Seasonal fruits and vegetables like cucumbers, tomatoes, and watermelon are the perfect antidotes to the excess heat that marks Summer body types. To balance heartburn and tame the manic Summer mind, cooling and refreshing salads are preferable over heavy dishes. Summer body types should focus on eating lots of fresh fruits and vegetables to soothe their overworked systems and keep their bodies light for the season's activities. Seafood, legumes, and tofu are ideal sources of protein since these foods tend to be lower in fat and have a more cooling thermal nature than meats. A vegetarian and low-salt diet is especially helpful in cases of hypertension. For Summer body types, cooking methods like steaming, blanching, and boiling can provide a moistening effect to foods and help to counteract any dryness in the body. To balance excess heat in the body, raw foods will typically provide the most cooling effect, though they should be eaten sparingly if there are signs of weakened digestion such as constipation, loose stool, abdominal pain, or bloating. Dairy foods can be helpful for moistening dryness and nourishing *yin*, but these foods should be minimized by individuals who have symptoms of excess phlegm, sinus congestion, arthritis, or edema.

It is also important for Summer types to limit their consumption of stimulants like coffee, alcohol, and spicy foods. While these foods may provide a temporary buzz or boost of energy, they can also serve to aggravate the heat conditions and insomnia that are common to this body type. Summer types require cool drinks and lots of them. Because of their cooler thermal natures, green and mint teas are preferable alternatives to coffee.

SUMMER BODY TYPE DIETARY PRINCIPLES

Emphasize:
» Cooling and refreshing foods
» Lots of fruits and vegetables
» Steaming, simmering, or boiling methods of cooking
» Some raw foods, if tolerable for digestion

Minimize:
» Fried and fatty foods
» Meats
» Spicy foods
» Stimulants (e.g. coffee and alcohol)

SUMMER BODY TYPE FOOD RECOMMENDATIONS

Grains
Amaranth
Barley
Buckwheat
Millet
Wheat
Wild rice

Legumes
Adzuki beans
Black beans
Black soybeans
Kidney beans
Mung beans
Yellow soybeans

Vegetables
Asparagus
Avocados
Broccoli
Celery
Cucumbers
Eggplants
Green beans
Lettuce
Mushrooms
Napa cabbage
Potatoes
Radishes
Spinach
Summer squash
Swiss chard
Tomatoes
Watercress

Fruits
Apples
Bananas
Figs
Grapefruits
Lemons
Limes
Mangoes
Oranges
Peaches
Pears
Pineapples
Plums
Tangerines
Watermelons

Seaweeds
Arame
Hijiki
Kombu
Nori
Wakame

Meats and Seafood
Clams
Crab
Octopus
Oysters
Pork

Eggs and Dairy*
Butter
Cheese
Eggs
Milk
Yogurt

Nuts and Seeds
Coconuts
Pine nuts
Sesame seeds

Herbs and Spices
Peppermint

*These foods should be minimized by individuals with symptoms of excess phlegm, congestion, arthritis, or edema.

INDIAN SUMMER

Sitting in the middle of the five-season cycle, Indian summer represents the perfect balance point of *yin* and *yang*, and the transition between two opposing extremes. The weather in this season is fickle: some days tease with the oncoming cool temperatures of fall, while others defiantly hang on to the warmth of summer. Indian Summer types are neutral and mild-mannered in personality, holding a space for contrast and change, but never pushing the boundaries or settling on the edge. These body types generally feel fatigued and have a weak digestive system; they can also be prone to worry and anxiety.

HEALING PRINCIPLES

Think

To achieve balance in their lives, Indian Summer body types must find ways to fortify themselves emotionally, physically, and spiritually. By strengthening their energetic connection to the universe around them, they can build a stable foundation for support. First and foremost, these body types must work on developing self-awareness and self-respect. Meditative practices that promote centering oneself and being present in the moment are suggested. Walking meditation, wherein one repeats a mantra while taking slow and deliberate steps, is one type of meditation practice they can use to increase awareness. It is essential for Indian Summer types to ground and balance their own individual energy before dedicating their resources to others. Although their altruistic nature makes them well-suited for careers in service, they will find their work to be of greatest value when they take the time to honor and care for their own needs first.

Because Indian Summer types often lack appreciation for themselves, they benefit from creating and engaging in a more positive belief system. Incorporating affirmations through journaling or self-talk will assist them in replacing their irrational worries and anxieties with thoughts that are more supportive and empowering. By acknowledging their unique contributions and abilities, and learning to accept recognition from others, Indian Summer types can build more confidence and respect for themselves. This would allow them to meet life's challenges with more balance, fortitude, and ease.

Do

For these body types, physical activity is important to help them create awareness of their bodies and focus on supporting themselves. Because they typically lack the energy levels needed to fully sustain their lifestyles, Indian Summer types should engage in activities that help to build and enhance *qi*, rather than expend it unnecessarily. Deep, abdominal breathing into the *dan tian*, or the body's center, is a fundamental practice for cultivating energy and vitality from within. (For a guide to deep breathing and *dan tian* breathing, see the activity boxes in Chapters 3 and 4.) Spending time outdoors in the fresh air and sunshine is also beneficial for these body types, allowing them the opportunity to absorb the infinite energy of the Earth and use it to replenish their own *qi*. By being in a natural environment, Indian Summer types can renew their connection to the Earth, grounding themselves and receiving support in ways they cannot get from other people. Activities like nature walks, hikes, and gardening are all excellent ways for them to strengthen and recharge their *qi*.

Bolstering the physical foundation and the body's center is key for Indian Summer types. These body types need to practice postural alignment and focus on strengthening their core. One option they can consider is the Feldenkrais system, which uses simple movements such as walking or bending as ways to expand self-awareness. (For more information on the Feldenkrais system, see the resource listing in the Appendix.) Building abdominal strength through activities like Pilates and yoga can also allow Indian Summer types to increase core strength and further support their bodies. Balance exercises like those performed on a balance board or through *tai chi* routines are beneficial for developing stability and building a sturdy foundation. In addition, higher-intensity activities which emphasize the core and torso muscles, like paddle boarding, surfing, and snowboarding, are recommended.

Eat

For Indian Summer types, eating foods which enhance *qi* and enrich the blood is essential. Fresh and vital foods provide the most nourishment, helping to boost energy and guard against lethargy. Organic foods and high-quality meats are especially recommended. In addition, fruits and vegetables should be prepared and eaten soon after they have been picked, since the fresher the produce, the more *qi* it has. This gives Indian Summer types an extra incentive to plant a garden and grow their own food. Whole grains and complex carbohydrates are important for these body types, providing them with sustainable, long-lasting sources of energy to support their activities throughout the day. Naturally sweet foods like beets, corn, and sweet potatoes can help to address their sweet cravings, and are preferable to the simple and refined sugars found in processed foods. For Indian Summer types, animal-source foods and dairy products can also have a beneficial place in the diet, due to their building, strengthening, and grounding energetic properties. Foods that are rich in iron like red meats and leafy greens are also helpful.

INDIAN SUMMER BODY TYPE DIETARY PRINCIPLES

Emphasize:

» Complex carbohydrates, grains, and staples

» Naturally sweet foods

» Fresh foods, preferably organic

» High-quality meats, seafood, and dairy products

» Chewing foods well and taking one's time when eating

Minimize:

» Raw foods

» Iced drinks and frozen desserts

» Refined sugars

» Foods with low-quality *qi* (e.g. processed, microwaved, or frozen foods)

Compared to the other seasonal types, Indian Summer types in particular require a sturdy physical center in order to live with self-assured initiative. Because they have characteristically weak digestive systems, they need to engage in dietary habits that support proper digestion. Generally, foods that are broken down by heat, chemical, or mechanical processes tend to be more easily digested than foods that are consumed raw. For example, foods that are well-cooked, cooked over long periods of time, or

INDIAN SUMMER BODY TYPE
FOOD RECOMMENDATIONS

Grains
Amaranth
Barley
Corn
Millet
Oats
Quinoa
Rice
Spelt
Wheat

Legumes
Adzuki beans
Black beans
Black soybeans
Garbanzo beans
Lentils
Peanuts
Yellow soybeans

Vegetables
Avocados
Beets
Cabbage
Carrots
Cauliflower
Corn
Eggplants
Fennel
Green beans
Kale
Mushrooms

Potatoes
Pumpkins
Spinach
Sweet potatoes
Swiss chard
Watercress
Winter squash

Fruits
Apples
Bananas
Cherries
Dates
Figs
Grapes
Lychees
Papayas

Meats and Seafood
Anchovies
Beef
Chicken
Eel
Lamb
Mackerel
Octopus
Oysters
Pork
Salmon
Sardines
Shrimp
Trout

Tuna
Turkey
Whitefish

Eggs and Dairy
Butter
Cheese
Eggs
Milk
Yogurt

Nuts and Seeds
Almonds
Chestnuts
Coconuts
Hazelnuts
Pine nuts
Sesame seeds
Sunflower seeds
Walnuts

Herbs and Spices
Caraway
Cardamom
Chamomile
Cumin
Fennel seeds
Ginger
Parsley
Peppermint
Thyme

fermented tend to be more beneficial for this body type, whereas raw foods or cold liquids tend to stress the digestive system further. Chewing foods well (i.e. twenty to thirty times per bite) can also ease the digestive process and enhance the body's absorption of nutrients. Indian Summer body types should take their time while eating and mindfully enjoy their food, instead of wolfing down their meals while reading or watching television. In terms of nutritional supplements, these types may find the support of probiotics or digestive enzymes to be helpful.

FALL

Fall is a time for harvesting, gathering, and storing in preparation for a long, cold winter. It is abundant with the smell of spices and baked foods, and its drying and aromatic ingredients are especially beneficial for Fall body types, who tend to experience a heavy, sluggish feeling that pervades throughout the mind and body. Fall body types are cautious and deliberate, and can also be prone to sadness.

HEALING PRINCIPLES

Think

To clear out the heavy fog and muzzy-headedness that they commonly feel, Fall types should consider adding some zest and fervor to their routines. These body types need to shift their focus away from their own inner ramblings and bring their attention to more carefree pleasures instead. Activities that are enjoyed in the company of others, like group hobbies or social clubs, are beneficial for these types. Engaging in the community by volunteering or taking on a mentoring role can also help them to enliven their spirits and bring more joy to their lives.

As Fall body types learn to lighten up their emotional outlook, they can begin to transform their feelings of heaviness, grief, and worry into a more lighthearted state of being. Practicing gratitude exercises and keeping a journal can help Fall types to better appreciate the mysteries of life and accept the full entirety of the human experience, both its joys and sorrows. Utilizing mind-body techniques like progressive relaxation and visualization can also benefit these types; by imagining their bodies and limbs progressively going from heavy to light, they can practice what it feels like to lighten and release in both their mental and physical realms. Fall types may also benefit from the Emotional Freedom Technique (EFT), an activity that uses a combination of acupressure and positive affirmations to encourage emotional healing. (For more information on EFT, see the resource listing in the Appendix.) By shedding the emotional clutter and baggage in their lives, these body types can make space for healing and recovery.

Do

Most Fall types benefit from the introduction or intensification of physical activity. Because these body types tend to feel cold and are prone to retaining fluids and excess phlegm, they need to find activities that both warm and dry their systems. Focusing on movement, especially of the aerobic variety, is essential. Aerobic exercise not only raises the heart rate and promotes the body's overall metabolism, it also encourages the release of excess moisture through sweating. Regular physical activity will also help Fall body types to burn off some of their feelings of heaviness and lose the excess weight they may be carrying. These types also benefit from regular massages, which promote movement and circulation in the body.

There are flowers everywhere, for those who bother to look.
– Henri Matisse

For Fall types, the most challenging part of developing a physical routine may be finding the motivation to get started. By seeking out activities that are fun and hold their interest, they can focus on the inherent pleasure that physical movement provides, instead of viewing exercise as a chore. Laughter yoga is one activity that promotes physical movement in a lighthearted way and also helps to clear out blocked emotions. Consisting of abdominal breathing, stretching, and simulated laughter exercises which lead to genuine, spontaneous laughter, laughter yoga is beneficial for relieving stress and improving one's mood. Fall body types may also consider adding some spice to their routines by participating in activities like salsa or belly dancing lessons. Playing team sports in tennis or softball leagues can also provide these types with some additional, external motivation, while offering them the social benefits and camaraderie found in group settings. In terms of volunteer work, these types might consider working at a community garden or building houses for the underprivileged; these kinds of activities not only engage them in a fun and physical way, but also provide a sense of social purpose and create meaningful ties to the community.

Eat

The diet of Fall body types should incorporate warming foods cooked with a bit of spice. Baked dishes and casseroles are recommended, as they help to warm and dry the latent cold and damp that is intrinsic to these body types. In contrast, raw or cooling foods tend to cool the body down even further. For Fall types, drying grains (e.g. barley, rye, and buckwheat) and foods with diuretic properties (e.g. corn, legumes, and lettuce) can be helpful for resolving the excess fluid, swelling, edema, and symptoms of arthritis that they experience.

As with Indian Summer body types, Fall types need to be mindful of encouraging optimal digestion. In order to generate the internal warmth and energy that they need, they must be able to absorb a food's *qi* and properly transform it for use by the body. It is important for these types to consume high-quality foods (e.g. minimally processed and organic foods) and chew them well. They should also minimize their consumption of fats and sweets, because these foods impair the gut's ability to digest and assimilate nutrients, and also hamper detoxification in the liver. Dairy products, although common in the Western diet, should also be minimized, as they tend to be too moistening and congestive for these types. In addition, Fall body types should avoid eating meals late at night. Although they may be inclined to turn to food for comfort in difficult times, it is preferable for them to engage in exercise instead; this allows for the release of endorphins that uplift both the body and mind.

FALL BODY TYPE DIETARY PRINCIPLES

Emphasize:

» Warming spices

» Whole, drying grains

» Baked dishes, casseroles, and slow-cooked foods

» Foods that promote diuresis and drain excess fluids

Minimize:

» Dairy products, especially ice cream

» Raw foods and iced drinks

» Unfermented soy products

» Refined sugars

» Fried and fatty foods

FALL BODY TYPE FOOD RECOMMENDATIONS

Grains

Amaranth

Barley

Buckwheat

Corn

Oats

Rice

Rye

Wild rice

Legumes

Adzuki beans

Black beans

Black soybeans

Garbanzo beans

Kidney beans

Lentils

Vegetables

Asparagus

Cabbage

Cauliflower

Celery

Corn

Green onions

Kale

Kohlrabi

Lettuce

Mushrooms

Mustard greens

Onions

Parsnips

Pumpkins

Radishes

Turnips

Winter squash

Fruits

Cherries

Grapes

Kumquats

Papayas

Quinces

Meats and Seafood

Anchovies

Chicken

Clams

Mackerel

Turkey

Herbs and Spices

Basil

Black pepper

Cardamom

Cinnamon

Cloves

Fennel seeds

Garlic

Ginger

Mustard seeds

Nutmeg

Thyme

WINTER

Winter's cold brings dormancy and decay. The sparse food supply primarily consists of hearty vegetables which store warmth, like roots and bulbs. Rich meats, proteins, and fats also offer nourishing sustenance and a source of *yang*. As the yearly cycle of seasons comes to an end, we slow down, conserve our energy, and find peace within. The coldest of all the body types, Winter types usually feel frigid, have cold hands and feet, and have difficulty keeping warm. They tend to be quiet and intuitive, but can also be insecure and fearful.

HEALING PRINCIPLES

Think

Although their physical realm is sedated and withdrawn, the mental life of Winter body types is active with dreams and ideas. However, fear often prevents them from taking steps toward actualizing those dreams. These body types need to seek inspiration to come out of their shells and leave their comfort zones, even if that means risking failure and rejection. By embracing the spirit of *yang*, Winter types can create some life fire for themselves and develop the courage needed to propel themselves forward. To boost self-confidence they can use affirmations, or words of encouragement spoken aloud to oneself in front of a mirror. Imagery and awareness exercises can also help these types to liberate and conquer their deep-rooted fears. By setting small, attainable goals for themselves and keeping track of their progress, Winter types can take action and move forward in ways that feel manageable.

Emotionally, these body types can feel strongly and deeply, so much so that they can become overwhelmed. Cognitive therapy can help them to manage and integrate their emotional sensitivity in a healthy, constructive way, and apply it toward personal, professional, and social success. Regular meditation practice is beneficial for increasing emotional awareness in these types and providing them with a safe space to experience and process the wide range of emotions that they feel. In alignment with the spirit of their season, Winter body types should relish the peace and solitude offered by the quieter, darker side of *yin*, but also be mindful not to withdraw too deeply within themselves.

Do

Like Fall body types, Winter types require regular physical activity to build warmth and increase their metabolism. It is essential for these types to keep the core of the body warm, especially the lower back and waist area. *Qi gong* techniques like light slaps to the back and sides can help to promote circulation and increase blood flow to cold extremities. Saunas, whirlpool baths, and massages in a warm setting are also beneficial for boosting body warmth.

Physical activity offers Winter types an ideal way to increase vigor, develop their *yang*, and light some fire from within. In order to shake off their year-long winter doldrums, these types should fully engage in the opportunities that life has to offer. Participating in races and athletic events will encourage them to set goals for themselves and help them to build confidence. Team sports are threefold in the benefits they offer: they get the body moving, they provide a social setting with playful interaction, and they develop a competitive spirit not usually seen in Winter types. These body types may also consider more adrenaline-pumping activities like whitewater rafting, rock climbing, sky diving, or competing in survival races. By pushing themselves in new and physical ways, these types can learn to overcome their fears and achieve goals they didn't think possible.

Eat

"Take a bite out of life" is the mantra that Winter body types should live by. In terms of diet, this means eating foods which provide more life-sustaining energy and nourishment, such as the complex carbohydrates found in this season's hearty root vegetables and squashes. These body types should consume foods which have a warming thermal nature, including energy-dense foods that have a higher fat content (e.g. certain animal products, fats and oils, and nuts). Examples of warming foods include meats like beef, chicken, and lamb, as well as oil-rich seafood like anchovies, salmon, and trout. Warming spices are also recommended for these body types, but they should be used in moderation in order to prevent the body from sweating too much and cooling down again.

Generally, Winter types should choose foods that warm, nourish, and protect the body from the season's elements. Consuming hearty soups, stews, roasts, and slow-cooked dishes will help these body types to sustain themselves through the cold. All foods should be cooked thoroughly, including any fruits (which are recommended only in moderate amounts because of their generally cooling nature).

WINTER BODY TYPE DIETARY PRINCIPLES

Emphasize:
- » Warming root vegetables and thick-skinned squash
- » Energy-dense foods, high-quality animal products and fats
- » Hearty soups and stews
- » Slow cooking methods (e.g. simmering, braising, roasting)
- » Warming spices, but not overly spicy foods

Minimize:
- » Raw fruits and vegetables
- » Cold foods
- » Iced drinks

WINTER BODY TYPE FOOD RECOMMENDATIONS

Grains
Oats
Quinoa
Rye

Legumes
Peanuts

Vegetables
Bell peppers
Brussels sprouts
Cabbage
Fennel
Green onions
Leeks
Onions
Parsnips
Winter squash

Fruits
Cherries
Dates

Meats and Seafood
Anchovies
Beef
Chicken
Lamb
Shrimp
Trout
Turkey

Nuts and Seeds
Chestnuts
Pine nuts
Walnuts

Herbs and Spices
Black pepper
Cayenne pepper
Chili pepper
Cinnamon
Cloves
Dill seeds
Fennel seeds
Garlic
Ginger

NOURISHING YOUR SEASONAL BODY TYPE

Balancing your body type involves choosing perspectives, activities, and foods that contrast with your thermal makeup. Summer body types benefit from embracing a cool, soothing, and inward-focused approach to balance their hot energy, while Winter types thrive by adopting the characteristics of summer. By emphasizing activities that oppose your *yin* or *yang* nature, you do not neutralize your individuality, but rather capitalize on the healthy aspects of your unique self. For a chart summarizing the five seasonal body types' characteristics and recommended healing principles, see the Appendix.

Everyone is prone toward a predominant seasonal body type based on the influences of genetic ancestry, living environment, and lifestyle choices. Although you may have a tendency toward more *yin* or more *yang* characteristics, you ideally will also harmonize along with the external seasons. For a Winter body type who generally feels cooler than others, this means warming up enough in the summertime to easily digest the raw salads and fruits of the season. Similarly, a Summer body type can engage in the thrills and excitement that he or she craves, and still desire to slow down and rest in the winter. Aligning with nature's cycles begins with first recognizing your health symptoms, tendencies, and characteristics within the context of your individual season, and then living along with the themes, spirit, and principles of all five seasons throughout the year.

INCORPORATING SEASONAL PRINCIPLES INTO YOUR DAILY PRACTICE

The healing principles in this book are intended to be suggestions and general recommendations; they work best when used in combination with your intuition. To incorporate the principles into your daily practice, there are three essential components to consider: eating, exercise, and mindfulness, each of which can be tuned with perfect synchronicity to your distinct body type and specific environment. As you take steps toward a healthier lifestyle, you will experience a life filled with less pain and resistance, and more joy and energy. There are three recommended ways to use the recipes and information found in this book: corrective (healing your seasonal body type), adaptive (living with the seasons), and intuitive (using your intuition in response to your daily condition).

CORRECTIVE

You may find it most helpful to begin by correcting the imbalance of your body type. Once you identify the seasonal body type or types that best describe you, you can start moving toward feeling your best. Follow the recommendations and healing principles from this chapter, and prepare the recipes from Chapters 11 through 15 that are specific to your season. If your body resembles the *yang* characteristics of Spring and Summer, use *yin* foods, recipes, and activities for balance. If you relate more to the *yin* of Fall and Winter, nourish your *yang* with warming foods and exercises. If you gravitate toward Indian Summer, focus on building and strengthening your core energy.

As you come into balance and move closer to your best self, you will notice your symptoms improve and become less clearly defined by any one body type. As your temperature becomes more adaptable to seasonal climate changes and your body becomes more neutral in character, you are becoming more balanced. When your aches and pains lessen, and your skin and sinuses show no ill response to the weather, you are coming more into balance. When your emotional responses become less extreme, and you have less to complain about and more to appreciate, you are also coming more into balance.

ADAPTIVE

Once you have restored balance to your seasonal body type, the repair work is done and maintenance can begin. At this point, let the seasons be your guide; eat from the bounty of each season, exercise according to its offerings, and embrace its theme and attitude. In the springtime, spend time in your garden, plant the seeds of change, and move forward to new goals; eat the leafy greens, herbs, and cleansing foods that are abundant in the season. Summer is for growth and expansion. To sustain the activity of the season, keep the body light and cool by eating fresh fruits and vegetables. Enjoy the long days of Indian summer outdoors, grounding yourself in nature and harmonizing your energy with naturally sweet foods and neutral staples. In the fall, as the pace of life begins to slow and home becomes the focus, express gratitude for the year's harvest and let the scent of baked goods and fragrant spices fill your kitchen. Finally, retreat inwards in the spirit of winter, and store up and strengthen your reserves as you wait for the cycle of seasons to begin again.

INTUITIVE

Each day, a variety of stressors and circumstances contribute to temporary imbalances in your state of health. As a result, you may find it necessary to fine-tune your diet depending on your daily health condition. Adjust your diet and activities to support your individual needs, and use your intuition to determine what it is that your body wants. Be conscious of how you are feeling, what your body is craving, and what recipes look appealing to you.

For example, if you are craving sweet flavors, try eating foods that are naturally high in sugar, like whole grains and fruits. If you are feeling low on energy, eat enriching foods like those found in the Indian Summer recipes. When you are feeling frustrated or stuck in a rut, eat the cleansing greens recommended for Spring body types. If you feel hot and overworked, or your heartburn is flaring up, eat the Summer recipes' cooling foods for soothing relief. If you are feeling under the weather, your body may require the comfort of a warming stew or chicken soup with ginger, like those presented in the Fall and Winter recipes. No matter what your seasonal body type is, you can use the seasonal healing principles to guide your food and activity choices on a daily basis. Your intuition will lead you to your body's most pressing needs and offer clear insights about your individual path toward optimal health.

Spring has its hundred flowers,
Autumn its moon,
Summer has its cooling breezes,
Winter its snow.
If you allow no idle concerns
To weight on your heart,
Your whole life will be one
Perennial good season.

– The Golden Age of Zen

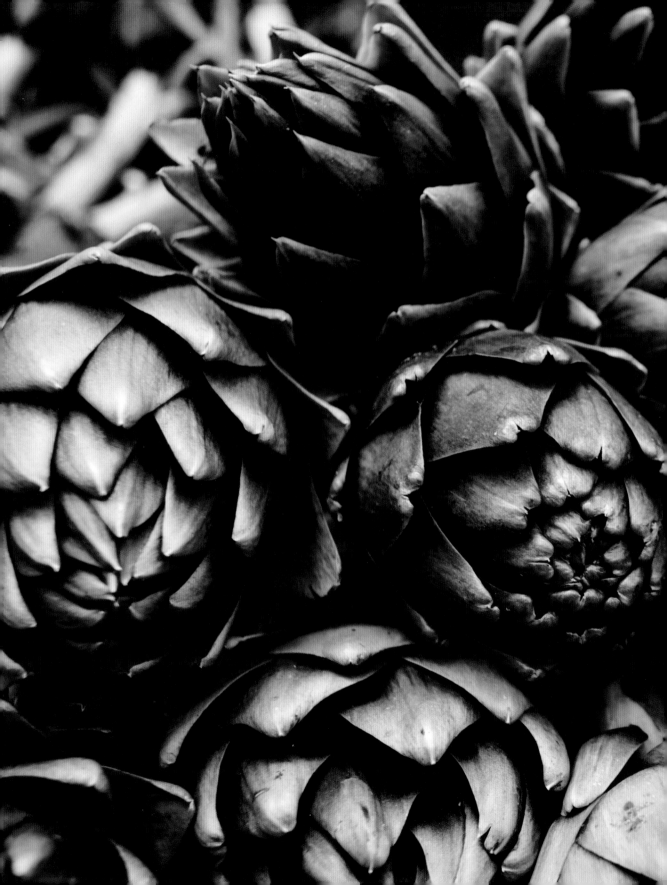

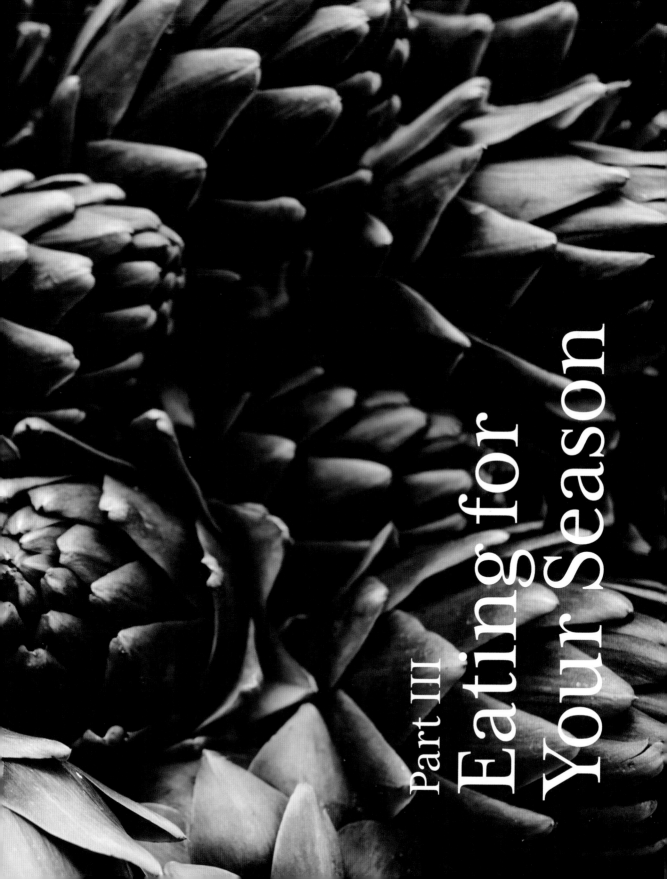

Part III
Eating for Your Season

Chapter 10
Foods and Ingredients: healing properties, seasonality, and selection

Using a combination of humoral, Traditional Chinese Medicine (TCM), and seasonal perspectives, this chapter lists the healing properties and medicinal uses of a variety of foods and ingredients. Each entry indicates the thermal nature of the food (cooling, neutral, or warming), as well as the seasonal body type or types for which each ingredient is most beneficial. Generally, foods which are higher in fat and calories, like meats and animal products, tend to build body mass and have a warming thermal nature. Plants which have a longer growing period or are grown under the soil, like cruciferous and root vegetables, are also warming. In contrast, plants which grow more quickly or are grown above the ground, like lettuces and leafy greens, tend to be more cleansing and cooling. Foods that are low in calories with a high water content (e.g. most fruits and vegetables) have a cooling thermal nature, while staples like grains, starches, and legumes tend to be thermally neutral.

Each entry also describes the beneficial health effects of the ingredient on the body in terms of its TCM properties and flavors. The five flavor designations from TCM (sour, sweet, salty, pungent, and bitter) indicate a food's medicinal use and beneficial action, but may not always correspond to the food's actual taste when eaten. In TCM dietary therapy, sour flavors are considered to have cleansing properties, sweet foods are building and nourishing, bitter foods help to dry excess fluids, pungent flavors encourage circulation, and salty foods are moistening.

Although you will be familiar with most of the ingredients listed in this chapter, some may be new additions to your daily cooking. For maximum nutritional benefit, emphasize seasonal foods in their whole or minimally processed forms. Be adventurous with your food and cooking. Visit your local farmers' markets and grocery stores for culinary inspiration; ask questions, engage your senses, and taste samples. By incorporating a variety of new ingredients into your diet, you can not only broaden your palate, but also take full advantage of the bounty of healing foods and flavors that nature has to offer.

GRAINS

Grains have been cultivated for thousands of years and have played a key role in the human diet since the beginning of civilization. Whole grains, which have their bran and germ layers intact, are preferable to refined and highly processed grains. In their whole form, grains contain all of the major nutrients that the body requires (i.e. carbohydrates, protein, fats, vitamins, minerals, and fiber). In particular, they provide high levels of B vitamins and dietary fiber. Their complex carbohydrates are slowly absorbed by the body, providing a steady and long-lasting source of energy. In general, grains have a neutral thermal nature, a sweet flavor as classified by TCM, and a strengthening action. They are building foods that form the foundation of the diet in most cultures. Whole grains are especially beneficial for Indian Summer body types, but they benefit the other body types as well.

Whole grains need to be cooked and chewed well for optimal digestibility. Before grains are cooked, they should be rinsed thoroughly under running water to remove any dirt or debris. Most whole grains can also be soaked in water for at least a few hours before cooking; doing so reduces their cooking time and makes them easier to digest. After discarding the soaking water, prepare the grains by adding 1 to 2½ cups of fresh water (or stock) per cup of uncooked grain. Bring the grains and liquid to a boil on the stovetop, cover, and simmer over low heat until the liquid is absorbed. Harder grains like buckwheat, spelt, and millet generally require a higher ratio of cooking liquid and a longer cooking time than softer ones, like barley, oats, and quinoa. Using an electric rice cooker or a steamer is also a convenient way to prepare whole grains.

AMARANTH

Body type(s): *Summer, Indian Summer, Fall*
Thermal nature: *neutral to cooling*

Once a sacred food of the Aztecs, amaranth contains all of the essential amino acids, is high in protein and calcium, and is gluten-free.

Amaranth helps to drain excess fluids and build energy. It is beneficial for pregnant women, children, and those who work in physically demanding environments. Amaranth has a nutty aroma and can be used in soups, porridges, breads, and cakes.

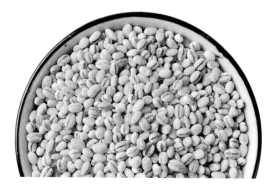

BARLEY

Body type(s): *Summer, Indian Summer, Fall*
Thermal nature: *cooling*

Whole barley has its bran layer intact and contains more fiber and nutrients than pearled barley, which is polished so that the bran is removed. Barley is a digestive aid and soothes the stomach and intestines. It nourishes *qi* within the body and has a diuretic effect. Whole barley has a chewy consistency and is a good source of dietary fiber, selenium, phosphorous, and copper. It adds heartiness to soups and stews, and can be used in whole-grain salads and pilafs.

BUCKWHEAT

Body type(s): *Spring, Summer, Fall*
Thermal nature: *neutral to cooling*

Technically neither a wheat nor a cereal grain, buckwheat is a pyramid-shaped seed with a robust, slightly bitter flavor. It is gluten-free and is a good substitute for wheat and other grains that contain gluten. Buckwheat helps to disperse fluid accumulations and increase circulation within the body. It is a good source of manganese and magnesium, and may help to lower blood pressure. Unroasted buckwheat comes in the form of groats, while toasted buckwheat is known as kasha. Kasha can be used as a substitute in rice dishes and stir-fries. Buckwheat flour is often used to make pancakes and soba noodles.

CORN

Body type(s): *Indian Summer, Fall*
Thermal nature: *neutral*

In its dried form, corn is classified as a grain. In its fresh form, it is used as a vegetable and is seasonally available in the late summer and early fall. Corn has a sweet flavor, is free of gluten, and is a fortifying and building food. It is beneficial for promoting diuresis and reducing edema. Corn silk (the hair-like tassels surrounding the ear of the corn) is a traditional remedy that is especially beneficial for this purpose. Corn is a good source of B vitamins, vitamin C, and manganese. Most corn crops in the U.S. are genetically engineered; for the highest-quality products, look for those with organic, GMO-free certifications.

MILLET

Body type(s): *Summer, Indian Summer*
Thermal nature: *cooling*

A member of the grass family, millet is gluten-free and has a sweet, nutty flavor. It has a light and fluffy texture similar to couscous, but can take on a porridge-like consistency when cooked with more liquid. Millet helps to soothe the stomach and gastrointestinal tract, and is good for those with weak digestion. It is rich in B vitamins, phosphorous, and magnesium. Millet can be used to thicken soups and is often eaten as a breakfast porridge; it can also be used in grain salads, baked goods, and granolas.

OATS

Body type(s): *Indian Summer, Fall, Winter*
Thermal nature: *warming*

Oats have a sweet yet slightly bitter flavor. They help to reduce cholesterol and stabilize blood sugar levels. Oats also help to tonify *qi* and drain excess fluids from the body. Whole oat groats and steel-cut oats (oat groats which have been cut into two or three pieces) retain their bran and germ layers, and are preferable over instant oatmeal products which are often laden with sugar and other additives. Rolled or old-fashioned oats are whole-grain oat groats which have been flattened and steamed. Oats are naturally gluten-free, but may become contaminated during processing by other grains that contain gluten.

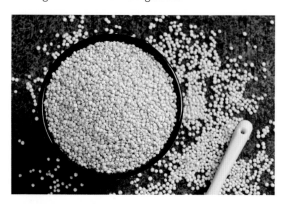

QUINOA

Body type(s): *Indian Summer, Winter*
Thermal nature: *warming*

Native to South America, quinoa is a seed that is commonly used as a grain. It is gluten-free, high in protein, and contains all eight essential amino acids. It is a good source of manganese, magnesium, phosphorous, iron, and B vitamins. Quinoa should be rinsed thoroughly since the seeds are naturally coated with saponins, chemical compounds that have a bitter taste and act as a bird and insect repellant. Quinoa can be prepared as a substitute for rice, as a cereal, and in salads and stuffings, and ground into flour for baked goods.

RICE

Body type(s): *Indian Summer, Fall*
Thermal nature: *neutral*

Rice is one of the most important food staples in the world. As a balanced food with a sweet flavor, rice strengthens the body and supplements *qi*. It is also gluten-free. Whole-grain varieties of rice come in colors like brown, black, red, and purple. Brown rice has its bran layer intact and contains more B vitamins than any other grain. White rice has been polished so that the germ and bran layers (and associated fiber and nutrients) have been removed. In Asia, rice is often simmered into a soft porridge (using one part rice to six parts water) as a remedy for weakness or illness.

RYE

Body type(s): *Spring, Fall, Winter*
Thermal nature: *neutral to warming*

Rye is a hardy grain with a bitter and sour flavor as classified by TCM. It helps to drain excess fluids from the body, increase circulation, build muscle, and boost endurance. It is a good source of dietary fiber and contains B vitamins, iron, and protein. Rye has the highest lysine content of any common grain. Because it is difficult to separate the bran and germ layers from rye, it is often sold in its whole-grain form as rye berries, cracked kernels, or rolled flakes. Rye berries can be used in grain salads and pilafs. Rye flakes and rye flour are often used to make breads and other baked goods.

SPELT

Body type(s): *Indian Summer*
Thermal nature: *warming*

Spelt is a variety of wheat, though it is higher in protein, fat, and fiber than common wheat. It is an ancient grain native to Europe with a sweet and nutty flavor. Spelt is beneficial for tonifying *qi* and strengthening immunity. Whole-grain spelt berries have a thick husk rich with nutrients. Like wheat berries, spelt berries can be cooked into grain salads or used as a substitute for rice. Spelt flour can be made into breads, cereals, crackers, and pastas.

WHEAT

Body type(s): *Summer, Indian Summer*
Thermal nature: *cooling*

A staple in many cultures, wheat is the primary grain eaten in the West. It is a building food that also helps to nourish *yin*. Wheat is a versatile grain that can be prepared in many forms. Wheat berries are de-hulled, whole-grain kernels with a chewy consistency. Whole wheat berries that have been steamed, dried, and cracked are called bulgur. Wheat is also milled into flour for the preparation of pastas and baked goods. Whole-grain wheat flours are sold as whole-wheat flour (made from traditional red wheat) or white whole-wheat flour (made from hard white spring wheat). White whole-wheat flour tends to be lighter in color and less bitter than traditional whole-wheat flour, but it still retains all of its original nutrients as a whole-grain product.

WILD RICE

Body type(s): *Summer, Fall*
Thermal nature: *cooling*

Wild rice is a type of grass and not technically a member of the rice family, though it is used as a grain. Native to North America, it is free of gluten and high in protein, B vitamins, and dietary fiber. Wild rice is beneficial for drying excess body fluids. With a black color and a hardy, nutty flavor, it is commonly used in rice pilafs and stuffings.

LEGUMES

The legume family includes foods like peas, beans, lentils, and peanuts. Legumes contain a variety of essential nutrients and are a good source of dietary fiber, potassium, iron, calcium, and B vitamins. They are high in protein, with some legumes containing more protein per calorie than meat. As a plant-source food, legumes are generally low in saturated fat and do not contain cholesterol. Diets that are rich in legumes may help to lower cholesterol levels, maintain healthy blood glucose levels, and prevent cardiovascular disease and cancer. From a TCM perspective, beans and legumes help to drain excess fluids from the body and nourish *yin*. According to TCM flavor classification, they have a sweet flavor. In general, legumes are beneficial foods for Summer and Fall body types.

For some individuals, beans and legumes may be difficult to digest and cause gas or bloating. This is due to the presence of certain oligosaccharides (a group of carbohydrates) which are indigestible by the human body. To prepare beans, first check for small rocks or debris, and then rinse under cold water. Soak the beans in water (3 to 4 cups of water per cup of dried beans) overnight and change the soaking water once or twice. Soaking beans before cooking helps to release their oligosaccharides, improve digestibility, and reduce cooking time. You may also use a quick-soak method by bringing the beans and water to a boil, removing the pot from the heat, covering, and soaking the beans for an hour in the hot water. For either method, drain the soaking water and rinse the beans with clean water before cooking. To cook the beans, add 3 to 4 cups of fresh water per cup of dried beans, cover, and bring to a boil for 10 minutes, skimming off any foam. Reduce the heat to low and simmer partially covered for 2 to 3 hours, or until beans are tender. Larger legumes, like kidney beans and soybeans, generally require a longer cooking time (4 to 5 hours) than smaller lentils and adzuki beans (1 to 2 hours). Adding a small piece of seaweed like kombu or kelp during cooking can also help to tenderize the beans and improve their digestibility. Using a slow cooker or crock pot is also convenient for preparing beans.

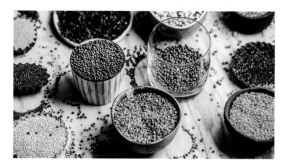

ADZUKI OR ADUKI BEANS

Body type(s): *Summer, Indian Summer, Fall*
Thermal nature: *neutral*

Native to Asia, adzuki beans have a dark red color and a sweet and sour flavor. They help to detoxify the body and drain edema and excess fluids. Adzuki beans are a good source of magnesium, zinc, potassium, iron, and B vitamins, and are easy to digest compared to other common beans. Adzuki beans are common in Asian desserts like mochi and red bean buns; they can also be used in savory recipes like soups and rice dishes.

BLACK OR BLACK TURTLE BEANS

Body type(s): *Summer, Indian Summer, Fall*
Thermal nature: *neutral to warming*

Originating from Central and South Americas, black beans are a staple in Latin cuisine. With a sweet flavor and a firm texture, black beans help to nourish *yin* and promote diuresis. They are a good source of protein, dietary fiber, iron, and folate; they are also rich in the antioxidants found in other darkly pigmented foods like red grapes and blueberries.

BLACK SOYBEANS

Body type(s): *Spring, Summer, Indian Summer, Fall*
Thermal nature: *neutral*

Black soybeans have a creamier texture and milder flavor than their yellow counterparts. They help to tonify *yin* and circulate blood. Black soybeans can also have a diuretic effect and help to remove toxins from the body. They are high in fiber and protein, and are a good source of iron. Black soybeans can be used in soups, chilis, and salads. Fermented soybeans are often served as an accompaniment to Asian dishes.

GARBANZO BEANS OR CHICKPEAS

Body type(s): *Indian Summer, Fall*
Thermal nature: *neutral*

Garbanzo beans were originally cultivated in the Middle East. With a sweet, nutty flavor and creamy texture, they are helpful for strengthening and supplementing *qi*. They also help to drain excess fluids from the body. Garbanzo beans are high in fiber, protein, folate, iron, and manganese; they are a source of polyunsaturated fats and help to lower cholesterol. They are used to make hummus and falafel, and are also good in soups, chilis, and stews.

KIDNEY BEANS

Body type(s): *Summer, Fall*
Thermal nature: *neutral*

Kidney beans have a hearty texture and absorb other flavors well, making them a good ingredient to use in simmered dishes like soups, stews, and chilis. They are helpful for supporting *yin* and reducing edema. High in fiber, protein, and folate, kidney beans are also a good source of the minerals manganese and molybdenum. Raw kidney beans have high levels of the toxin phytohemagglutinin; whether they are cooked in a slow cooker or over the stove, they should be boiled for a minimum of 10 minutes to destroy the toxin.

LENTILS

Body type(s): *Indian Summer, Fall*
Thermal nature: *neutral*

Popular in Indian cuisine, lentils are small legumes that are sold whole or split into halves. Lentils are available in a variety of colors, including green, brown, yellow, red, orange, and black. They are helpful for strengthening *qi* and draining excess fluids, and are rich in protein, fiber, B vitamins, and iron. Because of their small size, lentils do not need to be pre-soaked, though soaking can increase digestibility. Lentils take about 20 to 40 minutes to cook, depending on the variety. They are often simmered into dal, curries, and stews, and can be used in salads.

MUNG BEANS

Body type(s): *Summer*
Thermal nature: *cooling*

Mung beans are small, green legumes commonly eaten in Asian dishes and desserts. They supplement *yin*, clear excess heat, and cleanse and detoxify the body. Mung beans are a good source of B vitamins, magnesium, and phosphorous. Generally, they are easier to digest than other beans because of their low oligosaccharide content. The bean sprouts that are sold in grocery stores and eaten raw in salads are sprouted forms of the mung bean, and are more cooling than unsprouted mung beans. Mung beans are often used in soups, dal, and rice dishes. The flour from the mung bean can also be made into clear cellophane noodles.

PEANUTS

Body type(s): *Indian Summer, Winter*
Thermal nature: *neutral to warming*

Peanuts are legumes, but with a high fat and protein content, their characteristics are similar to tree nuts. They are a building food and help to strengthen *qi*. Peanuts are high in B vitamins like thiamine, niacin, and folate, as well as vitamin E, manganese, and iron. They are also a source of monounsaturated fats and the antioxidant resveratrol. Depending on their growing and storage conditions, peanuts may become contaminated by aflatoxin, a carcinogenic mold. To minimize aflatoxin contamination, purchase peanuts and peanut products from trusted sources and manufacturers, and store them in the refrigerator.

YELLOW SOYBEANS

Body type(s): *Spring, Summer, Indian Summer*
Thermal nature: *neutral to cooling*

Native to East Asia, yellow soybeans are high in complete protein. They are beneficial for alleviating excess heat, fortifying blood and *qi*, and increasing circulation in the body. A good source of manganese, molybdenum, iron, phosphorus, and dietary fiber, yellow soybeans also contain omega-3 fatty acids and isoflavones. Soybeans can also be eaten in their green, immature form known as edamame. In order to increase their digestibility, soybeans should be cooked well or fermented. Traditionally, yellow soybeans are cooked and ground to make soy milk and tofu. Tofu tends to be more cooling and moistening than whole soybeans, and more beneficial for clearing heat from the body. Yellow soybeans are fermented to make other traditional products like soy sauce, miso, natto, and tempeh; these soy foods are more easily digested than the beans themselves and are therefore recommended for individuals with weak digestion or digestive issues. Sprouted forms of soy products may be more digestible and have higher nutrient availability. Most soybean crops are genetically engineered and heavily sprayed with pesticides; for the highest-quality soy products, look for those with organic, GMO-free certifications.

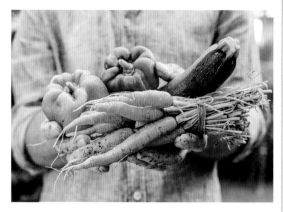

VEGETABLES

The most diverse of all of the food groups, vegetables have a wide range of health benefits and form an essential part of the daily diet for all body types. They provide an abundance of nutrients, including antioxidants, phytochemicals,

vitamins, minerals, and dietary fiber. In general, vegetables have a cleansing effect on the body and help to increase circulation and detoxify the blood. Raw vegetables tend to be more nutrient-rich, cleansing, and cooling than those that have been cooked. In contrast, cooked vegetables are more digestible, easier for the body to assimilate, and more warming and strengthening in terms of *qi*. Generally, raw vegetables are more appropriate for Spring and Summer body types, while cooked vegetables are recommended for Indian Summer, Fall, and Winter types, or any individuals with weakened digestive systems.

Leafy greens are the most cleansing of the vegetables, making them particularly beneficial for Spring types. Bulbs and members of the onion family (e.g. garlic, leeks, onions, and shallots) are also helpful for these body types; their pungent flavors, as classified by TCM, help to circulate *qi* and counteract stagnancy. Vegetables which grow in warmer climates, above ground, or over shorter periods of time tend to have a more cooling thermal nature. These include vegetables with high water content like cucumbers, lettuce, and celery, which are ideal for soothing excess heat found in Summer body types. On the other hand, vegetables which grow in cooler climates, below ground, or over longer periods of time tend to have a more warming thermal nature. Roots, tubers, and cruciferous vegetables generally store more energy as they grow and provide more warming sustenance than their quick-growing counterparts; consequently, they are more beneficial for the cooler Fall and Winter types. Vegetables with a neutral thermal nature and a naturally sweet flavor as classified by TCM (e.g. beets, corn, and pumpkins) are building foods and help to support *qi* within the body, making them ideal for Indian Summer types.

ASPARAGUS

Body type(s): *Summer, Fall*
Thermal nature: *neutral*

Although commonly available in the springtime, asparagus is beneficial for Summer and Fall body types, due to its slightly bitter flavor and diuretic properties. It contains the amino acid asparagine, which helps to reduce edema and water retention in the body. Asparagine is responsible for the characteristic odor present in urine when asparagus is consumed. Asparagus is also a good source of folate, iron, and vitamins A and K. It contains moderately high levels of purine, which should be minimized in the diets of those with gout or kidney inflammation.

AVOCADOS

Body type(s): *Summer, Indian Summer*
Thermal nature: *cooling*

Often used as a vegetable in culinary applications, avocado is technically a fruit. Most varieties of avocados are seasonally available in the spring and summer. Avocados have a rich, creamy texture and help to support *yin*. They are a very good source of monounsaturated fatty acids and are rich in potassium, B vitamins, vitamin E, and fiber.

BEETS

Body type(s): *Indian Summer*
Thermal nature: *neutral*

Beets are root vegetables with a sweet, earthy flavor. Their peak harvest season is during the summer and fall. Available in red, golden, and pink-and-white striped varieties, beets help to purify the blood and build *qi* within the body. Beets are a good source of fiber, folate, manganese, and potassium. They are often eaten raw, pickled, or roasted, and are also used in soups and salads. The leaves of beet plants are also edible; they are similar to Swiss chard, have a slightly bitter flavor, and are a good source of vitamin A, vitamin C, calcium, and iron.

BELL PEPPERS

Body type(s): *Spring, Winter*
Thermal nature: *warming*

Also known as sweet peppers, bell peppers have lower levels of the heat-producing capsaicin that is found in chili peppers. Although they are technically fruit, bell peppers are used as vegetables in cooking. They help to warm and circulate blood within the body and are rich in vitamins C, A, and K. Green bell peppers are less ripe and less sweet than yellow, orange, and red varieties. Red bell peppers contain the antioxidant lycopene.

BROCCOLI

Body type(s): *Spring, Summer*
Thermal nature: *cooling*

Broccoli is seasonally available in the spring through fall seasons. It is helpful for soothing heat, as well as moving and circulating *qi*. Broccoli is a member of the cruciferous family of vegetables, which are known for their high content of antioxidants and their role in cancer prevention. Broccoli is a good source of vitamins C, K, and A, several B vitamins, iron, and fiber.

BRUSSELS SPROUTS

Body type(s): *Winter*
Thermal nature: *warming*

The peak growing seasons for brussels sprouts are fall and winter. Brussels sprouts grow in bunches of twenty to forty sprouts per stalk. They are similar to cabbage and other cruciferous vegetables in terms of their nutritional benefits, providing a good source of iron, folate, and vitamins C and K. They are also a good source of omega-3 fatty acids. To minimize their bitter flavor, choose freshly picked sprouts with a bright-green color. Brussels sprouts are often served sautéed or roasted, and can be thinly sliced and used raw in salads.

CABBAGE

Body type(s): *Indian Summer, Fall, Winter*
Thermal nature: *neutral to warming*

Cabbage is a cool-season crop which benefits the stomach and digestive tract. Along with other cruciferous vegetables, it has been shown to protect against colorectal cancers. When prepared in pickled and fermented forms like sauerkraut and kimchi, cabbage has a cleansing and rejuvenating effect on the digestive system. Cabbage is a good source of iron, several B vitamins, and vitamins C and K. Compared to green cabbage, the red variety contains high levels of anthocyanins, which provide anti-inflammatory and antioxidant benefits.

CARROTS

Body type(s): *Spring, Indian Summer*
Thermal nature: *neutral*

Carrots are root vegetables with a naturally sweet flavor. They tonify and circulate both *qi* and blood; cooked carrots are beneficial for those with weakened digestion. Carrots are an excellent source of antioxidants and are one of the richest food sources of beta-carotene and vitamin A. They are also a good source of dietary fiber, potassium, and vitamins C and K.

CAULIFLOWER

Body type(s): *Indian Summer, Fall*
Thermal nature: *neutral*

Seasonally available in the summer and fall, cauliflower has a sweet and slightly bitter flavor as classified by TCM. It has many of the same nutritional benefits as broccoli, cabbage, and other cruciferous vegetables, including anti-cancer and antioxidant properties. Cauliflower is high in vitamins C and K, and is a good source of B vitamins, potassium, and manganese.

CELERY

Body type(s): *Summer, Fall*
Thermal nature: *cooling*

Celery is available all year round, but is at its best during the summer and fall months. It is beneficial for draining excess fluids, reducing inflammation, and alleviating arthritis. According to TCM flavor classification, celery has a bitter flavor; this bitterness is thought to help with appetite control. Celery is high in silicon, which helps to renew connective tissue. It also provides a good source of dietary fiber and vitamins A and K. For Fall body types, celery should be eaten in its cooked form to reduce its cooling effect on the body.

CUCUMBERS

Body type(s): *Summer*
Thermal nature: *cooling*

A summer crop which grows on a vine, cucumbers have one of the highest water contents of any fruit or vegetable. Their cooling nature makes them helpful for soothing excess heat, quenching thirst, and relieving inflammation. Cucumbers also remove toxins and have a mild diuretic effect on the body. They are a good source of potassium and vitamins K and C.

EGGPLANTS

Body type(s): *Spring, Summer, Indian Summer*
Thermal nature: *cooling*

Also known as aubergines, eggplants belong to the nightshade family and are at their peak during summer and fall. Eggplants have a sweet and slightly bitter flavor, and are helpful for enriching the blood, clearing excess heat, and moving stagnant *qi*. They also provide a good source of dietary fiber, potassium, manganese, copper, and several B vitamins, including folate.

FENNEL

Body type(s): *Spring, Indian Summer, Winter*
Thermal nature: *warming*

Fennel is very aromatic and has a flavor similar to anise and licorice. The whole fennel plant can be used in cooking, from its bulb, stalk, and leaves to its seeds. Fennel helps to circulate and tonify *qi*, aid the digestive system, and nourish *yang* within the body. It is also a good source of vitamin C, folate, potassium, manganese, and fiber. Fennel is often eaten raw in salads, or roasted and braised for a mellower flavor.

GARLIC

Body type(s): *Spring, Fall, Winter*
Thermal nature: *very warming*

A member of the onion family, garlic is beneficial for circulating *qi* and nourishing *yang*. It is rich in sulfur-containing compounds, which are responsible for its pungent flavor, aroma, and many health benefits. A good source of manganese and vitamins B6 and C, garlic has antibacterial, anti-parasitic, and antiviral properties. It also has shown the potential to enhance the immune system, prevent cancer, and protect the liver.[1,2] Garlic can be eaten raw or cooked; when steamed or roasted, it develops a milder, sweeter flavor and loses some of its protective benefits.

GREEN BEANS

Body type(s): *Summer, Indian Summer*
Thermal nature: *neutral*

Also known as string beans, green beans are the immature pods of the common bean plant which produces other varieties of beans, including black, kidney, and pinto beans. Like dried beans, green beans are a type of legume, though they are more commonly used as a fresh vegetable in cooking. They are at their seasonal peak during the summer and early fall. With a mild, sweet flavor, they are beneficial for strengthening both *yin* and *qi*. Green beans contain antioxidants like carotenoids and flavonoids; they are a good source of vitamins C, K, and A, manganese, and fiber.

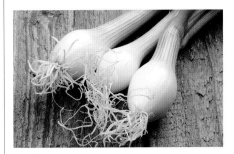

GREEN ONIONS

Body type(s): *Spring, Fall, Winter*
Thermal nature: *warming*

Also known as spring onions or scallions, green onions have a milder flavor compared to other members of the onion family. They are cultivated for their hollow green leaves and stalks rather than their bulbs. Green onions have warming, diuretic, and detoxifying effects on the body. They have healing properties similar to garlic, but to a milder degree. Green onions are rich in vitamins A, C, and K, and B vitamins.

KALE

Body type(s): *Indian Summer, Fall*
Thermal nature: *warming*

Kale is a member of the cabbage family and is available in a range of varieties, including curly, ornamental, and dinosaur kale. A cool season crop, kale has a slightly bitter flavor which tends to sweeten after a frost. It is rich in phytonutrients and chlorophyll, and it enriches the blood. Kale is an excellent source of vitamins K, C, and A; it also provides a good source of manganese, calcium, and dietary fiber. It can be served raw in salads and smoothies, simmered into soups, sautéed, and dried in the oven to make kale chips.

KOHLRABI

Body type(s): *Spring, Fall*
Thermal nature: *neutral to warming*

Seasonally available in the winter and spring, kohlrabi is a vegetable from the cabbage family and is available in green and purple varieties. Kohlrabi improves the circulation of *qi* in the body and drains excess fluids. The large bulb of the vegetable has a crunchy texture and a flavor similar to broccoli stems; its leaves are also edible and can be cooked in a similar manner as kale or mustard greens. Kohlrabi is a good source of vitamins C and A, potassium, and fiber. It is often eaten raw as a salad or slaw, boiled and mashed with other root vegetables, or roasted.

LEEKS

Body type(s): *Spring, Winter*
Thermal nature: *warming*

Leeks are related to onions and garlic, but are milder in flavor and pungency. A leek resembles a large green onion, with dark green leaves and a thick, white base. The white and light green parts of the leaves are the main edible portions of the plant. Leeks help to warm the body and circulate *qi*, though their healing effect is more moderate than other members of the onion family. They are a good source of vitamins K, A, and C, manganese, and folate. Leeks should be washed well before using since dirt becomes trapped in the white leaf base as the plant grows; cut the leeks into pieces and rinse in a strainer until the water is clear. They can be used as a substitute for onions, sautéed in stir-fries, and added to soups and stews.

LETTUCE

Body type(s): *Summer, Fall*
Thermal nature: *cooling*

Grown in moderate temperatures, lettuce is available in several varieties. It has a bitter flavor as classified by TCM and drains excess fluids from the body; it also has a sedative effect and can help to soothe the nerves. Lettuce is rich in folate and vitamins K, A, and C. Varieties like romaine lettuce and arugula, which have a bitterer flavor and darker green leaves, tend to be richer in nutrients and antioxidants than those with lighter-colored leaves. While lettuce is typically eaten raw in the West as salad greens, it is often cooked in the East; for Fall body types, lettuce should be eaten in its cooked form to reduce its cooling effect.

MUSHROOMS

Body type(s): *Summer, Indian Summer, Fall*
Thermal nature: *cooling*

The high levels of glutamate in mushrooms give them their rich, umami flavor. Available in several different varieties, mushrooms help to clear excess mucus and strengthen the immune system; they are also used medicinally to prevent cancer and inhibit tumor growth.[3] Shiitake mushrooms, in particular, are beneficial for nourishing *qi* and enhancing immunity. Mushrooms are an excellent source of B vitamins and minerals like selenium, copper, and phosphorus.

MUSTARD GREENS

Body type(s): *Spring, Fall*
Thermal nature: *warming*

Seasonally available in the winter and spring, mustard greens have a spicy and pungent flavor. They are beneficial for improving circulation and reducing phlegm. Mustard greens are an excellent source of folate and vitamins K, A, and C; they are also a good source of manganese, vitamin E, calcium, and fiber. The leaves of young plants can be used raw in salads, while the leaves of more mature plants are usually steamed, sautéed, or boiled.

NAPA CABBAGE

Body type(s): *Summer*
Thermal nature: *neutral to cooling*

Often used in Asian cuisine, napa cabbage has a higher water content and is more lettuce-like than common cabbage. It also has a more cooling thermal nature and milder flavor. Napa cabbage helps to clear heat and promote diuresis in the body. It is a good source of folate and vitamins C and A. Similar to common cabbage varieties, napa cabbage can be cooked, pickled (e.g. kimchi), or used raw in slaws and salads.

ONIONS

Body type(s): *Spring, Fall, Winter*
Thermal nature: *warming*

Onions have a strong, pungent flavor that is tempered with cooking. They stimulate the circulation of blood and *qi* within the body, and also treat the common cold and other sinus conditions by draining mucus and loosening phlegm. Rich in sulfur and phytonutrients, onions have antibacterial, antifungal, and antiviral properties. They also provide a good source of vitamin C, B vitamins, and dietary fiber.

PARSNIPS

Body type(s): *Fall, Winter*
Thermal nature: *warming*

Relatives of the carrot, parsnips are root vegetables that are seasonally available in the fall and winter. They have a creamy white color, a nutty flavor, and a sweetness which is enhanced after frosty weather. Parsnips help to dry excess fluids in the body and can benefit individuals with rheumatism and arthritis. They are a good source of manganese, vitamins C and K, folate, and dietary fiber. Often roasted or cooked into soups or stews, parsnips should be used soon after being harvested, or else their flavor can become bitter and overpowering.

POTATOES

Body type(s): *Summer, Indian Summer*
Thermal nature: *neutral*

Belonging to the nightshade family, potatoes are starchy tubers and one of the primary staple crops worldwide. They are rich in carbohydrates and easy to digest. Potatoes are beneficial for nourishing *yin* and reducing inflammation; in addition, they are a building food which fortifies *qi* in the body. Potatoes provide a good source of potassium and vitamins C and B6; when they are eaten in their whole form with their skins, they are also a good source of dietary fiber.

PUMPKINS

Body type(s): *Indian Summer, Fall*
Thermal nature: *neutral to warming*

Pumpkins are a type of squash, planted in the summer and harvested in the fall. They have a sweet flavor which helps to nourish *qi*. They are also beneficial for reducing edema and swelling in the body. Pumpkins provide a very good source of vitamin A, and a good source of vitamin C, manganese, potassium, and fiber. Their seeds are rich in zinc and are helpful for eliminating intestinal parasites.

RADISHES

Body type(s): *Spring, Summer, Fall*
Thermal nature: *cooling*

Radishes are rapid-growing root vegetables with a crisp texture and pungent flavor. There are several different varieties of radishes, ranging from the small, red globe radishes common in North America to the large, white daikon radishes originally from Asia. In general, radishes help to increase circulation, detoxify the body, and resolve heat and excess mucus. They are a good source of vitamin C, folate, potassium, and fiber. Radishes are often pickled or served raw in salads and sandwiches.

SPINACH

Body type(s): *Summer, Indian Summer*
Thermal nature: *cooling*

Grown in temperate climates, spinach is at its peak during spring and early summer. Its dark green leaves are rich in chlorophyll and iron, making them beneficial for fortifying the blood. Spinach also helps to nourish *yin*. A powerhouse of nutrients and antioxidants, spinach is an excellent source of vitamins K and A, and a good source of vitamins C and E, B vitamins, calcium, potassium, fiber, and omega-3 fatty acids.

SUMMER SQUASH

Body type(s): *Summer*
Thermal nature: *cooling*

A member of the gourd family, summer squash is in season from the summer through early fall. Squash varieties that have a thin, edible skin and are harvested when immature are known as summer squash; those that have a thick rind and are harvested when fully mature are known as winter squash. Some popular varieties of summer squash include zucchini, crookneck, and patty-pan. Summer squash tends to have a higher water content and a more cooling thermal nature than winter squash; it is helpful for supporting *yin*. It is also a good source of vitamins C and B6, manganese, and potassium.

SWEET POTATOES

Body type(s): *Indian Summer*
Thermal nature: *neutral*

Seasonally available in the fall and winter, sweet potatoes are starchy tubers that help to strengthen *qi* and enrich the blood. Their naturally sweet flavor and complex carbohydrates make them a building food. Sweet potatoes are available in a variety of colors, including white, yellow, orange, and purple; in the U.S., the orange-fleshed varieties are often mislabeled as yams. The shoots and leaves of the sweet potato plant are also edible. Sweet potatoes are an excellent source of vitamin A, and a good source of vitamins C and B6, manganese, potassium, and dietary fiber.

A SPECTRUM OF COLORS AND NUTRIENTS

Fruits and vegetables are abundant in essential nutrients and antioxidants. By eating a wide variety of different plant-source foods and creating a "rainbow" of colors on your plate, you can nourish your body, promote health, and prevent chronic disease. The colors or pigments of a plant-source food indicate some of the types of phytonutrients it contains.[4] Phytonutrients have an antioxidant effect on the body, helping to prevent cellular damage and support immune function.[5]

» **Red fruits and vegetables** – contain antioxidants like lycopene and anthocyanins, which have been shown to reduce the risk of prostate cancer and heart disease.[6,7] Examples include beets, cherries, red peppers, strawberries, and tomatoes.

» **Orange and yellow fruits and vegetables** – are rich in carotenoids like beta-carotene and zeaxanthin, which are beneficial for reducing the risk of macular degeneration, cardiovascular disease, and certain cancers.[8,9] Examples include apricots, carrots, mangoes, oranges, papayas, squash, and sweet potatoes.

» **Green fruits and vegetables** – have high levels of chlorophyll and lutein, which protect against cancer, benefit vision health, and support the immune system.[10,11] Examples include avocados, broccoli, dark leafy greens, green peppers, kiwis, and peas.

» **Blue and purple fruits and vegetables** – contain anthocyanins, which protect against inflammation and show preventive effects on heart disease, type 2 diabetes, and cancer.[12] Examples include blueberries, eggplants, grapes, plums, and red cabbage.

» **White fruits and vegetables** – are colored by anthoxanthins and contain chemicals like allicin and quercetin, which may help to lower cholesterol and reduce the risk of heart disease and some cancers.[13,14] Examples include bananas, cauliflower, mushrooms, onions, pears, and potatoes.

SWISS CHARD

Body type(s): *Summer, Indian Summer*
Thermal nature: *cooling*

Swiss chard belongs to the same family as beets and spinach, and is seasonally available in the summer and fall. It helps to clear excess heat and enrich the blood. Both the leaves and stems of the plant are edible. As a dark green leafy vegetable, Swiss chard is rich in phytonutrients; it is an excellent source of vitamins K, A, and C, and a good source of magnesium, manganese, iron, potassium, vitamin E, and fiber. Swiss chard can be sautéed, added to soups, or baked in casseroles.

TOMATOES

Body type(s): *Summer*
Thermal nature: *cooling*

Botanically considered a fruit but used as a vegetable in cooking, tomatoes are seasonally available in the summer through early fall. They are members of the nightshade family, along with potatoes, eggplants, and peppers. Tomatoes are beneficial for nourishing *yin* and detoxifying the body. They contain the antioxidant lycopene, and are a good source of vitamins C, A, and K, potassium, and manganese.

TURNIPS

Body type(s): *Spring, Fall*
Thermal nature: *neutral*

Turnips are members of the cruciferous family of vegetables with a seasonal peak in the fall and winter. They help to circulate *qi* and blood, and drain excess fluids. The root bulbs of the turnip plant have a white flesh with a white, red, purple, or green skin. They are a good source of vitamin C, manganese, and potassium. Turnips are often pickled, cooked into soups and stews, boiled and mashed, or roasted. The leaves of the turnip plant are also edible, providing an excellent source of folate and vitamins K, A, and C.

WATERCRESS

Body type(s): *Spring, Summer, Indian Summer*
Thermal nature: *cooling*

Watercress is a member of the cabbage family and a relative of mustard greens. It has a pungent, peppery flavor and a stimulating effect on the body. It helps to tonify *yin*, enrich and cleanse the blood, and promote diuresis. It is a good source of chlorophyll, vitamins A, C, and K, and calcium. Like collard greens, kale, and many other greens, watercress can be eaten raw or cooked. It is often used in salads, sandwiches, soups, and stir-fries.

WINTER SQUASH

Body type(s): *Indian Summer, Fall, Winter*
Thermal nature: *warming*

Seasonally available in the fall through early spring, winter squash includes varieties like acorn, butternut, kabocha, pumpkin, and spaghetti squash. Winter squash is beneficial for nourishing *qi* and draining excess fluids from the body. It is a good source of complex carbohydrates and dietary fiber, as well as vitamins A and C, B vitamins, manganese, and potassium.

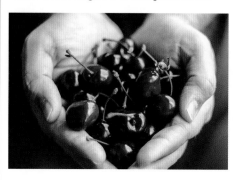

FRUITS

Like vegetables, fruits are rich in phytochemicals, antioxidants, and dietary fiber, and they also provide a good source of vitamin C and potassium. Fruits commonly have sweet and sour flavors as classified by TCM, and a cooling, refreshing effect on the body. As a food group, they nourish *yin* and are beneficial for soothing the overworked and overheated body types. They also have a mildly cleansing effect, which can help to balance a meal or diet of rich, heavy foods.

The majority of fruits have a cooling thermal nature; fruits with high water content, like melons and citrus, are especially cooling. A few fruits, like cherries and peaches, have a warming effect; however compared to other foods, that effect tends to be shorter lasting and less intense. Generally, fruits have a more cooling and cleansing action when they are eaten raw. Fruits in their raw form are beneficial for Spring and Summer body types, but should be minimized by colder body types or those with weakened digestion, like Indian Summer, Fall, and Winter body types.

Dried or cooked fruits, which are more warming and *yang*-like, are more appropriate for these types.

The natural sugars in fruits offer a preferable alternative to the refined sugars found in processed foods and sweets. However for some individuals, overconsumption of sweet foods can have a negative effect on health, even when those sugars come from natural sources. People who are sensitive to sugar, are prone to yeast infections, or have diabetes should moderate their intake of certain fruits, especially those with a very sweet flavor like bananas and dates. Because the sugars in dried fruits and fruit juices tend to be highly concentrated, those foods should be eaten in moderation as well.

APPLES

Body type(s): *Summer, Indian Summer*
Thermal nature: *cooling*

Grown in subtropical and temperate climates, apples are in season from late summer to early winter; however, they are generally available all year round because they store well. With a sweet and sour flavor, apples are beneficial for soothing heat and nourishing *yin* and *qi*. They have also been shown to help lower the risk of heart disease. When eaten whole with their skins, they are a good source of dietary fiber, vitamin C, and antioxidants.

BANANAS

Body type(s): *Summer, Indian Summer*
Thermal nature: *very cooling*

Bananas are a staple crop grown in tropical regions. Their cooling, moistening nature helps to clear excess heat and support *yin*. Bananas are easy to digest and helpful in cases of digestive weakness, constipation, and diarrhea. They provide a very good source of vitamin B6 and a good source of vitamin C, manganese, fiber, and potassium.

CHERRIES

Body type(s): *Spring, Indian Summer, Fall, Winter*
Thermal nature: *warming*

Stone fruits grown in temperate climates, cherries are at their seasonal peak during the summer. They help to improve circulation of the blood, strengthen *qi*, and defend against the cold. They also have an anti-inflammatory effect and are beneficial for relieving gout and arthritis pain. Cherries are a good source of vitamin C and antioxidants; they also contain iron, vitamin A, and dietary fiber.

DATES

Body type(s): *Indian Summer, Winter*
Thermal nature: *warming*

Dates are the very sweet fruit of the date palm and a staple food in the Middle East. They are beneficial for building and tonifying *qi*. Naturally low in moisture, fresh dates are harvested in the fall and winter, and include soft, semi-dry, and dry varieties. Dates are also sold in a dried, dehydrated form, which is more concentrated in flavor than a fresh date. Dates are often used in desserts, as well as in tagines and couscous dishes. They provide a good source of magnesium, manganese, potassium, B vitamins, copper, and dietary fiber.

FIGS

Body type(s): *Summer, Indian Summer*
Thermal nature: *neutral*

Native to the Middle East, figs are available fresh in the summer and early fall. Because figs have a fragile skin and are difficult to transport, they are commonly available dried. Figs are beneficial for fortifying both *qi* and blood. They are a highly alkaline food and may help to balance the acid-forming foods common in the Western diet. Fresh figs are high in dietary fiber. In their dried form, they are also a concentrated source of vitamins and minerals such as calcium, iron, potassium, and B vitamins. Figs can be used in salads and breads, and are often paired with cheese or honey.

GRAPES

Body type(s): *Indian Summer, Fall*
Thermal nature: *neutral*

Seasonally available in the fall, grapes are primarily grown for the production of wine, but they are also commonly consumed fresh, or in their dried form as raisins. They help to fortify *qi* and blood, as well as promote diuresis. Grape skins contain several phytonutrients, including resveratrol, an antioxidant that helps protect against cancer, cardiovascular disease, and stroke. Red wine has higher resveratrol levels than white wine, due to the presence of grape skins during the wine fermentation process. Grapes are a very good source of manganese and vitamins K and C, while raisins are high in iron and potassium.

GRAPEFRUITS

Body type(s): *Summer*
Thermal nature: *very cooling*

Grown in tropical and subtropical regions, grape-fruits have a tart and slightly bitter flavor, and a seasonal peak in the winter and spring. Like other members of the citrus family, grapefruits are helpful for cooling excess heat and quenching thirst. They are high in vitamins C and A; varieties with pink and red flesh also contain the antioxidant lycopene. The bitter extract of grapefruit seeds is used medicinally for its antibiotic and antifungal properties. Individuals who take pharmaceuticals should consume grapefruits and grapefruit juice with caution, since those foods have been shown to interact with certain medications and increase their potencies.

KUMQUATS

Body type(s): *Spring, Fall*
Thermal nature: *warming*

Native to Asia, kumquats resemble small, bite-size oranges with an oval shape. They are seasonally available in the winter through spring. Kumquats are beneficial for circulating *qi* within the body and resolving excess mucus. Their thin peels are edible and have a sweet flavor, while their flesh is juicy and tart. High in vitamin C, kumquats are often served fresh in salads, or preserved and prepared as candied fruit, jams, or jellies.

LEMONS/LIMES

Body type(s): *Spring, Summer*
Thermal nature: *cooling*

Lemons and limes are at their peak from the late spring to early fall. They have a sour flavor and are high in citric acid; limes tend to be less acidic than lemons. Both lemons and limes have the ability to relieve thirst, clear excess heat, and support *yin*. They increase circulation and help to cleanse the body. With antiseptic and anti-bacterial properties, these fruits are useful in treating colds, coughs, and flus. They are an excellent source of vitamin C and a good source of potassium and B vitamins.

LYCHEES

Body type(s): *Spring, Indian Summer*
Thermal nature: *neutral to warming*

Native to Asia, the lychee is a fruit that is grown in tropical and subtropical climates and is seasonally available in the summer. Lychees have a rough, red, inedible shell which surrounds a white and juicy flesh. They are helpful for increasing circulation and fortifying both *qi* and blood. Lychees are rich in vitamin C and provide a good source of copper, phosphorus, and potassium. They are often served in salads, desserts, and drinks.

MANGOES

Body type(s): *Summer*
Thermal nature: *cooling*

Mangoes are fragrant stone fruits native to South Asia. Grown in tropical and subtropical climates, several varieties are seasonally available in the spring and summer. Mangoes are beneficial for supporting and tonifying *yin*, and are rich in antioxidants and vitamins C, A, and B6. While red, yellow, and orange varieties are typically eaten raw as cooling fruits, green varieties can be cooked, pickled, and prepared in savory recipes.

ORANGES

Body type(s): *Spring, Summer*
Thermal nature: *cooling*

Belonging to the citrus family, oranges are available in several varieties and are grown for both their flesh and juice. They are at their seasonal peak during the winter and spring, depending on the variety. Like lemons and limes, oranges are beneficial for soothing heat, quenching thirst, and nourishing *yin*. Both the flesh and peel of the orange are helpful for increasing circulation. Oranges are an excellent source of

vitamin C, and a good source of dietary fiber, B vitamins, potassium, and calcium.

PAPAYAS

Body type(s): *Indian Summer, Fall*
Thermal nature: *neutral*

Papayas are tropical fruit with a seasonal peak in summer and fall. They have a soft, yellow-orange flesh and edible, round, black seeds which have a bitter, peppery flavor. Papayas help to build *qi*, benefit the digestive system, and resolve excess mucus. They contain the digestive enzyme papain, which helps to break down proteins and tenderize meat. Papayas provide an excellent source of vitamins C and A, and a good source of folate, potassium, and dietary fiber. They are often eaten fresh or made into salads, and can also be dried, baked, or roasted.

PEACHES

Body type(s): *Spring, Summer*
Thermal nature: *neutral to warming*

Seasonally available in the summer, peaches are stone fruits native to Asia. They belong to the same family as nectarines, with the main difference lying in the texture of their skins. Peaches are beneficial for increasing the circulation of *qi* and nourishing *yin*. They are a good source of vitamins C and A, dietary fiber, and potassium.

PEARS

Body type(s): *Summer*
Thermal nature: *cooling*

Pears are grown in temperate climates and are harvested in the summer and fall, though some varieties are available in the winter. They help to tonify *yin* and resolve excess mucus in the body. Pears are a good source of vitamins C and K;

FRUITS AND VEGETABLES TO BUY ORGANIC

When purchasing fruits and vegetables, it is important to consider the environmental conditions in which those foods are grown. Unlike conventional farming methods, organic methods exclude the use of synthetic fertilizers, pesticides, and chemicals. Pesticide use may have an adverse effect not only on the health of the people who consume those crops, but also on the health of farms, farm workers, and the environment.[15] To minimize your consumption of pesticides and your exposure to toxic chemicals, choose fruits and vegetables that have been sprayed with fewer pesticides, tend to retain less pesticide residue on their skins, or are organically grown.

The Environmental Working Group (EWG) analyzes data from the U.S. Department of Agriculture and the Food and Drug Administration to create a list of foods with the highest levels of pesticide residue. This annual Dirty Dozen list includes twelve fruits and vegetables that tend to be heavily sprayed with pesticides, have thin skins or flesh that more readily absorb chemical contamination, or are grown in countries with fewer restrictions on pesticide use. For more information on the EWG, see the resource listing in the Appendix.

The following fruits and vegetables have been included on the EWG's advisory list in the past several years. Eat organic versions when possible. If you are unable to purchase organic forms of these fruits and vegetables, consider substituting them with conventionally grown produce not on this list that have lower levels of pesticides.

» Apples	» Grapes	» Pears
» Bell peppers	» Green beans	» Potatoes
» Blueberries	» Hot peppers	» Spinach
» Carrots	» Kale/collard greens	» Strawberries
» Celery	» Lettuce	» Summer squash
» Cherries	» Nectarines	» Tomatoes
» Cucumbers	» Peaches	

when eaten whole with their skins, they are also a good source of dietary fiber.

PINEAPPLES

Body type(s): *Summer*
Thermal nature: *neutral to cooling*

Native to South America, pineapples are grown in tropical regions with a seasonal peak from late spring to early summer. With a sweet and sour flavor, pineapples are beneficial for clearing excess heat and supporting *yin*. They contain the enzyme bromelain, which has anti-inflammatory properties and works as a digestive aid. Pineapples are an excellent source of vitamin C and manganese, and a good source of B vitamins, copper, and dietary fiber.

PLUMS

Body type(s): *Spring, Summer*
Thermal nature: *neutral*

Plums are stone fruit that are related to peaches, cherries, and almonds. They are in season from the late spring to early fall with a peak in mid-summer. Plums help to circulate *qi*, nourish *yin*, and soothe heat in the body. Plums are a good source of vitamins C, A, and K, and a moderate source of potassium and dietary fiber. Dried plums, also known as prunes, can have a laxative effect.

QUINCES

Body type(s): *Fall*
Thermal nature: *neutral to warming*

A relative of apples and pears, quinces are seasonally available in the fall and early winter. They have a hard texture and are high in tannins, making their taste astringent and unpleasant when eaten raw. Quinces have a drying effect and can help to reduce swelling in the body. Most often cooked into jams, jellies, preserves, or desserts, they are a good source of vitamin C, copper, and iron.

TANGERINES

Body type(s): *Spring, Summer*
Thermal nature: *cooling*

Tangerines belong to the mandarin orange family along with clementines and satsumas. They are small citrus fruit that are easy to peel, with a seasonal peak in the winter and spring. Tangerines help to circulate *qi* within the body as well as soothe excess heat. They provide a good source of vitamins C and A.

WATERMELONS

Body type(s): *Summer*
Thermal nature: *very cooling*

One of the most cooling fruits, a watermelon contains over 90% water by weight. Watermelons are at their seasonal peak in the summer. They are beneficial for quenching thirst and tonifying *yin*, and they also have a mild diuretic effect. Watermelons provide a good source of potassium and vitamins C and A. Red-fleshed varieties are also high in the antioxidant lycopene.

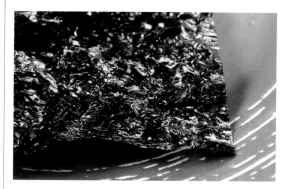

SEAWEEDS

Also sometimes called sea vegetables, seaweeds are edible forms of algae which are available in red, brown, green, and blue-green varieties. Seaweeds are some of the most highly nutritious foods found on Earth, providing an extremely concentrated source of minerals and trace elements needed for human health. They are a staple food in coastal regions and Asian diets. High in iodine, iron, calcium, and magnesium, some varieties of seaweeds offer over ten times the minerals of plant-source foods that are grown on land. They are also a good source of protein and several B complex vitamins.

Seaweeds have a cooling thermal nature and offer numerous healing properties. According to TCM flavor classification, their rich and salty flavor helps to enrich both *yin* and blood. With a detoxifying effect on the body, they also help to remove heavy metals, toxins, and radioactive substances from the blood. Seaweeds are beneficial for shrinking tumors, masses, and swellings; they also promote diuresis and reduce edema.[16,17] In addition, they help to regulate thyroid function, counteract inflammation, reduce blood cholesterol, and manage body weight.[17,18] Because seaweeds are cooling and cleansing in nature, they are suitable for the warmer Spring and Summer body types. They should be eaten sparingly by colder body types or those with weak digestion.

Most commercially available seaweeds are known by their Japanese names, due to their widespread production and consumption in Japan. Some seaweeds are sold fresh, while others are dried and may need to be rehydrated before use. Fresh and reconstituted seaweeds are often used in salads or soups. Seaweeds that are processed into dried sheets or flakes can be used for wrapping sushi or sprinkling over food as a topping. Seaweeds can also be simmered with beans to help break down the dietary fibers of the beans and increase their digestibility. When purchasing seaweeds, it is important to consider their source and growing environment. Like other foods, seaweeds grown in polluted environments can absorb contamination from their surroundings; this includes heavy metals like arsenic and lead that may be found in polluted bodies of water.

ARAME

Body type(s): *Spring, Summer*
Thermal nature: *very cooling*

Arame is a type of brown algae with dark, thin, lace-like fronds. Because it has a sweet and mild flavor, arame is more versatile than other seaweeds and can be a good option for those who are introducing seaweeds into their diets. Arame helps to soften masses in the body. Rich in iodine, it also benefits the thyroid. It is also a good source of vitamin A, calcium, and magnesium. Sold in a dried form, arame should be soaked for 5 to 10 minutes in water before using. It can be prepared in a variety of dishes, including whole grains, stir-fries, pastas, salads, soups, and stuffings.

HIJIKI

Body type(s): *Spring, Summer*
Thermal nature: *very cooling*

A variety of brown algae, hijiki is stronger in flavor than arame and has a slightly nutty taste. It grows in long, thin strands and looks like black, wiry pasta noodles when dried. Hijiki has a diuretic and detoxifying effect; it also helps to resolve excess mucus in the body. Compared to other types of seaweeds, hijiki contains very high amounts of calcium and iron. When hijiki is rehydrated from its dried form, it can expand to three times its original volume. It is often used in broths and salads, or sautéed with vegetables.

KOMBU

Body type(s): *Spring, Summer*
Thermal nature: *very cooling*

Kombu is a type of kelp with large leaves that can grow to over twenty feet in length. It is beneficial for nourishing *yin*, promoting diuresis, improving edema and arthritis, and reducing the growth of tumors. Kombu is a good source of iodine, magnesium, and calcium. It also contains glutamic acid, which adds a natural umami flavor. Kombu is often sold dried and cut into strips, to be used in soup stocks and broths.

A small piece can be added to beans or grains during the cooking process, to both increase digestibility and infuse minerals into the dish. It is also available in flake and powder forms, or in tablet form as a dietary supplement.

NORI
Body type(s): *Spring, Summer*
Thermal nature: *very cooling*

Also known as laver in the United Kingdom, nori is a type of red algae. In Japan, it is traditionally used to wrap sushi, and in Wales, it is used in oatmeal cakes. Nori is one of the most easily digested seaweeds. It tonifies *yin* and drains excess fluids. Rich in protein, nori also provides a good source of vitamin A, iron, iodine, and B vitamins. It is mostly available pressed and dried into crisp, paper-like sheets, which can be rolled into sushi or eaten on their own as a snack. Dried nori can also be crumbled over salads, grains, soups, or stir-fries.

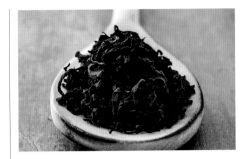

WAKAME
Body type(s): *Spring, Summer*
Thermal nature: *very cooling*

Wakame is a type of brown algae with tender leaves that is commonly available in dried strips or pre-cut pieces. It fortifies both *yin* and blood, and also has a diuretic effect. Additionally, wakame helps to reduce excess phlegm and soften masses. It is high in calcium, magnesium, manganese, and iron, and provides a good source of B vitamins and vitamin E. It is often used in miso soup and salads. Dried wakame should be rinsed and soaked in water for 10 minutes before using.

GENETICALLY MODIFIED FOODS

Genetically modified (GM) or genetically engineered (GE) foods are foods which have been altered through the addition or deletion of genetic material in order to produce a desired trait. These foods fall under the broad category of genetically modified organisms (GMOs). GM foods are engineered for purposes like increasing disease and pest resistance, improving crop yield and growth characteristics, and enhancing nutritional value. However, the safety and long-term health risks associated with consuming GM foods are not yet clear. Some researchers suggest that GM foods may contribute to allergies and toxicity in humans, increased pesticide use on farms, and damage to local eco-systems.[19,20,21] In the United States, the majority of soybean, corn, sugar beet, and cotton crops are genetically modified. The production of GM foods is highly regulated or restricted in most developed countries. To avoid GM foods, buy products that are 100% organic; organic certifications prohibit the use of genetic engineering and genetically engineered ingredients, including their use in animal feed. Food products that are certified by the Non-GMO Project are also free of GMOs. For more information on non-GMO foods, see the resource listings in the Appendix.

MEATS AND SEAFOOD

Foods that are derived from animals tend to be both building and energizing in nature. They offer high levels of protein and can also provide a good source of B vitamins and minerals like zinc, iron, and magnesium. Generally, meats and poultry help to warm the body, supplement *qi*, and nourish *yang*. Useful for strengthening the body and supporting its recovery from physical exertion, meats and poultry tend to be more appropriate for Indian Summer, Fall, and Winter body types. Fish and seafood, on the other hand, tend to be more nourishing toward *yin*; they are generally lower in calories than meats and have higher levels of polyunsaturated fats, including omega-3 fatty acids. Varieties of fish and seafood which are lower in fat and have a cooling thermal nature are more beneficial for the robust Summer body types, who are characterized by excess heat and *yang*. Other varieties which are more oil-rich and warming (e.g. salmon, tuna, anchovies, and mackerel) tend to be more similar to meats, and are more appropriate for boosting the fatigued or colder body types.

Animal-source foods play a very prominent role in many Western diets. Although the energy-boosting characteristics of animal products can be beneficial for some individuals, overconsumption of these foods can have a negative effect on health. Many foods from animal sources are rich in fat. Fatty and heavy foods help to boost energy and warm the body, but they can also congest the system, contributing to excess heat and *yang*, and feelings of stagnancy and heaviness. Consumption of animal products is also associated with an increased risk for heart disease, type 2 diabetes, and some cancers. For most people, a plant-based diet with small amounts of animal-source foods is more appropriate and healthful. Some may even benefit from a vegetarian or vegan diet, depending on their individual health requirements.

Animal-source foods should be eaten in moderation; the recommended serving size for meats and seafood is three to four ounces, which is approximately the same size as a deck of cards. It is also important to select high-quality meats and seafood because of their benefits to both consumer and environmental health. Animals which are raised free-range, without hormones or antibiotics, and with organic feed are higher in quality than conventionally produced meats.[22,23,24,25] Similarly, seafood should be sustainably caught or farmed in waters that have minimal pollution and low levels of toxins and heavy metals.

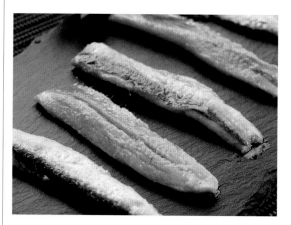

ANCHOVIES

Body type(s): *Indian Summer, Fall, Winter*
Thermal nature: *warming*

Anchovies are small, salt-water fish that are helpful for strengthening *qi* and warming the body. Rich in omega-3 fatty acids, anchovies store oils throughout their tissue and flesh. They provide a good source of protein, niacin, selenium, iron, and calcium. Often preserved in salt and oil, or pickled in vinegar, commercially prepared anchovies can have a strong flavor and are typically used in small quantities. Anchovies and anchovy paste can be used to add flavor to salad dressings, pastas, and meat and fish dishes.

BEEF

Body type(s): *Indian Summer, Winter*
Thermal nature: *warming*

Beef helps to fortify both *qi* and blood in the body. It is also beneficial for building muscle and strengthening tendons and bones. An excellent source of protein, beef also provides several B vitamins, as well as selenium, zinc, phosphorous, and iron. Lean cuts of beef (e.g. round, strip, or flank) have lower levels of saturated fat and total fat than other cuts. Compared with grain-fed beef, grass-fed beef tends to contain less fat and more omega-3 fatty acids, beta-carotene, and vitamin E.[26]

CHICKEN

Body type(s): *Spring, Indian Summer, Fall, Winter*
Thermal nature: *warming*

Chicken is a building food that is especially beneficial for weak, ill, or elderly individuals. It helps to enrich *qi* and blood, increase circulation, and reduce edema. High in niacin, protein, and selenium, chicken also provides a good source of vitamin B6 and phosphorus. For the highest-quality products, choose organically raised chickens that are raised without the use of antibiotics and growth hormones. Their feed does not contain animal by-products or pesticides, and they are allowed access to the outdoors in a pasture setting.

CLAMS

Body type(s): *Summer, Fall*
Thermal nature: *cooling*

Clams are shellfish with a salty flavor and chewy texture. With a cooling thermal nature, they counteract heat and nourish *yin* within the body. They also are beneficial for draining excess fluids and edema. Clams are rich in iron, vitamin B12, and protein, and they also provide a good source of omega-3 fatty acids, zinc, manganese, and selenium. When purchasing live clams, choose ones with tightly closed shells for optimal freshness. For Fall body types, clams should be prepared with warming spices like ginger and garlic to moderate their cooling thermal nature.

CRAB

Body type(s): *Spring, Summer*
Thermal nature: *very cooling*

A member of the crustacean family, crab is beneficial for tonifying *yin*, increasing the circulation of blood, and cooling the body. It is a very good source of lean protein, vitamin B12, selenium, copper, and zinc. Crab also offers a good source of phosphorus, magnesium, vitamin B6, and folate. Common varieties include blue, Dungeness, king, snow, and stone crabs.

EEL

Body type(s): *Spring, Indian Summer*
Thermal nature: *warming*

Eels are found in both fresh and salt water. The freshwater varieties are commonly used in Japanese cuisine and are known as unagi. As a building food, eel helps to strengthen *qi* and enrich the blood. It offers a very good source of vitamins A, D, and B12, and a good source of vitamin E, phosphorus, and omega-3 fatty acids. Eel is often smoked or grilled. Due to the current lack of sustainable farming options, caution is recommended when purchasing and consuming eel.

LAMB

Body type(s): *Indian Summer, Winter*
Thermal nature: *very warming*

One of the most warming animal-source foods, lamb energizes and fortifies both blood and *qi* in the body. It also helps to defend against weakness and excess cold. A good source of protein, selenium, niacin, vitamin B12, zinc, and phosphorus, lamb also contains omega-3 and omega-6 fatty acids. Grass-fed lamb has been shown to contain significantly higher levels of omega-3 fatty acids and a lower ratio of omega-6 to omega-3 fatty acids than conventionally raised lamb.[27] Sheep tend to be raised on grass pasture and given fewer antibiotics than cattle; this makes lamb a good alternative to beef.

MACKEREL

Body type(s): *Indian Summer, Fall*
Thermal nature: *neutral*

Mackerel is a dark, oily fish in the same family as tuna. It nourishes *qi*, drains edema and excess fluids, and benefits rheumatism. It is rich in vitamins B12 and D, niacin, selenium, and protein, and also provides a good source of magnesium, phosphorus, and omega-3 fatty acids. Mackerel can be eaten fresh, but because it tends to spoil quickly, it is often pickled or preserved with salt. It can be smoked, baked, grilled, or fried.

OCTOPUS

Body type(s): *Summer, Indian Summer*
Thermal nature: *cooling*

Belonging to the mollusk family, octopi are relatives of squid. They are beneficial for cooling excess heat and enriching *qi* and blood. Low in saturated fat, octopus provides a good source of vitamin B12, selenium, iron, and protein. Common in Mediterranean and Asian cuisines, octopus is often simmered, grilled, or served in salads. It can become tough and chewy if overcooked.

OYSTERS

Body type(s): *Summer, Indian Summer*
Thermal nature: *neutral*

Oysters are bivalve mollusks with a sweet and briny flavor. They are moistening and help to enrich *yin*, *qi*, and blood. A very good source of vitamin B12, zinc, copper, iron, selenium, and protein, oysters also provide a good source of niacin and phosphorus. Oysters are available year round and can be eaten either raw or cooked.

PORK

Body type(s): *Summer, Indian Summer*
Thermal nature: *neutral to cooling*

Unlike other meats, pork tends to have a neutral to cooling thermal nature. It helps to support *yin* and fortify *qi* and blood. Pork is a good source of protein, selenium, thiamin, niacin, and vitamins B6 and B12. Cuts like tenderloin, center loin, and rib chops tend to be leaner than the shoulder, belly, and leg.

SALMON

Body type(s): *Indian Summer*
Thermal nature: *warming*

Salmon is rich in oils and omega-3 fatty acids, particularly eicosapentaenoic acid (EPA) and docosahexaenoic acid (DHA). It is a building food and is beneficial for fortifying *qi* and blood. Salmon is a very good source of vitamin B12, niacin, and selenium, as well as a good source of protein, vitamin B6, and phosphorous. Compared to farmed salmon, wild-caught Pacific salmon has been found to contain lower levels of environmental contaminants like dioxins and polychlorinated biphenyls (PCBs).[28]

SARDINES

Body type(s): *Spring, Indian Summer*
Thermal nature: *neutral*

Sardines are small, oily fish with soft bones. They help to enrich *qi* and blood in the body. Rich in omega-3 fatty acids, they are also a good source of vitamins B12 and D, niacin, selenium, phosphorous, calcium, and protein. As forage fish that are low on the food chain, sardines tend to contain lower levels of environmental contaminants than larger, predatory fish. Sardines are often preserved and canned in oil or water. They are commonly served in pastas and salads, and can be grilled or broiled.

SHRIMP

Body type(s): *Spring, Indian Summer, Winter*
Thermal nature: *warming*

Members of the crustacean family, shrimp are relatives of crab and lobster. They increase blood circulation, strengthen *qi*, warm the body, and tonify *yang*. Shrimp provide a very good source of selenium, protein, and vitamin B12, and a good source of niacin, phosphorous, copper, iron, and omega-3 fatty acids. They are also a low-calorie food.

TROUT

Body type(s): *Indian Summer, Winter*
Thermal nature: *warming*

Relatives of salmon, trout are oil-rich, freshwater fish. Beneficial for supplementing *qi*, trout also help to defend against cold and nourish *yang*. They are a very good source of protein, vitamin B12, and niacin, and also offer a good source of phosphorous and selenium. Common varieties include rainbow or steelhead trout, which are typically farmed sustainably in the U.S.

TUNA

Body type(s): *Indian Summer*
Thermal nature: *neutral to warming*

Tuna is an oily, saltwater fish which fortifies *qi* and blood. When eaten fresh, it is a good source of omega-3 fatty acids. Tuna is high in selenium, niacin, and vitamins B12 and B6. As a predatory fish that is high on the food chain, tuna can become contaminated with mercury and can pose a health risk to humans, especially children and pregnant women. Due to high demand and overfishing, several species of tuna have become endangered, including populations of bluefin, yellowfin, and albacore.

TURKEY

Body type(s): *Indian Summer, Fall, Winter*
Thermal nature: *warming*

Turkey is a type of poultry that is native to the Americas. It is a building food which helps to nourish and strengthen *qi*. Turkey is a very good source of protein, selenium, and tryptophan, and a good source of niacin, vitamin B6, phosphorous, and zinc. Because pasture-raised turkeys are allowed to forage on a variety of vegetation and nutrients, they tend to contain higher levels of omega-3 fatty acids than conventionally raised turkeys.

ANIMAL-SOURCE FOOD LABELING

The quality of animal-source foods depends on the health, living conditions, and treatment of animals throughout the rearing process. Conventional production methods for animal-source foods may include the use of confinement systems, feedlots, antibiotics, and hormones, as well as feeds that contain ingredients not found in the animal's natural diet. The following describes several production methods and terms that you may see on animal-source food labels. While some of these terms are regulated by the U.S. Department of Agriculture (USDA), others may be used for marketing purposes without enforcement by a regulatory body.

» **Natural (meats, poultry, eggs)** – products which are minimally processed without the use of artificial ingredients, colorings, flavorings, brines, or preservatives. This term only applies to processing after the animal has been slaughtered, not during the raising of the animal.

» **No hormones administered, rBGH-free (cattle, dairy)** – animals that have been raised without the use of hormones. By law, the USDA prohibits the use of hormones in poultry and pork. However, conventionally raised cattle may be given hormones such as recombinant bovine growth hormone (rBGH) to accelerate growth and increase milk production.

» **No antibiotics added (meats, poultry)** – animals that have been raised without the use of antibiotics.

» **Free-range (poultry, eggs)** – products from animals that have been allowed access to the outdoors, without specifications regarding the amount of time outdoors or the size of the outdoor space.

» **Pasture-raised (poultry, eggs)** – products from animals that are raised outdoors and allowed to forage on pasture.

» **Grass-fed (cattle, sheep, bison)** – animals that have continuous access to pasture and have been fed a 100% grass diet (freshly grazed or stored grasses) without grain or grain by-products.

» **USDA organic (meats, poultry, dairy, eggs)** – animals and products from animals that live in conditions accommodating their natural behaviors, have access to pasture, are fed a 100% organic diet free of pesticides, chemicals, or animal by-products, and are raised without the use of antibiotics or growth hormones.

» **Certified humane (meats, poultry, dairy)** – animals that are reared in accordance with voluntary standards for animal welfare that require humane treatment and slaughter, access to the outdoors, and cage-free living; the use of antibiotics and growth hormones is also prohibited.

SUSTAINABLE SEAFOOD

As global demand for fish and seafood has increased, wild fish populations are in decline due to overfishing, unregulated fishing, bycatch issues, and the destruction of natural habitats. Farm-raised seafood (i.e. animals that are commercially raised in tanks or enclosures) alleviates the overfishing of wild seafood (i.e. animals that spend their entire lives in the wild and are caught in the wild). Over half of the seafood sold in the U.S. is now farmed. However, sustainability is an issue for both wild and farm-raised seafood. Environmental contamination from toxic chemicals like mercury, dioxins, dichlorodiphenyltrichloroethane (DDT), and polychlorinated biphenyls (PCBs) is a concern, especially in large, predatory fish that reside at the top of the food chain. Some fish farming and aquaculture practices can also lead to overcrowding, pollution, ecological damage, disease, and a decline in the populations of smaller wild fish that are used as feed. Both the health of seafood populations and the health of the planet's oceans depend upon sustainable fishing practices and management. For more information on sustainable seafood choices, see the resource listings in the Appendix. Look for products certified by the Marine Stewardship Council and reference the Seafood Watch list published by the Monterey Bay Aquarium.

WHITEFISH

Body type(s): *Indian Summer*
Thermal nature: *neutral*

Compared to oily fish, whitefish are low in fat and have a mild flavor. Some examples of whitefish include cod, haddock, pollock, halibut, and sole. Whitefish are beneficial for the digestive system and for harmonizing *qi*. They offer a good source of lean protein, phosphorous, selenium, vitamin D, and several B vitamins, including B6, B12, and niacin.

DAIRY AND EGGS

Animal products like milk, yogurt, butter, cheese, and eggs are energy-boosting foods that help to build *qi* and defend against weakness. According to TCM, they have a sweet flavor and a moistening effect on the body, and they are nourishing toward *yin*. In general, dairy products and eggs have a neutral thermal nature; exceptions include yogurt which tends to be more cooling, and butter which is more warming. Providing a good source of nutrients like vitamin B12, riboflavin, calcium, phosphorous, and protein, these foods can also offer a good source of energy and animal-source nutrition for vegetarians who choose not to consume meat or seafood. Like other animal-source foods, certain products in this food group (e.g. butter, cheese, and eggs) are also rich in saturated fat.

Eggs and dairy products are most appropriate for nourishing Summer body types and strengthening energy-deficient Indian Summer body types, but should be eaten in moderation or avoided by other body types. For individuals who are prone to symptoms like excess phlegm, sinus problems, arthritis, fluid retention, and edema, the moistening and congestive qualities of dairy products can further aggravate these conditions. Many dairy products, particularly cow's milk, are mucus forming and can be difficult to digest. Raw milk, which is unpasteurized and not homogenized, is sometimes better tolerated. When milk is fermented or cultured into products like yogurt, buttermilk, and kefir, it also tends to be more easily digested by the body. Another alternative is goat's milk, which is generally less mucus forming and more digestible than cow's milk. Goat's milk tends to be richer in certain nutrients, since it typically is produced by animals raised entirely on grass pasture and is less processed than cow's milk.

Like other animal-source foods, dairy products and eggs should be eaten in moderation. While these foods may be beneficial for individuals who show signs of weakness, they are often eaten in excessive amounts in the Western diet. When consuming dairy products and eggs, small amounts of high-quality products are recommended. Products which are in their whole form or are minimally processed are preferred; for example, whole milk and full-fat yogurt are preferable over low-fat and skim products. The healthy fats in dairy products can increase satiety, reducing the amount of food that we need to eat in order to feel full. They may also support the absorption and utilization of fat-soluble vitamins. Like other refined foods, reduced-fat dairy products are missing many of the essential fats and nutrients found in their whole and unprocessed forms. Processed dairy products can also contain oxidized cholesterol, a substance which can lead to atherosclerosis.[29,30]

When choosing dairy products and eggs, consider their source. What were the animals fed? Were they allowed access to pasture? Were they treated with hormones or antibiotics? With unpasteurized dairy products like raw milk, it is particularly important to know the supplier and their standards. The lack of pasteurization at high heat can lead to the presence of both beneficial and harmful bacteria alike; consequently, any nutritional advantages should be considered along with concerns for food safety.

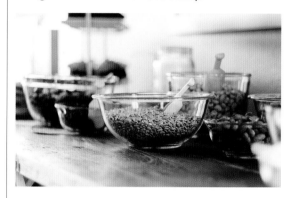

NUTS AND SEEDS

Nuts and seeds are some of the most energy-dense plant-source foods available. With a rich flavor and high levels of fat and protein, they are building and strengthening foods. Most nuts and seeds are neutral to warming in thermal nature and have a sweet flavor as classified by TCM. In general, they enrich both *qi* and blood, and are beneficial for balancing Indian Summer body types. Some of the more warming nuts like chestnuts and walnuts also help to support *yang*, making them ideal for Winter body types. Because they are rich and concentrated foods, nuts and seeds should be eaten in small amounts. Their oily nature can have a congestive effect on the body. While they tend to be beneficial for boosting weak and cold body types, they should be minimized by individuals with signs of excess heat or phlegm.

Rich in antioxidants, fiber, and essential fats, nuts and seeds exhibit protective, immune-enhancing, and anti-inflammatory effects on the body. They are good sources of several vitamins and minerals, including B vitamins, vitamin E, copper, manganese, phosphorus, and magnesium; some varieties also provide good sources of calcium, iron, and zinc. They also contain beneficial fats. Flax seeds, chia seeds, and walnuts are particularly good sources of unsaturated fats and omega-3 fatty acids. Coconuts, brazil nuts, and macadamia nuts are rich in saturated fats compared to other plant-source foods, but their levels are lower than those found in animal-source foods.

The oil-rich nature of nuts and seeds makes them easily susceptible to rancidity and the accumulation of toxins. Rancid products can be even more congestive to the body and difficult to digest. To minimize rancidity and the deterioration of essential nutrients, purchase nuts and seeds that have their protective hulls and shells when possible. Organic products which have not been sprayed with herbicides or pesticides are preferred. Nuts and seeds should also be stored in cool and dark locations, like the refrigerator or freezer, to help preserve their essential nutrients. To increase their digestibility, nuts and seeds may be soaked, sprouted, or roasted before eating. Roasting them also increases their warming effect on the body. To freshly roast nuts and seeds, place them in an oven or on the stovetop over low heat, stirring frequently to prevent them from burning.

HERBS AND SPICES

With their fragrant aromas and strong flavors, herbs and spices are used to preserve foods and enhance their taste. Herbs are derived from the leaves of plants and are used in both their fresh and dried forms. Spices are taken from other parts of the plant, including the roots, bark, seeds, fruit, and berries, and are most often used dried.

Traditionally, herbs and spices have played a role in both culinary and medicinal applications. They are used as natural remedies in herbalism and aromatherapy. Generally, herbs and spices are good sources of phytochemicals and antioxidants, as well as nutrients like vitamin K, manganese, iron, copper, calcium, and dietary fiber. Their high antioxidant levels make them beneficial for boosting immunity. Several herbs and spices also have anti-microbial and anti-inflammatory properties. Some also act as digestive aids, helping to improve the digestibility of foods and soothe the gastrointestinal system.

According to TCM, most herbs and spices have a warming thermal nature and a pungent or bitter flavor. In general, their warming energy is most appropriate for bringing balance to colder Fall and Winter body types. For Fall body types, warming herbs and spices that help to reduce symptoms of congestion and the accumulation of fluids are recommended; these include basil, black pepper, cardamom, cinnamon, cloves, fennel seeds, garlic, ginger, mustard seeds, nutmeg, and thyme. For Winter types, spices that warm and support *yang*, like black pepper, cayenne pepper, chili pepper, cinnamon, cloves, dill seeds, and fennel seeds, are ideal. Some herbs and spices also have the ability to improve the circulation of *qi* and blood within the body, making them beneficial for Spring body types; these foods include caraway seeds, cardamom, cayenne pepper, chili pepper, cinnamon, fennel seeds, garlic, and turmeric. Parsley and thyme fortify *qi* and blood, and are helpful for Indian Summer types; these body types can also reap benefits from caraway seeds, cardamom, chamomile, cumin, fennel seeds, ginger, and peppermint, which are beneficial for digestion. Mint, one of the most cooling herbs, is helpful for soothing the excess heat of Summer body types.

Although herbs and spices can be used in their fresh or dried forms, their properties differ somewhat in each. Fresh herbs tend to taste more delicate and refreshing, while dried herbs are more intense and concentrated in flavor. Dried herbs and spices may lose their potency over time and should be stored in a cool, dark location; they tend to keep longer when they are stored in their whole form, rather than already ground. To grind dried herbs and spices, use a mortar and pestle or an electric coffee grinder. Herbs and spices can also be toasted to release more of their aromatic flavors and essential oils. Herbs can be directly added to foods, used as essential oils or extracts, or made into teas. Some herbal teas are particularly helpful for soothing the digestive system and can be made by steeping the fresh or dried herbs in hot or boiling water.

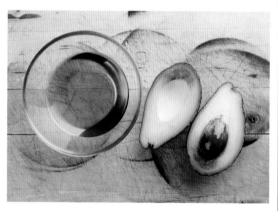

FATS AND OILS

Fats and oils are high in caloric energy and are extracted from foods like nuts, seeds, plants, and animal products. Generally speaking, fats are solid at room temperature, while oils are liquid. Fats are necessary for building cells, tissues, and nerves, insulating the organs, and supporting skin and hair growth. Fats and oils sustain the body with warmth and energy; they are beneficial for boosting internal heat and for strengthening weak and thin individuals. However, because of their heavy, grounding nature, they can also have a congestive quality and should be minimized in those with signs of excess heat, mucus congestion, or fluid retention.

Each dietary fat is comprised of both unsaturated and saturated fats. Both types are necessary for health. Most Western diets tend to include more saturated fats than monounsaturated and polyunsaturated fats. Saturated fats are found in animal products like meats, eggs, cheese, and butter; some plant-source foods like coconut, cottonseed, and palm oils are also concentrated in saturated fats. These fats are more stable at room temperature and less likely to become rancid than unsaturated fats. Research into the health effects of saturated fat consumption is evolving. Saturated fat has previously been associated with an increased risk of cardiovascular disease, but some studies suggest that the ratio of polyunsaturated fats to saturated fats in the diet may be the more important factor.[31,32] Furthermore, recent studies show no association between saturated fat intake and cardiovascular disease and an inverse association with stroke.[33,34] Saturated fats play a beneficial role in the diet, particularly for deficient body types and in unrefined, whole food forms.

Monounsaturated fats are common in the Mediterranean diet and are found in high quantities in foods like nuts, avocados, olive oil, and canola oil. Polyunsaturated fats are found in dark green leafy vegetables, walnuts, seeds (e.g. flax, chia, hemp, and pumpkin), and seafood (e.g. salmon, mackerel, and sardines). Polyunsaturated oils provide two essential fatty acids that the body cannot produce on its own: alpha-linolenic acid (ALA), an omega-3 fatty acid, and linoleic acid, an omega-6 fatty acid. ALA is converted by the body to produce eicosapentaenoic acid (EPA) and docosahexaenoic acid (DHA), two important omega-3 fatty acids which help to regulate cholesterol and fat levels in the blood, aid in brain development, and reduce inflammation.

Due to their chemical structures, unsaturated oils are easily susceptible to oxidation and rancidity. Exposure to light, oxygen, and heat can all lead to the degradation of oil products. Consequently, the ways in which oils are processed, stored, and used in cooking affect their quality and stability. Rancid and poor-quality fats are more congestive to the system and more difficult for the liver to process. Hydrogenated oils and trans fats, products which have been chemically modified to increase shelf stability, are particularly damaging to health. Most common vegetable oils available in grocery stores have been chemically extracted at high heat; these products should be used with caution because they are highly processed and refined, and they have already developed some degree of oxidation or rancidity before they are even opened.[35,36]

For most individuals consuming a Western diet high in animal products and processed foods, an overall reduction of poor-quality fats and oils is recommended. However, moderate quantities of high-quality fats can be beneficial. Saturated fats should be minimized and unsaturated forms should be emphasized, especially polyunsaturated fats high in omega-3 fatty acids. In general, fats and oils that are consumed in whole foods, like nuts, seeds, plants, meats, and seafood, are preferable to oils that have been refined or extracted. If oils are needed for cooking, choose products that have been mechanically extracted at low heat or those that are cold-pressed. Extra-virgin oils are produced from the first pressing and are usually processed at lower temperatures without the use of chemical solvents. Additionally, look for products that are labeled as unrefined and unfiltered, as they tend to retain more of the original food's nutrients, minerals, and flavor than their refined counterparts. For all oils, check for signs of rancidity, such as discoloration, foul odor or taste, or other inconsistencies. To reduce oxidation, oils should be stored in air-tight containers that are opaque or made of dark glass, and placed in a cool and dark location. Fresh, cold-pressed polyunsaturated oils such as flax seed, chia seed, pumpkin seed, and walnut oils can be used as a dietary supplement and a source of omega-3 fatty acids. In order to preserve their nutritional value, these oils should be stored in the refrigerator and should not be heated; they can be used fresh as a dressing for salads or poured directly over foods right before serving.

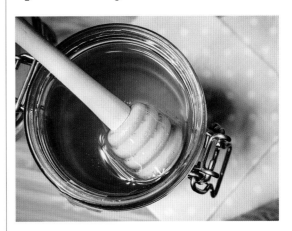

SWEETENERS

Like most fats and oils, sweeteners are found in excess in the standard American diet. The consumption of large amounts of added sugars and sweeteners may have far-reaching implications on health, including an increased risk of obesity, type 2 diabetes, and heart disease.[37,38,39] Refined sugars can have an addictive quality and cause significant fluctuations in blood sugar and insulin levels. When these sweeteners are consumed, they quickly enter the bloodstream, spike blood sugar levels for a short boost of energy, and trigger the secretion of insulin and the uptake of glucose. The resulting drop in blood sugar levels leads to a dip in energy and further, cyclic sugar cravings.

For some body types, especially the weaker and fatigued Indian Summer types, sweet foods can be beneficial and therapeutic. These foods are helpful for building energy and fortifying both *qi* and blood. However, naturally sweet foods are generally sufficient for meeting the body's needs. Eating whole foods is preferable to adding refined sugars, highly concentrated sweeteners, and artificial sugars to the diet. The sugars in whole foods like fruits, carrots, squash, sweet potatoes, and whole grains are naturally balanced with vitamins, minerals, and dietary fiber. Because complex carbohydrates, like those found in whole grains, are absorbed into the bloodstream more slowly than simple sugars, they are less likely to cause rapid fluctuations in blood sugar levels.

When choosing sweeteners or added sugars, look for products that have been minimally processed, are as close to their whole food form as possible, and still retain some of their original nutrients and flavors. While all sweeteners are refined or processed to some extent, some products can be appropriate in small quantities. Molasses, sucanat, and brown sugar are preferred over white granulated sugar, as they tend to have a richer flavor and more trace minerals from the original sugar cane. Although raw, unpasteurized honey is refined and concentrated by bees, it

contains several vitamins, minerals, and beneficial enzymes; it also has antibacterial and antifungal properties, as well as a therapeutic effect on coughs and lung conditions. Compared to the 99% sucrose content found in white sugar, maple syrup contains just 65%; it is made from the sap of maple trees and contains minerals like manganese and zinc. Agave nectar is a natural sweetener derived from a type of cactus plant; it has a mild flavor and a lower glycemic index (GI) than other sweeteners. As a measure of a food's effect on blood sugar level, the glycemic index ranks carbohydrate-containing foods based on how much of the food is converted to glucose by the body. Foods with a high GI are digested quickly and can cause significant spikes in blood sugar levels, while foods with a low GI are digested more slowly and cause a less significant rise in blood sugar. Some sweeteners are made from the complex carbohydrates and whole grains of rice and barley; these malted grain syrups tend to be less processed than white sugar and more slowly absorbed by the body. Another option is the leaves of the stevia plant, which are almost thirty times sweeter than cane sugar; they are low in calories, inhibit oral bacteria and tooth decay, and may be beneficial for regulating blood sugar levels. When using stevia, choose green powders or whole leaf products which retain the natural phytonutrients of the whole plant, rather than white powders or extracts.

Authors' Notes on the Recipes and Ingredients

In the following chapters, we present recipes that incorporate our seasonal approach to health along with dietary principles from Traditional Chinese Medicine (TCM). For each season's recipes, we emphasize foods that are especially beneficial for that seasonal body type, as well as ingredients that are available within that growing season. Readers who identify with the characteristics of a specific seasonal body type should prepare and eat from the recipes for that season; Spring body types should eat from the Spring recipes, Summer body types from the Summer recipes, etc. Once your body is in balance, is more thermally neutral, and does not exhibit the chronic symptoms and characteristics of one seasonal body type, you should eat along with the seasons and align with nature's offerings throughout the year; prepare the Spring recipes and foods in the spring season, then move on to the other foods and recipes as the seasons progress.

The cooking methods that we recommend reflect the spirit of the season and are appropriate for addressing the body's needs at different times of the year. Dishes that are raw, steamed, or lightly cooked tend to be more cooling and are generally recommended for the warmer Spring and Summer body types and seasons. Dishes which involve longer cooking times like stews and braises, or use high-heat methods like roasting and grilling, tend to have a more warming effect on the body and are more appropriate for the cooler seasonal body types and latter seasons of the year.

Generally, we recommend the use of whole foods whenever possible; this means consuming whole grains that are minimally processed, fruits and vegetables with their skins and peels intact, full-fat dairy products, etc. Our intention is to retain as many of the original nutrients, minerals, dietary fiber, and flavors which are present in a food's natural state but often stripped away during processing. When the recipes do call for processed foods such as flours, noodles, sweeteners, or condiments, we recommend using products that are minimally refined. For example, several recipes include the use of white whole-wheat flour, which is a whole-grain product that is milled from a softer variety of wheat and has a lighter, less bitter taste than traditional whole-wheat flours. When a recipe calls for the use of liquid sweeteners, we generally choose honey for its beneficial energetic properties or agave nectar for its clean, neutral flavor profile. We also prefer molasses and brown sugar over white sugar, because they tend to retain more of the trace minerals and depth of flavor from the original sugar cane.

Our dietary approach focuses on incorporating more plant-based foods like whole grains, vegetables, legumes, and nuts. In an effort to offer balance to the standard American diet which commonly includes a high proportion of meats and animal products, we have included several vegetarian and vegan recipes, even for the cooler seasons and body types. In addition to legumes and tofu, seafood provides a lighter alternative to meat and can be substituted into many of the recipes. Vegetable broth can also be substituted for chicken broth throughout. For dairy product alternatives, consider using rice or nut milks instead of cow's milk.

Our recipes were developed to minimize the consumption of poor-quality fats and added oils. When cooking oil is used, we prefer unrefined, cold-pressed extra-virgin olive oil for most applications, especially in dishes that are minimally cooked or served raw, like salads. For high-heat cooking methods like grilling, we typically use vegetable oil because it has a higher smoke point than olive oil and is less prone to burning. We also suggest the use of cooking sprays for recipes where only small amounts of oil are required to prevent the food from sticking. As a good source of unsaturated fatty acids, olive oil can also be used as a substitute for butter in baked goods.

In terms of seasonings, we generally prefer kosher salt, because its coarser grain is easy to handle and its taste tends to be milder and less metallic than table salt. High-quality sea salt is ideal when the flavor of the salt is more prominent, e.g. for the finishing of dishes or for simple recipes with very few ingredients. Generally, sea salts that are harvested by hand and produced using traditional methods, like Maldon sea salt from England and *fleur de sel*, tend to be higher in quality than those produced by industrial methods. Also look for high-quality sea salts that may be produced in your local region. For spices like black pepper, we prefer freshly ground versions as they tend to be more flavorful and aromatic than pre-ground alternatives. For recipes that call for the use of curry powder, the product you choose can have a significant influence on the overall flavor of the dish. We generally use S&B Oriental curry powder in our cooking; it is a Japanese product with a well-rounded balance of spices suitable for a wide variety of recipes. For soy sauce, we recommend using products made from organic, non-GMO soybeans when available. Tamari is a good alternative for individuals looking to minimize gluten in their diet; it is a type of soy sauce that is produced with little or no wheat.

In each of the following chapters, the recipes progress from soups, salads, and appetizers to main dishes and entrées, and finally, to desserts. The recipes are intended to offer general guidelines based on our seasonal approach to health and our professional experience. They are recommendations, rather than requirements. Experiment and adjust the recipes while taking into consideration convenience, cost, your style of cooking, your individual needs and preferences, and the ingredients that are available in your area. Most importantly, be flexible; use nature's seasons as your guide, follow your intuition, and enjoy the process of creating healthful and nourishing meals for yourself and your family.

GUIDE TO THE RECIPE FORMAT

You may find the recipe layout to be a bit different than what you are accustomed to. The table format was designed to make the recipes clearer and easier to follow. Instead of listing the ingredients above the cooking steps, the ingredients are listed alongside their corresponding steps. Before making each recipe, fully read through both the ingredients and steps, in order to familiarize yourself with the general procedure and techniques that will be used. If extra time is needed to prepare any of the ingredients beforehand, it is noted at the beginning of the recipe.

Ingredients are grouped together and listed on the left

2 teaspoons extra-virgin olive oil

2 cups chopped leeks, white parts, rinsed thoroughly (about 4 medium leeks)

2 cups chopped fennel bulb

2 cloves garlic, minced

In a medium pot, heat oil over medium heat. Sauté leeks and fennel for 7 to 10 minutes, or until leeks are translucent and fennel is slightly caramelized. Add garlic and cook for 1 minute.

Corresponding steps for each group of ingredients are listed on the right

4 medium potatoes, peeled and cut into chunks (about 2 pounds)

¾ cup low-sodium vegetable broth

1¼ cups water

1½ teaspoons kosher salt

⅛ teaspoon freshly ground black pepper

Add potatoes, broth, water, salt, and black pepper, and bring to a boil over high heat. Reduce heat to low and simmer for 30 minutes, or until potatoes are tender.

Remove pot from heat and purée the soup. If using an immersion blender, the soup can be directly blended in the cooking pot. If using a countertop blender, purée the soup in small batches and combine before serving.

As you work through the steps on the right, reference the quantities for each ingredient on the left

KEY TO RECIPE SYMBOLS

Look for the following symbols at the top of each recipe to indicate if the dish is prepared without meats, animal-source products, dairy, or gluten:

(V)   Vegetarian

(V+)   Vegan

(DF)   Dairy-free

(GF)   Gluten-free*

* The recipes that include oats and buckwheat are designated as gluten-free (GF). Note that although these grains are naturally free of gluten, they often become cross-contaminated with wheat gluten during processing. The recipes that include soy sauce are not designated as GF. For a gluten-free preparation of those recipes, use a gluten-free soy sauce or tamari product.

Spring is when life's alive
in everything.
– Christina Rossetti

Chapter 11
Spring Recipes: moving and cleansing

The spring themes of birth and renewal are reflected throughout the season, from the sprouting of vibrant greens to the initiation of activities like cleaning house, playing outdoors, and planting a garden. As the weather begins to thaw after a cold winter, the body also begins its own reawakening. Consuming pungent and warming foods will encourage this process, while also balancing the mild external climate.

Nutrient-rich, leafy greens are the highlight of spring, promoting movement and light cleansing within the digestive system. With their spicy and peppery flavors, watercress and mustard greens are particularly helpful for stimulating the circulation of *qi* within the body. For an invigorating effect, consume pungent aromatics like garlic, ginger, and members of the onion family, as well as sour flavors like vinegar and lemon. Herbs also play an important role in the spring recipes by keeping the dishes fresh and flavorful.

Requiring minimal preparation, these recipes are ideal for quick, weeknight meals. Light and simple, they embody the refreshing approach of the season. As the start of the seasonal cycle, spring represents an opportunity to let go of the old and usher in the new; its lively attitude encourages us to look forward and welcome the year that lies ahead.

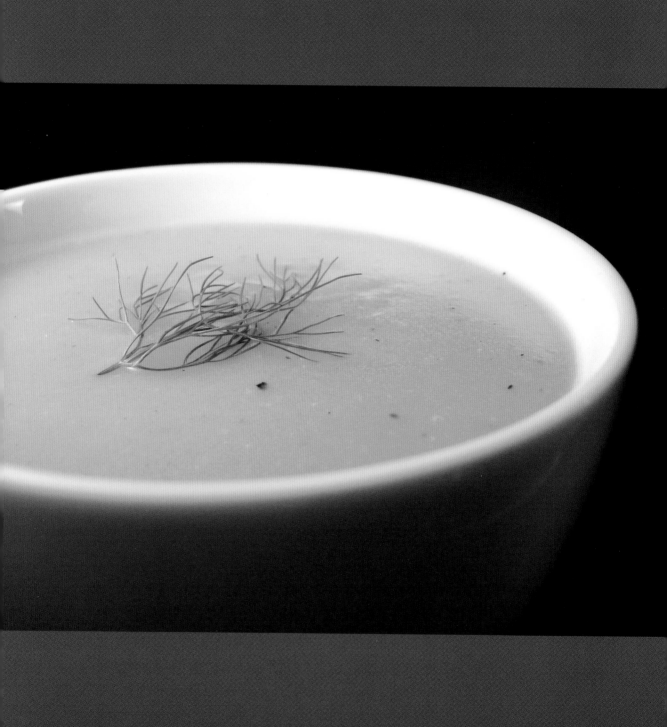

POTATO, LEEK, AND FENNEL SOUP

SERVES 4

Caramelized fennel and delicate leeks combine with potatoes to create a light, yet flavorful soup. Blend the ingredients together to achieve a creamy texture in this vegan, dairy-free recipe.

2 teaspoons extra-virgin olive oil

2 cups chopped leeks, white parts, rinsed thoroughly (about 4 medium leeks)

2 cups chopped fennel bulb

2 cloves garlic, minced

In a medium pot, heat oil over medium heat. Sauté leeks and fennel for 7 to 10 minutes, or until leeks are translucent and fennel is slightly caramelized. Add garlic and cook for 1 minute.

4 medium potatoes, peeled and cut into chunks (about 2 pounds)

¾ cup low-sodium vegetable broth

1¼ cups water

1½ teaspoons kosher salt

⅛ teaspoon freshly ground black pepper

Add potatoes, broth, water, salt, and black pepper, and bring to a boil over high heat. Reduce heat to low and simmer for 30 minutes, or until potatoes are tender.

Remove pot from heat and purée the soup. If using an immersion blender, the soup can be directly blended in the cooking pot. If using a countertop blender, purée the soup in small batches and combine before serving.

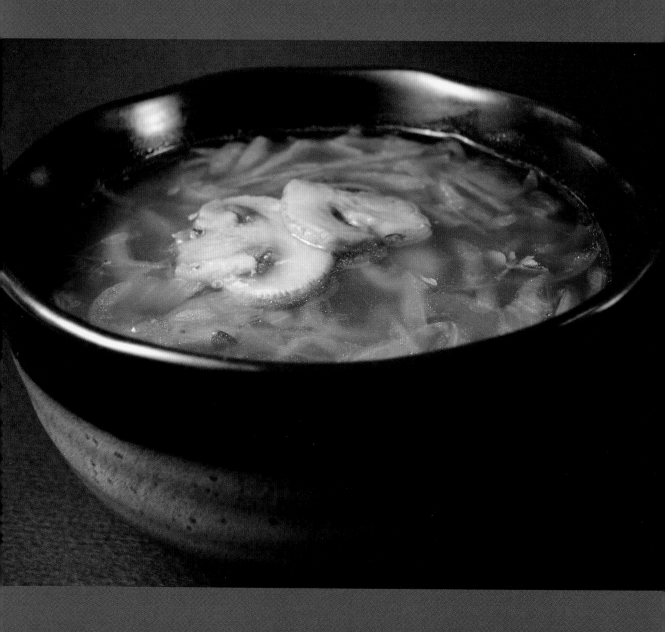

THREE ONION SOUP

SERVES 3 TO 4

Use a broth made from fresh and dried mushrooms for this vegetarian version of French onion soup. Slowly cooking the onions over low heat results in a deep, caramel flavor. With a warming thermal nature, onions are beneficial for increasing the circulation of *qi* within the body.

1 tablespoon extra-virgin olive oil

1 cup sliced yellow onions (about 1 small onion)

1 cup sliced white onions (about 1 small onion)

1 cup sliced red onions (about 1 small onion)

1 teaspoon kosher salt

1 clove garlic, minced

In a medium pot, heat oil over low heat. Add yellow onions, white onions, red onions, and salt to the pot. Caramelize onions for 45 to 50 minutes, stirring often. Add garlic and cook for 1 minute.

4 cups water

½ ounce dried mushrooms (such as porcini or shiitake)

½ cup sliced button mushrooms

While the onions are caramelizing, bring water to a boil in a separate pot over high heat. Add dried and button mushrooms, reduce heat to medium-low, cover, and simmer for 5 minutes. Strain mushrooms and reserve the mushrooms and cooking liquid.

Deglaze the pot of onions by adding the reserved mushroom liquid and scraping the caramelized bits from the bottom of the pot with a wooden spoon until dissolved.

1 cup water

2 teaspoons soy sauce

1 dried bay leaf

2 sprigs fresh thyme

1 teaspoon kosher salt

⅛ teaspoon freshly ground black pepper

Add water, soy sauce, bay leaf, thyme, salt, and black pepper, and simmer for 15 to 30 minutes.

Add reserved mushrooms. Remove bay leaf and thyme sprigs before serving.

CARROT GINGER SOUP

SERVES 6

This light and simple recipe is an ideal start to any spring menu. Freshly grated ginger adds a spicy kick that balances the natural sweetness of the carrots.

¼ teaspoon extra-virgin olive oil

½ cup diced white or yellow onions (about ½ of a small onion)

In a medium pot, heat oil over medium-low heat. Add onions and cook for 3 minutes, stirring occasionally.

8 medium carrots, cut into chunks (about 1½ pounds)

2½ cups water

2 cups low-sodium vegetable broth

1¾ teaspoons kosher salt

1 pinch freshly ground black pepper

Add carrots, water, vegetable broth, salt, and black pepper, and bring to a boil over high heat. Reduce heat to medium-low, cover, and simmer for 30 to 45 minutes, or until the carrots are tender.

2 teaspoons finely minced or grated ginger

Add ginger and cook for 5 minutes.

Remove pot from heat and purée the soup. If using an immersion blender, the soup can be directly blended in the cooking pot. If using a countertop blender, purée the soup in small batches and combine before serving.

If a thinner consistency is desired, strain and push the soup through a sieve, or add a little more vegetable broth.

1 tablespoon chopped fresh chives (optional)

Garnish with chives before serving, if desired.

SAUTÉED GREENS WITH WHITE BEANS AND GARLIC

SERVES 4

Mustard greens have a pungent flavor and are especially beneficial for the season, but they can be substituted with other leafy greens like kale or chard.

1 teaspoon extra-virgin olive oil

¾ cup sliced white or yellow onions (about ½ of a medium onion)

¼ teaspoon dried oregano

¼ teaspoon crushed red pepper flakes

2 cloves garlic, sliced

In a large skillet, heat oil over medium heat. Sauté onions for 1 minute. Add oregano, red pepper flakes, and garlic, and cook for 1 minute.

2 bunches mustard greens, chopped

1 cup (or about ½ of a 15-ounce can) cooked cannellini beans, drained

¼ cup low-sodium vegetable broth

1 teaspoon kosher salt

⅛ teaspoon freshly ground black pepper

Add mustard greens, cannellini beans, vegetable broth, salt, and black pepper, and cook over low heat for 2 to 4 minutes, or until greens are tender.

SCALLION PANCAKES

MAKES 4 PANCAKES

Special equipment (optional): stand mixer with dough hook

1 cup white whole-wheat flour

1 cup all-purpose flour

½ teaspoon kosher salt

⅔ cup boiling water

½ teaspoon sesame oil

½ teaspoon extra-virgin olive oil

1 cup chopped fresh green onions

4 tablespoons chopped fresh cilantro

1 teaspoon kosher salt

⅛ teaspoon freshly ground black pepper

With a crisp crust and chewy interior, these savory Chinese pancakes make for a great appetizer or snack. A hint of sesame oil complements the flavors of fresh cilantro and scallions (also known as green onions).

If making the dough with an electric stand mixer, combine the white whole-wheat flour, all-purpose flour, and salt in the bowl of the mixer. With a dough hook attached and the mixer on low speed, gradually add the water to the flour mixture. Mix the dough for about 5 to 6 minutes, or until the dough is smooth and elastic.

If making the dough by hand, combine the white whole-wheat flour, all-purpose flour, and salt in a medium bowl. Gradually stir in the water until the mixture is cohesive. Remove the dough from the bowl and knead on a floured surface for about 12 to 15 minutes, or until the dough is smooth and elastic.

Cover the dough with plastic wrap and allow it to rest for 30 minutes.

Prepare the filling by mixing together sesame oil, olive oil, green onions, cilantro, salt, and black pepper.

Divide the dough equally into four balls. With a rolling pin, roll out one ball into a 9-inch circle. Spread one-quarter of the filling mixture over the surface of the dough. Roll the dough up tightly into a thin log, starting with the edge closest to you and working your way up. Curl the tube of dough around itself into a snail-like shape. Gently flatten the dough with the palm of your hand until the pancake is about 6 inches in diameter and ⅛ inch thick.

Repeat with the remaining three balls of dough.

2 teaspoons extra-virgin olive oil, divided

In a medium nonstick skillet over medium heat, pan-fry the pancakes one at a time. Heat about ½ teaspoon of oil and add one pancake to the pan. Using a spatula, flatten the pancake as it begins to cook. Pan-fry the pancake for 3 to 4 minutes on each side, or until the surface is golden brown and crispy and the dough is cooked through.

Repeat with the remaining oil and pancakes. Cut each pancake into 4 to 6 wedges before serving.

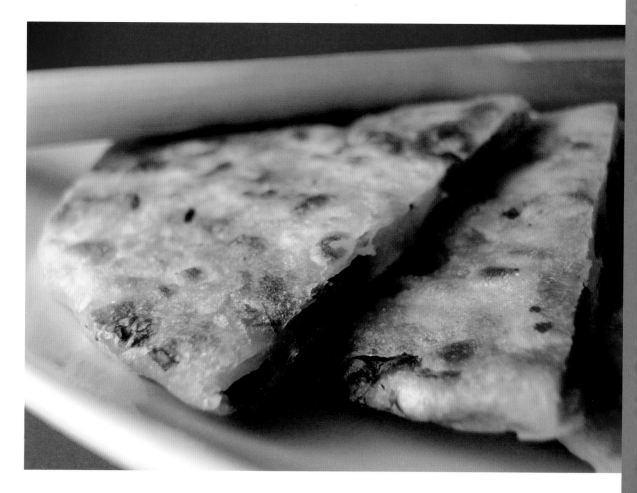

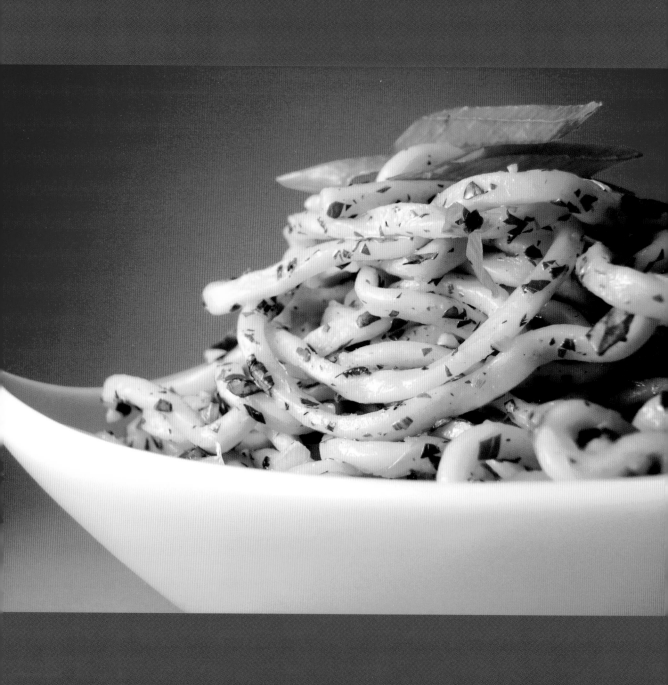

GARLICKY HERB NOODLES

SERVES 4 TO 6

Vietnamese crab noodles serve as the inspiration for this garlicky dish. The combination of herbs, onions, and garlic livens up the flavor of the chewy noodles and helps to circulate *qi* within the body.

1 pound fresh egg noodles

Cook noodles according to package directions and drain.

4 tablespoons extra-virgin olive oil

2 cloves garlic, sliced

3 cloves garlic, minced

In a large skillet, heat oil over low heat. Add sliced garlic and cook for 2 minutes, being careful not to burn the garlic. Add minced garlic and remove the skillet from the heat; allow the oil to infuse with the garlic for 5 minutes.

¼ cup chopped leeks, white parts, rinsed thoroughly (about 1 small leek)

Place the skillet over medium heat, add leeks, and cook for 1 to 2 minutes.

½ cup chopped fresh green onions

2 teaspoons dried minced onions

½ teaspoon garlic salt

¼ cup packed chopped fresh cilantro

¼ cup packed chopped fresh Italian parsley

¼ teaspoon crushed red pepper flakes

½ teaspoon kosher salt

¼ teaspoon freshly ground black pepper

Add cooked noodles, green onions, dried onions, garlic salt, cilantro, parsley, red pepper flakes, salt, and black pepper. Toss until well incorporated and cook for 1 minute.

OAT-CRUSTED CHICKEN

SERVES 3 TO 4

This recipe is a healthy, yet equally delicious alternative to deep-fried chicken tenders. Coating the chicken with whole-grain oats gives this dish a satisfying crunch.

¼ cup rolled oats

1½ tablespoons packed fresh Italian parsley

¾ teaspoon fresh thyme leaves

½ teaspoon kosher salt

⅛ teaspoon freshly ground black pepper

Pulse rolled oats, parsley, thyme, salt, and black pepper in a food processor (preferable) or blender until fine.

2 tablespoons rolled oats

In a small bowl, mix together ground oat mixture with additional rolled oats.

8 chicken tenders (or 2 boneless, skinless chicken breasts, cut into 8 strips)

½ teaspoon kosher salt

⅛ teaspoon freshly ground black pepper

Season chicken pieces with salt and black pepper. Roll the chicken in the oat mixture to coat.

2 teaspoons extra-virgin olive oil

In a medium skillet, heat oil over medium-high heat. Lightly pan-fry the chicken for 1 to 2 minutes on each side, or until crust is golden brown and chicken is cooked through.

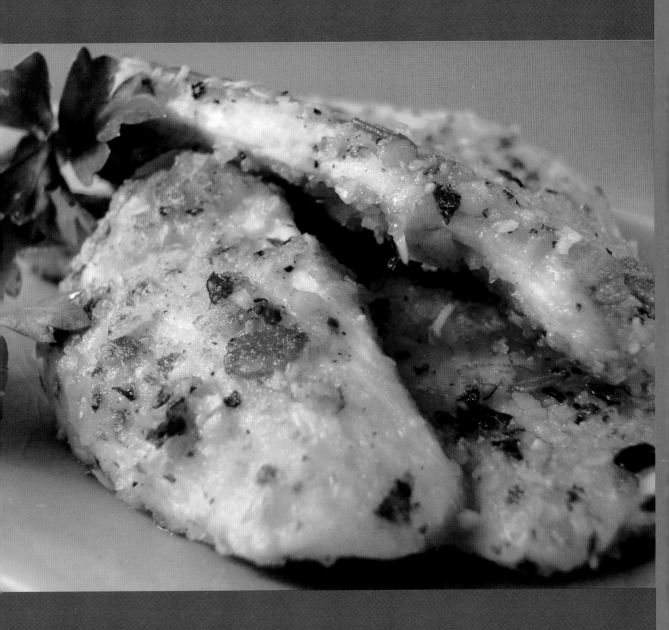

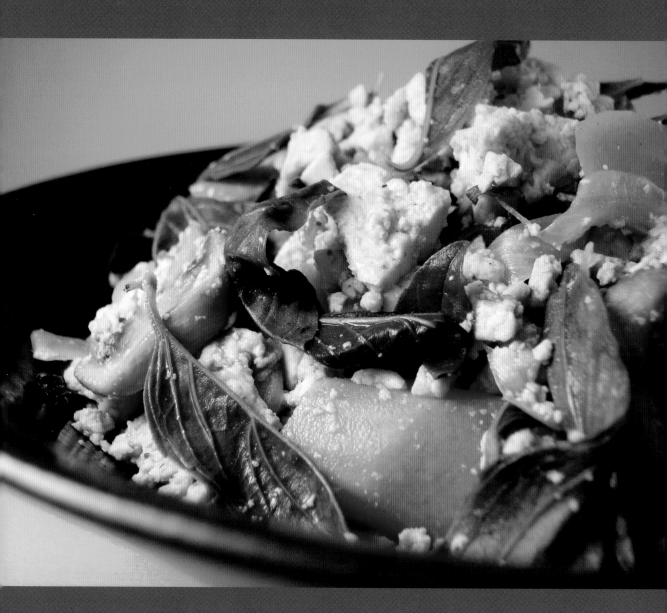

THAI BASIL TOFU

SERVES 4

Sweet Thai basil (*bai horapa*) and seasonal vegetables are the highlights of this stir-fry. Traditionally, this dish is made with ground beef, chicken, or pork, but this recipe uses tofu for a low-fat, vegan version.

2 teaspoons extra-virgin olive oil

¾ cup sliced yellow onions (about ½ of a medium onion)

3 cups sliced button mushrooms

In a wok or large skillet, heat oil over medium-high heat. Add onions and cook for 1 minute, then add mushrooms and cook for 1 minute.

2 cloves garlic, minced

1 teaspoon minced ginger

16 ounces extra-firm tofu

Add garlic and ginger and cook for 1 minute.

Using a fork, gently mash the extra-firm tofu. Add mashed tofu to the wok and cook for 1 minute.

½ cup water

4 teaspoons soy sauce

3 tablespoons hoisin sauce

In a small bowl, mix together water, soy sauce, and hoisin sauce, and pour mixture into the wok.

1 medium carrot, sliced

½ teaspoon chopped fresh jalapeño pepper, seeds and membranes removed

¼ teaspoon crushed red pepper flakes

1 teaspoon kosher salt

⅛ teaspoon freshly ground black pepper

Add carrots, jalapeño peppers, red pepper flakes, salt, and black pepper, and cook for 1 to 2 minutes.

1 cup fresh Thai basil leaves

Remove from heat and stir in the basil leaves.

INDIAN CHICKEN KEBABS

SERVES 3 TO 4

(DF) (GF)

Special equipment: eight wooden or metal skewers

¾ cup chopped white or yellow onions (about ½ of a medium onion)

½ cup packed fresh mint leaves

½ cup packed fresh cilantro

½ cup packed fresh Italian parsley

¼ teaspoon chopped fresh jalapeño pepper, seeds and membranes removed

1 clove garlic

1 teaspoon extra-virgin olive oil

1 teaspoon lemon juice

2 teaspoons kosher salt

¼ teaspoon ground cumin

⅛ teaspoon ground coriander

⅛ teaspoon ground turmeric

8 chicken tenders (or 2 boneless, skinless chicken breasts, cut into 8 strips)

Cooking spray or vegetable oil

Fresh green herbs like mint, parsley, and cilantro play off of traditional Indian spices in this recipe. The kebabs can be served as an appetizer or a main course.

Blend together onions, mint, cilantro, parsley, jalapeño peppers, garlic, oil, lemon juice, salt, cumin, coriander, and turmeric in a food processor (preferable) or blender.

Coat chicken with marinade, place in a covered container, and marinate in the refrigerator for at least 1 hour.

If using wooden skewers, soak them in enough water to cover for 10 minutes to prevent them from burning on the grill. Remove chicken from refrigerator. Thread chicken onto the skewers.

Spray outdoor grill or indoor grill pan with cooking spray, or wipe with oil. Grill skewers over medium heat for about 2 minutes on each side, or until chicken is cooked through.

FILIPINO ADOBO

SERVES 4 TO 6

This simple recipe is often considered the national dish of the Philippines. The chicken is braised in soy sauce, vinegar, and spices until it falls off the bone. The sour flavor of the vinegar is ideal for this season because of its cleansing effect and its ability to circulate *qi*.

6 chicken leg pieces (drumsticks and/or thighs), bone-in, skin removed and trimmed

1¾ cups water

¾ cup white vinegar

½ cup soy sauce

2 dried bay leaves

2 cloves garlic, sliced

⅛ teaspoon freshly ground black pepper

¼ teaspoon whole black peppercorns

In a medium pot, bring chicken, water, vinegar, soy sauce, bay leaves, garlic, ground black pepper, and whole peppercorns to a boil over medium-high heat. Reduce heat to low, cover, and simmer for 1 hour.

½ cup sliced yellow onions (about ½ of a small onion)

Add onions and simmer for 30 minutes.

1 tablespoon chopped fresh green onions or Italian parsley (optional)

Remove bay leaves before serving. If desired, serve chicken over rice with a small amount of the cooking liquid and garnish with green onions or parsley.

CHINESE-STYLE STEAMED FISH

SERVES 2

Traditionally, celebratory meals in Chinese culture include a whole steamed fish for good luck. This simple recipe uses individual fish fillets prepared in the same manner to yield a moist, tender, and aromatic meal.

Special equipment: steamer

---

2 fish fillets (such as mahi-mahi, red snapper, halibut, or sea bass, about 4 to 6 ounces each)

⅛ teaspoon kosher salt

1 pinch freshly ground black pepper

Prepare the steamer by placing a bamboo or metal steamer basket over the top of a pot, or place a metal cake rack inside a deep skillet. Add about 1 inch of water to the pot or skillet, making sure the water level is below the bottom of the steamer basket or cake rack.

Season both sides of the fish fillets with salt and black pepper. Place the fish in a single layer on a heatproof dish that will fit inside the steamer basket or skillet.

¼ cup julienned carrots (about ½ of a medium carrot)

1 cup sliced fresh shiitake mushroom caps (about 2 large mushrooms)

¼ inch ginger, peeled and julienned

½ stalk green onion, thinly sliced on the diagonal (about ¼ cup)

6 sprigs fresh cilantro

Layer the carrots, mushrooms, ginger, green onions, and cilantro over top of the fish.

---

2 teaspoons soy sauce

1 teaspoon extra-virgin olive oil

½ teaspoon rice vinegar

⅛ teaspoon sesame oil

In a small bowl, stir together soy sauce, olive oil, rice vinegar, and sesame oil. Drizzle sauce over top of the fish and vegetables. Marinate for 10 minutes.

While the fish is marinating, bring the water in the pot or skillet to a boil over medium heat.

Carefully place the dish into the steamer. Reduce heat to medium-low, cover, and steam over simmering water for 8 to 10 minutes, or until fish is just cooked through and flakes apart with a fork.

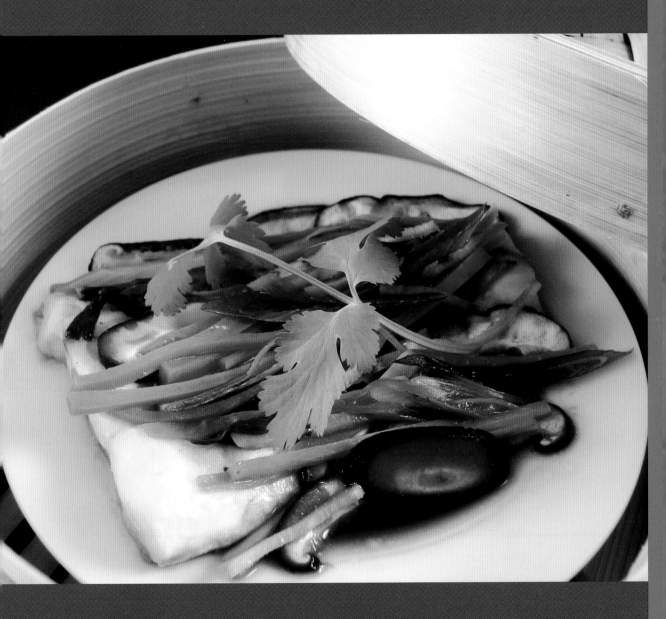

ASIAN CHICKEN AND WATERCRESS SALAD

SERVES 2 TO 4

Ginger-marinated chicken and fresh watercress combine with a sweet and tangy dressing for a light spring meal. Watercress's pungent and peppery flavor makes it beneficial for regulating and circulating *qi* within the body.

1 clove garlic, minced

¼ teaspoon minced ginger

2 tablespoons soy sauce

1 teaspoon honey

1 tablespoon chopped fresh green onions

8 ounces boneless, skinless chicken breasts

PREPARE THE CHICKEN:
In a shallow bowl, make the marinade by combining garlic, ginger, soy sauce, honey, and green onions.

Add the chicken and marinate covered in the refrigerator for at least 1 hour.

Cooking spray or vegetable oil

Spray outdoor grill or indoor grill pan with cooking spray, or wipe with oil. Grill chicken over medium heat for about 3 minutes on each side or until cooked through. When chicken is cooked through, remove it from the grill and allow it to rest on a plate. Collect 1 teaspoon of juice from the plate and reserve.

1 tablespoon lemon juice

1 tablespoon honey

¼ teaspoon soy sauce

1½ tablespoons minced shallots

½ teaspoon finely minced or grated ginger

1½ teaspoons kosher salt

⅛ teaspoon freshly ground black pepper

3 tablespoons extra-virgin olive oil

MAKE THE DRESSING:
In a small bowl, whisk together reserved juice from the cooked chicken, lemon juice, honey, soy sauce, shallots, ginger, salt, and black pepper. Add the oil in a steady stream, whisking until emulsified.

2 cups packed watercress, stems trimmed (about 2 bunches)

1 cup mung bean sprouts

¼ cup sliced fresh green onions

½ cup sliced water chestnuts

ASSEMBLE THE SALAD:

Slice chicken into ¼-inch strips. In a medium bowl, combine the watercress, bean sprouts, green onions, and water chestnuts with the chicken, and toss with enough dressing to coat lightly.

Extra dressing can be served on the side.

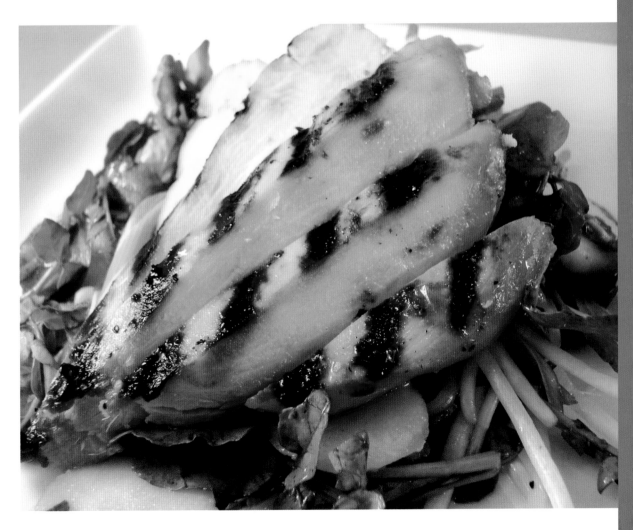

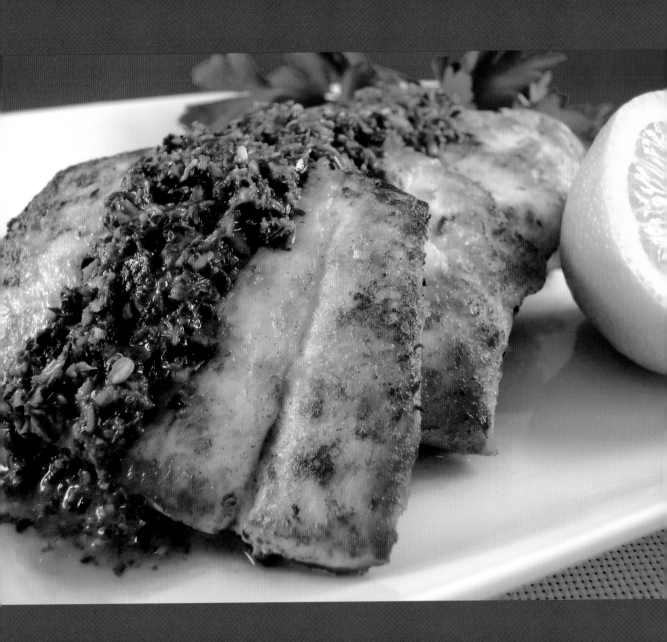

FISH WITH ARGENTINEAN CHIMICHURRI SAUCE

SERVES 4

This fresh herb sauce is traditionally served with grilled steak, but is equally delicious over fish.

2 cups packed fresh Italian parsley (about 1 bunch)

4 cloves garlic

1 tablespoon chopped shallots

1 teaspoon dried oregano

½ teaspoon grated lemon zest

1 tablespoon lemon juice

1 tablespoon red wine vinegar

½ teaspoon crushed red pepper flakes

1 teaspoon kosher salt

⅛ teaspoon freshly ground black pepper

3 tablespoons extra-virgin olive oil

2 tablespoons water

MAKE THE CHIMICHURRI SAUCE:

In a food processor (preferable) or blender, blend together parsley, garlic, shallots, oregano, lemon zest, lemon juice, red wine vinegar, red pepper flakes, salt, black pepper, oil, and water, until mixture reaches a sauce-like consistency.

4 fish fillets (such as mahi-mahi, red snapper, halibut, or sea bass, about 4 to 6 ounces each)

¼ teaspoon kosher salt

⅛ teaspoon freshly ground black pepper

PREPARE THE FISH:

Reserve ¼ cup of chimichurri sauce for topping.

Put fish and the remaining chimichurri sauce in a bowl and marinate for 15 to 20 minutes.

Remove fish from the marinade and season with salt and black pepper.

2 teaspoons extra-virgin olive oil

Heat oil in a nonstick skillet over medium heat. Pan-fry the fish for 3 to 4 minutes on each side, or until cooked through. (Generally, the cooking time for fish is 8 to 10 minutes per inch of thickness.)

Top the fish with reserved chimichurri sauce.

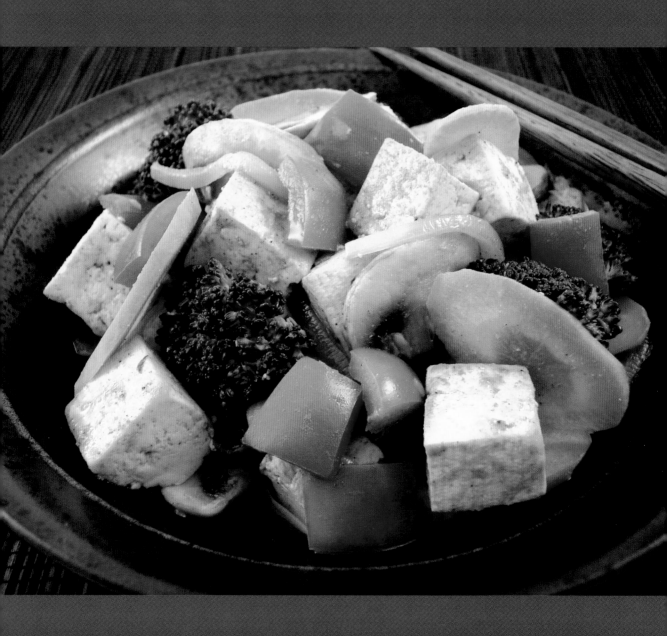

CURRY IN A HURRY

SERVES 3 TO 4

A touch of curry transforms this simple spring medley of vegetables into a tasty and satisfying meal.

1 tablespoon extra-virgin olive oil

¾ cup sliced yellow onions (about ½ of a medium onion)

1 clove garlic, minced

1 teaspoon minced ginger

1 tablespoon curry powder

In a wok or large skillet, heat oil over medium heat. Add onions and sauté for 1 minute. Add garlic and ginger and cook for 1 minute. Add curry powder and toast for 30 seconds, stirring continuously to prevent the spices from burning.

14 ounces regular or firm tofu, cubed

2 cups sliced button mushrooms

½ cup low-sodium vegetable broth

2 teaspoons soy sauce

Increase heat to medium-high; add tofu, mushrooms, vegetable broth, and soy sauce, and cook for 2 minutes.

½ cup sliced carrots

2 cups broccoli florets

½ cup chopped red bell pepper

½ cup chopped green bell pepper

1 teaspoon kosher salt

⅛ teaspoon freshly ground black pepper

Add carrots, broccoli, red and green bell peppers, salt, and black pepper, and cook for 1 to 2 minutes, or until vegetables are cooked through but still crunchy.

CANDIED KUMQUAT AND TANGERINE CRÊPES

SERVES 2 TO 3

Kumquats are small, oval-shaped citrus fruit with sweet rinds and tart centers. The complex carbohydrates from the oat and white whole-wheat flours give the crêpes a natural sweetness.

1 tablespoon agave nectar

½ cup water

6 kumquats with peels intact, sliced about ⅛ inch thick, and seeds removed

---

1 tangerine, zest grated, fruit peeled, and cut into pieces

¼ teaspoon lemon juice

1 fresh basil leaf, sliced thin (chiffonade)

½ cup oat flour

¼ cup white whole-wheat flour

1½ teaspoons brown sugar

¾ cup unsweetened almond milk

1 egg

2 tablespoons extra-virgin olive oil

Cooking spray

MAKE THE SAUCE:
In a small skillet over low to medium heat, dissolve the agave nectar in the water. Add kumquats and simmer for about 15 to 20 minutes, or until sauce is reduced to a thin, syrupy consistency.

Reserve the tangerine zest for the crêpe batter. Remove the sauce from the heat and stir in the tangerine pieces, lemon juice, and basil.

MAKE THE CRÊPES:
While the sauce is reducing, stir together oat flour, white whole-wheat flour, brown sugar, and reserved tangerine zest in a medium bowl.

Add almond milk, egg, and oil, and whisk until well combined.

Lightly coat a medium nonstick skillet with cooking spray and place over medium heat. Pour ¼ cup of the crêpe batter into the skillet; immediately tilt the skillet and swirl the batter to evenly coat the surface. Cook for about 1 minute or until the bottom is lightly browned. Loosen the edges of the crêpe with a spatula, turn the crêpe over, and cook for 1 minute. Fold the crêpe in half, then in half again, and transfer to a plate. Wipe the skillet with a paper towel. Repeat cooking process with remaining batter.

Spoon the sauce over top of the folded crêpes before serving.

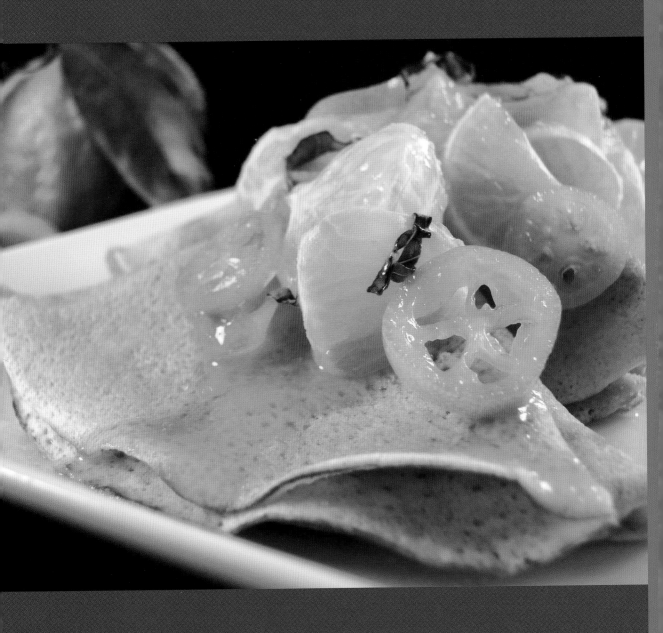

LEMON OLIVE OIL CAKE

SERVES 4

Special equipment: 6-inch or 7-inch cake pan, parchment paper (optional)

This recipe uses olive oil instead of butter for a light and moist dessert. The lemon and ginger in the cake help to promote circulation and improve digestion, making it the perfect finish to a springtime meal.

Olive oil cooking spray

Preheat oven to 350°F.

Spray the bottom of a 6-inch or 7-inch cake pan with cooking spray. If desired, add parchment paper to the bottom of the pan to prevent the cake from sticking.

½ cup white whole-wheat flour

⅛ teaspoon ground ginger

In a small bowl, combine the flour and ginger and reserve.

---

2 eggs, separated

2 tablespoons lightly packed light brown sugar

Reserve the egg whites. In a large bowl, beat together 2 egg yolks and brown sugar until the mixture is thick and pale.

---

6 tablespoons extra-virgin olive oil

1 teaspoon grated lemon zest

1½ teaspoons lemon juice

2 tablespoons honey

Add oil, lemon zest, lemon juice, and honey and mix until just combined. The mixture may appear separated.

Mix in the reserved flour and ginger mixture until just combined, being careful not to over-mix.

¼ teaspoon kosher salt

1½ tablespoons lightly packed light brown sugar

In a clean large bowl, beat the reserved 2 egg whites with salt until bubbles begin to form. Gradually add brown sugar and continue beating until the egg whites hold soft peaks.

Stir one-third of the egg white mixture into the yolk mixture to lighten the batter. Gently fold remaining whites into the batter until just combined, being careful not to over-mix or the cake will become dense.

Pour batter into the cake pan. Gently tap the pan to release any large air bubbles. Bake for 30 minutes, or until golden brown and a toothpick inserted into the center of the cake comes out clean.

Place pan on a rack to cool for 15 minutes. Loosen the cake from the pan by running a knife between the cake and the sides of the pan. Invert the pan over a plate and gently unmold the cake. Remove parchment paper if used and flip the cake right-side up onto a serving dish. Allow the cake to cool. Serve with fresh berries if desired.

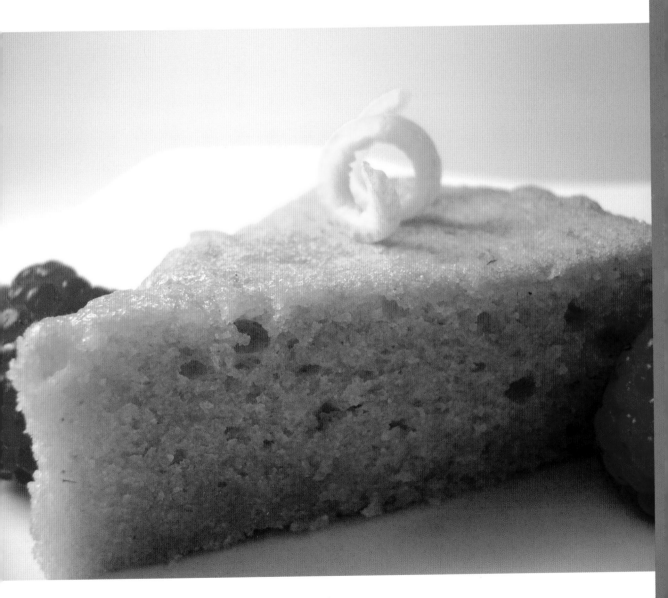

*Summertime is always the best
of what might be.*
– Charles Bowden

Chapter 12
Summer Recipes:
cooling and refreshing

The blazing summer sun represents the peak of *yang* within the cycle of the seasons. With its flourishing growth and bounty of fresh fruits and vegetables, summer encourages us to play outdoors and enjoy our surroundings. By keeping our bodies light and agile, we can fully engage in the season's activity and excitement. Requiring minimal preparation time, these simple recipes cool the body and offer a refreshing respite from the heat.

Juicy fruits and vegetables are the highlight of the season, from tomatoes and cucumbers to lettuces and watermelons. These cooling, *yin* foods provide the ideal balance for those with a hot and flushed, *yang*-dominant Summer body type. Dishes like salads help to calm and restore an overworked system. Emphasis is placed on vegetarian sources of protein, like legumes and tofu, instead of meats. To further enhance the cooling nature of these foods, the summer dishes are lightly cooked or served raw. However, raw foods should be minimized if there are signs of weak digestion, such as bloating, gas, constipation, or loose stool.

Embracing the spirit of summer means taking risks and experiencing life to its fullest. However, keeping up with the energetic pace of the season is impossible without appropriate rest and relaxation. Just as a cool evening breeze tempers a long summer day, the light, fresh foods of this season offer us a chance to refresh and recharge our bodies.

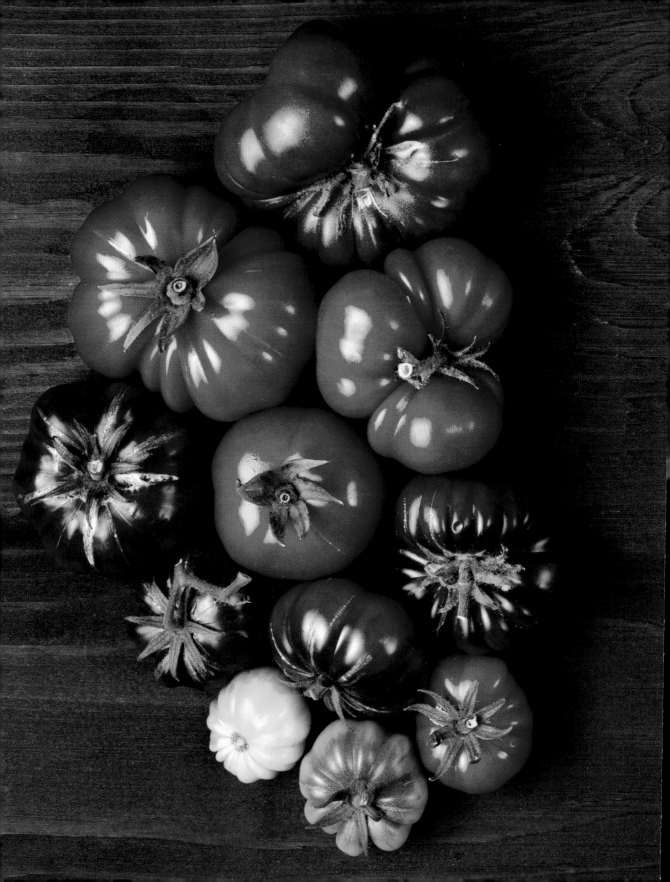

HEIRLOOM TOMATO SALAD

SERVES 4

This is a simple but elegant summer salad that refreshes the senses with a burst of colorful tomatoes and fragrant basil.

---

1 cup packed fresh basil leaves

¾ cup extra-virgin olive oil

⅛ teaspoon kosher salt

Blend together basil leaves, oil, and salt in a blender (preferable) or food processor, then strain through a fine sieve.

---

6 to 8 heirloom tomatoes of varying colors, cut into wedges or slices

Arrange tomatoes on a plate and drizzle 1 to 2 tablespoons of basil oil over top.

¼ teaspoon high-quality sea salt

⅛ teaspoon freshly ground black pepper

3 to 4 fresh basil leaves, sliced thin (chiffonade)

Sprinkle sea salt and black pepper over top of the tomatoes and garnish with basil.

Remaining basil oil can be stored in the refrigerator for up to 1 week.

CUCUMBER SEAWEED SALAD

SERVES 4 TO 6

This recipe combines two cooling foods, lightly pickled cucumber and wakame seaweed, for a simple and refreshing salad. With a bright, clean taste, it is the ideal side dish to complement an Asian-inspired meal.

(V) (V+) (DF) (GF)

2 tablespoons packed dried wakame seaweed

Soak seaweed in enough water to cover for 5 to 10 minutes or prepare according to package directions. Drain and rinse the seaweed, then cut into bite-sized strips.

1 English cucumber, cut into thin slices

½ teaspoon kosher salt

In a small bowl, toss cucumbers with salt and let sit for 10 to 15 minutes. Gently squeeze cucumbers and discard excess liquid.

4 teaspoons lemon juice

4 teaspoons agave nectar

In a small bowl, mix together seaweed, cucumber slices, lemon juice, and agave nectar. Cover and refrigerate for 3 to 4 hours.

½ teaspoon white sesame seeds

Sprinkle with sesame seeds before serving.

ROASTED EGGPLANT SPREAD

MAKES 2 CUPS

With a hint of lemon and garlic, this Mediterranean-inspired recipe is great as a spread for sandwiches or as a dip for vegetables and crackers.

3 medium eggplants, stems removed, halved lengthwise

2 tablespoons extra-virgin olive oil

½ teaspoon kosher salt

Preheat oven to 400°F.

Place eggplants on a baking sheet skin-side down, drizzle oil over top, and sprinkle with salt. Bake for 45 minutes or until tender, and allow to cool.

---

4 tablespoons extra-virgin olive oil

2 cloves garlic, sliced

While the eggplants are roasting, heat oil in a small skillet over low heat. Add garlic and cook for 1 to 2 minutes, or until golden.

---

1 tablespoon lemon juice

1½ tablespoons chopped fresh Italian parsley, divided

1½ teaspoons kosher salt

⅛ teaspoon freshly ground black pepper

In a food processor (preferable) or blender, purée roasted eggplant, garlic and oil mixture, lemon juice, 1 tablespoon parsley, salt, and black pepper until smooth.

Garnish with remaining ½ tablespoon parsley before serving.

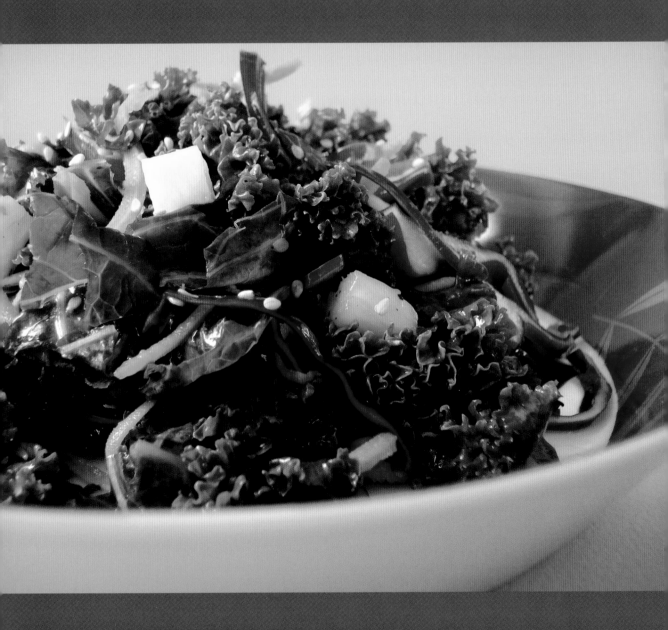

KALE SALAD WITH PINEAPPLE DRESSING

SERVES 4

This colorful salad incorporates fresh pineapple into a naturally sweet and tangy dressing. Massage the kale by hand to break down the greens and take the opportunity to reflect and be grateful for summer's bounty.

3 tablespoons chopped pineapple

¼ teaspoon honey

3 tablespoons extra-virgin olive oil

⅛ teaspoon sesame oil

⅛ teaspoon kosher salt

1 pinch freshly ground black pepper

MAKE THE DRESSING:
Blend together pineapple, honey, olive oil, sesame oil, salt, and black pepper in a blender or food processor.

1 bunch kale, stems removed and leaves torn into bite-sized pieces (about 3 cups)

¾ teaspoon kosher salt

1 tablespoon lemon juice

ASSEMBLE THE SALAD:
In a medium bowl, gently massage kale with salt for 1 minute.
Add lemon juice and massage for 1 minute.

¾ cup shredded carrots

1½ cups thinly sliced red cabbage

1½ cups chopped pineapple

1 tablespoon flaxseed oil (optional)

Add carrots, red cabbage, pineapple, and flaxseed oil to the kale.

Toss dressing into kale mixture and allow salad to sit for at least 1 hour in the refrigerator.

½ teaspoon white sesame seeds

Sprinkle with sesame seeds before serving.

AVOCADO LEMONGRASS SALAD WITH GRILLED CHICKEN

SERVES 4

Traditionally used in Thai recipes, lemongrass adds a distinct citrus aroma and zesty flavor. Here, the lemongrass is infused into a creamy avocado dressing to contrast with crisp jicama and mixed greens.

2 tablespoons lime juice

4 teaspoons extra-virgin olive oil

2 teaspoons minced lemongrass, pale green parts

2 teaspoons soy sauce

½ teaspoon minced ginger

1 pound boneless, skinless chicken breasts

PREPARE THE CHICKEN:

In a small bowl, make the marinade by mixing together lime juice, oil, lemongrass, soy sauce, and ginger.

Add the chicken, coat, and marinate covered in the refrigerator for at least 30 minutes.

Cooking spray or vegetable oil

½ teaspoon kosher salt

⅛ teaspoon freshly ground black pepper

Spray outdoor grill or indoor grill pan with cooking spray, or wipe with oil. Season both sides of the chicken with salt and black pepper. Grill chicken over medium heat for about 3 to 4 minutes on each side, or until cooked through. Allow chicken to cool, then cut into ¼-inch strips.

¼ of an avocado

1 teaspoon chopped lemongrass, pale green parts

½ teaspoon chopped shallots

2 tablespoons extra-virgin olive oil

2½ tablespoons water

2 teaspoons lime juice

1 teaspoon honey

1 teaspoon fresh cilantro

MAKE THE DRESSING:

Blend together avocado, lemongrass, shallots, oil, water, lime juice, honey, cilantro, salt, and black pepper in a food processor (preferable) or blender.

½ teaspoon kosher salt

⅛ teaspoon freshly ground
black pepper

2 cups mixed greens

½ of a tomato, cut into wedges

¼ of an avocado, cut into chunks

¼ cup sliced jicama

ASSEMBLE THE SALAD:

When ready to serve, combine mixed greens, tomatoes, avocado, jicama, and chicken strips in a large bowl and toss with enough dressing to coat lightly.

Leftover dressing can be served on the side.

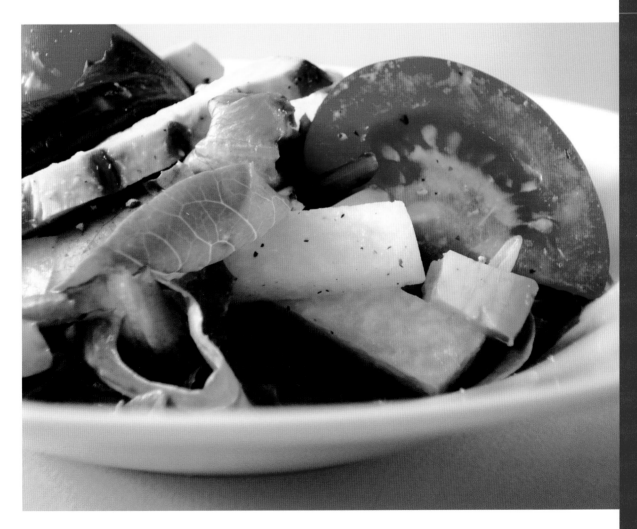

GRILLED TOFU PINEAPPLE SKEWERS

SERVES 4

Special equipment: four wooden or metal skewers

In this recipe, caramelized pineapple and a citrus-mint marinade add a fresh twist to traditional, summer grill fare.

---

2 teaspoons chopped fresh mint

2 tablespoons extra-virgin olive oil

1 teaspoon lime juice

½ teaspoon kosher salt

⅛ teaspoon freshly ground black pepper

In a large bowl, mix together mint, oil, lime juice, salt, and black pepper.

---

6 ounces extra-firm tofu, cubed

½ of a medium zucchini or yellow squash, cut into 1-inch chunks (about 1 cup)

¼ of a medium red onion, cut into 1-inch chunks (about ⅓ cup)

4 medium button mushrooms, halved

½ cup grape tomatoes

Add tofu, zucchini or yellow squash, red onions, mushrooms, and tomatoes to the bowl, toss together, and marinate for 30 minutes.

1½ cups cubed pineapple

If using wooden skewers, soak them in enough water to cover for 10 minutes to prevent them from burning on the grill.

Thread the marinated ingredients and the pineapple onto the skewers. Using an outdoor grill or indoor grill pan, grill skewers over medium heat for approximately 3 to 4 minutes, then turn over and cook for 3 minutes, or until vegetables are cooked through and caramelized.

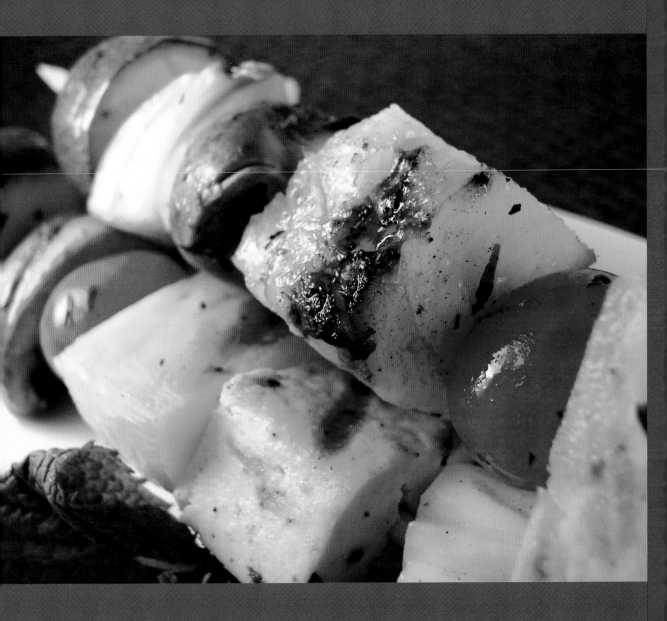

GLASS NOODLE SALAD

SERVES 4

Chewy noodles, crunchy vegetables, and roasted peanuts complement each other in this simple and light summer dish. Popular in Asian cooking, these translucent noodles are usually made from the starch of green mung beans or rice.

4 tablespoons water

2 tablespoons extra-virgin olive oil

2 teaspoons lime juice

2 teaspoons soy sauce

¼ teaspoon sesame oil

MAKE THE DRESSING:
In a large bowl, whisk together water, olive oil, lime juice, soy sauce, and sesame oil.

4 ounces dried mung bean noodles

PREPARE THE NOODLE SALAD:
Soak the mung bean noodles in enough cold water to cover for 5 to 10 minutes, then drain.

2 quarts water

3 teaspoons kosher salt

In a medium pot, bring water to a boil over high heat. Reduce the heat to medium-high, add the salt and noodles, and simmer for 5 minutes, or until the noodles are soft and appear clear. Drain noodles, soak in enough cold water to cover to keep them from sticking together, and reserve.

1 tablespoon extra-virgin olive oil

2 cloves garlic, minced

2 teaspoons minced ginger

In a large skillet, heat oil over medium heat. Add garlic and cook for 1 minute, then add ginger and cook for 1 minute.

2 cups sliced fresh shiitake mushroom caps (about 4 large mushrooms)

¼ teaspoon kosher salt

2 teaspoons water

1 cup sugar snap peas, thinly sliced on the diagonal

Add mushrooms, salt, and water, and cook for 3 to 4 minutes. Add snap peas and cook for 2 minutes.

½ cup shredded carrots

⅔ cup mung bean sprouts

2 tablespoons chopped fresh cilantro

4 teaspoons chopped fresh mint

¾ teaspoon kosher salt

¼ teaspoon freshly ground black pepper

Remove skillet from heat and add carrots, bean sprouts, cilantro, mint, salt, and black pepper.

Drain the reserved noodles, add them to the dressing along with the vegetable mixture, and toss together.

¼ cup chopped roasted peanuts

Garnish with chopped peanuts before serving.

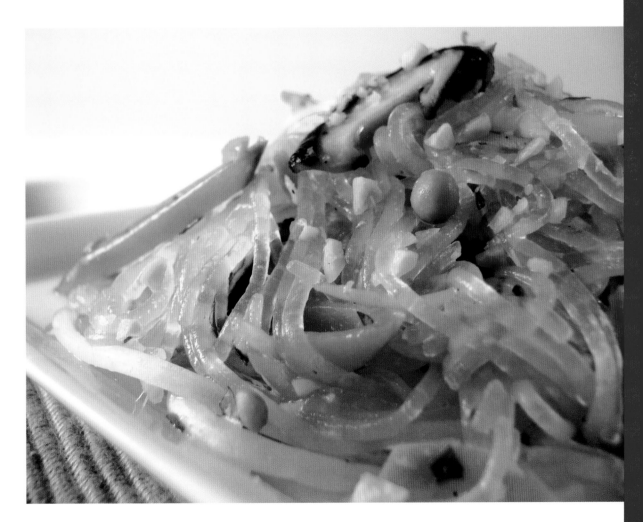

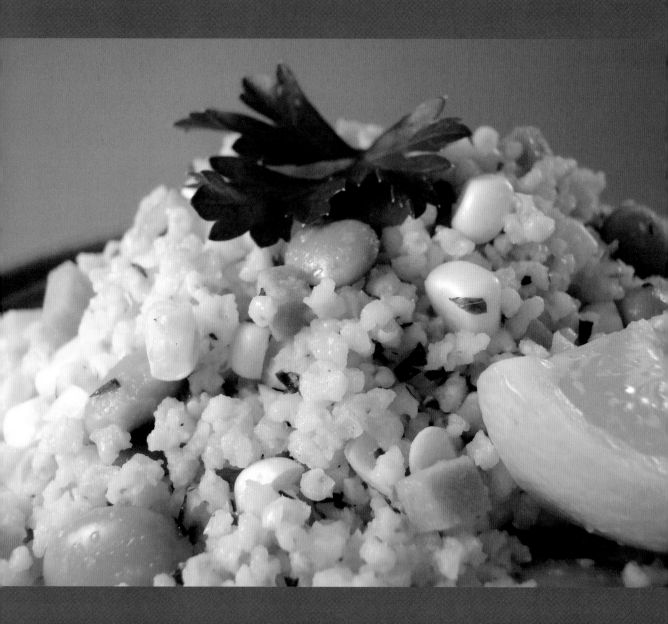

TOASTED MILLET SALAD

SERVES 6 TO 8

Fresh lemon and parsley brighten up this salad made of millet, a cereal grain with a texture similar to couscous. The extra step of toasting the millet enhances its nutty flavor.

1 cup millet, rinsed and drained

1 teaspoon extra-virgin olive oil

PREPARE THE MILLET:
In a medium pot, toast millet in oil over medium heat for 10 minutes or until golden in color, stirring occasionally to prevent from burning.

1 cup water

1 cup low-sodium vegetable broth

¾ teaspoon kosher salt

Add water, vegetable broth, and salt, and bring to a boil over high heat. Reduce heat to low, cover, and simmer for 18 to 20 minutes, or until the liquid is almost absorbed. Remove from heat and allow millet to sit covered for 5 minutes. Transfer millet to a large bowl, fluff gently with a fork, and allow it to cool.

1 teaspoon grated lemon zest

2 tablespoons lemon juice

1 tablespoon water

2 teaspoons minced shallots

¾ teaspoon kosher salt

⅛ teaspoon freshly ground black pepper

4 tablespoons extra-virgin olive oil

MAKE THE DRESSING:
While the millet cools, combine lemon zest, lemon juice, water, shallots, salt, and black pepper in a small bowl.

Add the oil in a steady stream, whisking until emulsified.

½ cup diced carrots

1 cup fresh corn kernels (from about 1 ear)

½ cup cooked and shelled edamame

4 teaspoons chopped fresh Italian parsley

ASSEMBLE THE SALAD:
Add carrots, corn, edamame, and parsley to the cooled millet. Add dressing and gently toss together.

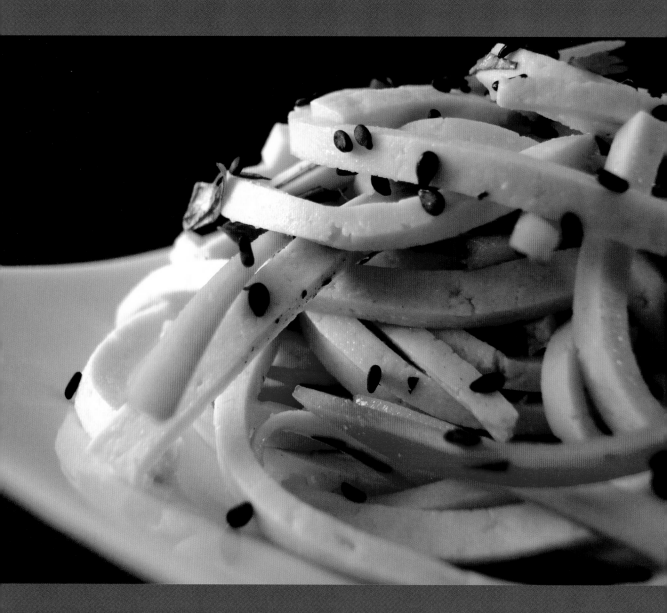

TOFU NOODLE SALAD

SERVES 4

Julienned vegetables, thinly cut noodles of protein-rich tofu, and a dash of sesame oil make up this cooling dish. Black sesame seeds are also added due to their beneficial *yin*-nourishing properties.

16 ounces firm or extra-firm tofu, sliced into long, thin strips

1 medium carrot, julienned

1 celery stalk, julienned

1 tablespoon chopped fresh cilantro

½ teaspoon kosher salt

⅛ teaspoon freshly ground black pepper

In a medium bowl, combine tofu, carrots, celery, cilantro, salt, and black pepper.

2 teaspoons extra-virgin olive oil

⅛ teaspoon sesame oil, or more to taste

In a small bowl, whisk together olive oil and sesame oil. Pour over top of tofu mixture and gently toss together. Cover and refrigerate for at least 1 hour.

½ teaspoon black sesame seeds

Sprinkle black sesame seeds over top before serving.

NOT EXACTLY CHICKEN SALAD

SERVES 2 TO 4

Note: overnight preparation is recommended for this recipe.

A lighter alternative to the classic chicken salad, this recipe combines grilled tofu, crunchy apples, and a creamy vegan dressing.

---

16 ounces firm or extra-firm tofu, cut into ½-inch strips

1 teaspoon extra-virgin olive oil

PREPARE THE TOFU:

Coat tofu with oil. Using an outdoor grill or indoor grill pan, grill over medium heat for 2 to 3 minutes on each side, or until grill marks are achieved. Allow tofu to cool.

---

5 ounces firm tofu

1 tablespoon extra-virgin olive oil

1 teaspoon lemon juice

1 teaspoon Dijon mustard

½ teaspoon water

1 teaspoon kosher salt

MAKE THE VEGANNAISE DRESSING:

While the grilled tofu cools, blend together tofu, oil, lemon juice, mustard, water, and salt in a blender or food processor until smooth.

---

1 medium apple, diced

¼ cup shredded carrots

¼ cup diced celery

1 teaspoon chopped fresh Italian parsley

½ teaspoon kosher salt

⅛ teaspoon freshly ground black pepper

ASSEMBLE THE SALAD:

When the tofu is cool, cut into ½-inch cubes.

In a medium bowl, toss together grilled tofu, apples, carrots, celery, parsley, salt, black pepper, and ½ cup of vegannaise dressing. Chill completely. The salad's flavors come together best if chilled overnight.

Remaining vegannaise dressing can be stored in the refrigerator for up to 1 week.

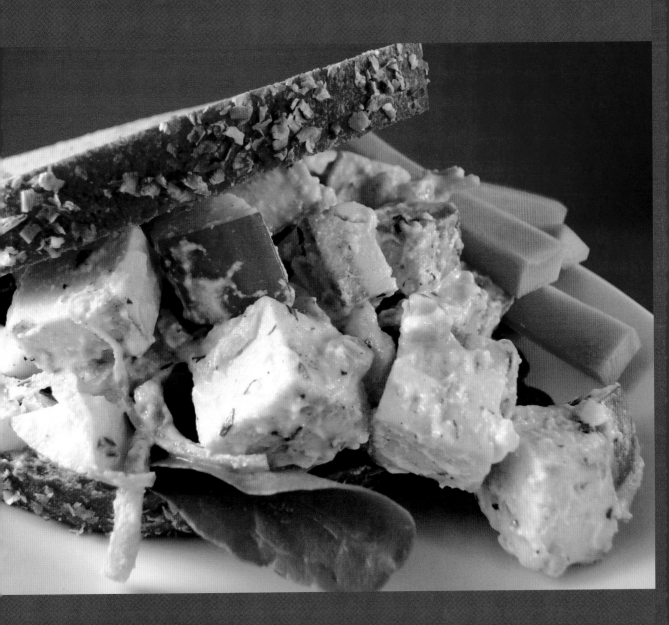

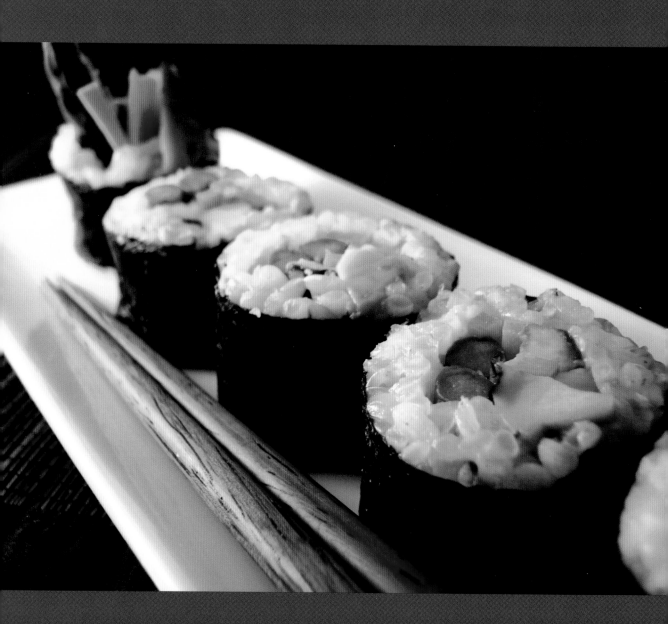

BROWN RICE VEGETABLE SUSHI

MAKES 4 ROLLS

Special equipment: sushi mat or sushi roller

Note: this recipe uses cooked brown rice, which should be prepared beforehand.

Make these portable rolls with whole-grain brown rice and any seasonally available fillings. Use freshly grated wasabi for a complex flavor not found in artificially colored, pre-packaged versions.

---

1 quart water

1 tablespoon kosher salt

8 asparagus spears

Prepare a medium bowl of ice water.

In a medium pot, bring 1 quart of water to a boil over high heat. Add salt and blanch asparagus in the boiling water for 2 minutes, or until bright green. Immediately place them in the ice water to stop the cooking process. Drain asparagus and pat dry.

---

1 teaspoon extra-virgin olive oil

2 cups sliced fresh shiitake mushroom caps (about 4 large mushrooms)

In a small skillet, heat oil over medium heat. Sauté mushrooms for 3 to 5 minutes, or until tender.

---

4 sheets dried nori

3 to 4 cups cooked short-grain brown rice, divided

½ of a medium carrot, julienned, divided

½ of a medium cucumber, julienned, divided

½ of an avocado, cut into slices, divided

Line a sushi mat or sushi roller with plastic wrap. Place one sheet of nori on top of the plastic wrap and spread ¾ to 1 cup of cooked brown rice over the bottom two-thirds of the nori surface. Place two asparagus spears, one-quarter of the sautéed mushrooms, one-quarter of the carrots, one-quarter of the cucumbers, and one-quarter of the avocado slices in a line along the center of the rice.

Starting with the edge closest to you, roll the sushi up, firmly tucking in the roll as you go to get it as tight as possible. When you get to the end of the roll, moisten the edge of the nori with a small amount of water and press lightly to seal.

Repeat with the remaining sheets of nori and filling. Cut the rolls into bite-sized pieces, approximately ¾ inch thick.

---

1 tablespoon grated fresh wasabi (optional)

Soy sauce (optional)

Mix together fresh wasabi and soy sauce for a dipping sauce, if desired.

SUMMER SQUASH "SPAGHETTI"

SERVES 4

For this raw "pasta" dish, use thin strips of any seasonal squash, such as zucchini, crookneck, or patty pan. The vegetables can also be blanched or lightly cooked. The simple sauce incorporates sun-dried tomatoes and fresh basil for an antioxidant-rich dish that is perfect for summer.

Special equipment (optional): spiral slicer

2 tablespoons sun-dried tomatoes

½ cup water

MAKE THE SAUCE:

In a small pot, heat the water over high heat until just boiling. Remove from heat and soak the sun-dried tomatoes in the water for 30 minutes. Strain and reserve the tomatoes and 2 tablespoons of the soaking liquid.

1 medium tomato, chopped

1 tablespoon extra-virgin olive oil

½ teaspoon lemon juice

1 tablespoon packed fresh basil

1 tablespoon packed fresh Italian parsley

¼ teaspoon dried oregano

¾ teaspoon kosher salt

⅛ teaspoon freshly ground black pepper

Purée soaked sun-dried tomatoes, reserved liquid, chopped tomatoes, oil, lemon juice, basil, parsley, oregano, salt, and black pepper in a blender (preferable) or food processor for 30 to 45 seconds, or until sauce reaches your desired consistency.

2 zucchini

2 yellow squash

1 carrot

MAKE THE "PASTA":

If using a spiral slicer, cut zucchini, yellow squash, and carrot into long, thin strips.

If using a knife, cut each vegetable lengthwise into slices about ¼ inch thick. Stack vegetable slices on top of each other. Cut slices again lengthwise to make ¼-inch strips that resemble spaghetti.

Blanch or lightly cook the vegetables, if desired.

1 small tomato, diced

½ teaspoon kosher salt

⅛ teaspoon freshly ground black pepper

In a large bowl, toss together the zucchini, yellow squash, carrots, diced tomatoes, salt, and black pepper.

Serve with tomato sauce over top.

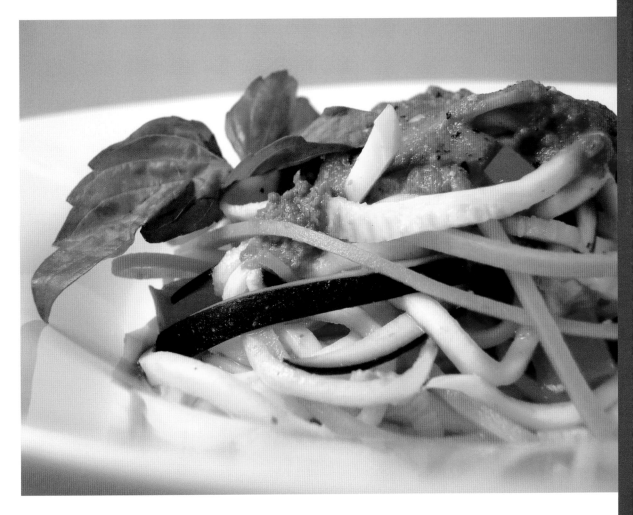

CRAB CAKES WITH FRUIT SALSA

MAKES 6 TO 7 CRAB CAKES

Fresh lump crab meat is the star of this simple summer dish. The sweet flavor and cooling nature of the crab is enhanced by the addition of a refreshing fruit salsa.

1 cup dried bread crumbs, divided (or 4 to 5 slices whole-wheat bread if making from fresh)

⅛ teaspoon kosher salt

⅛ teaspoon freshly ground black pepper

MAKE THE CRAB CAKES:

If making your own bread crumbs, pulse enough bread slices in a food processor (preferable) or blender to measure 2 cups fresh bread crumbs. In a small skillet, toast the bread crumbs over medium heat for 5 minutes until light golden brown, stirring continuously. Let cool. The toasted bread crumbs should measure about 1 cup.

Reserve ½ cup of toasted or store-bought bread crumbs for the crab mixture. Place remaining ½ cup bread crumbs on a plate and mix in salt and black pepper for the coating.

1 teaspoon extra-virgin olive oil

½ cup diced yellow onions (about ½ of a small onion)

In a small skillet, heat oil over medium heat. Add onions and cook for 2 minutes.

2 cups cooked lump crab meat

¼ cup diced red bell pepper

¼ cup diced celery

1 tablespoon chopped fresh Italian parsley

2 teaspoons lemon juice

1 egg, beaten

¾ teaspoon kosher salt

⅛ teaspoon freshly ground black pepper

In a medium bowl, mix ½ cup reserved bread crumbs, sautéed onions, crab meat, bell peppers, celery, parsley, lemon juice, egg, salt, and black pepper.

Divide crab mixture into ⅓ cup portions and lightly form into individual patties about 1 inch thick. Coat crab cakes with seasoned bread crumb mixture on all sides. Place crab cakes on a large plate, cover, and allow to rest in refrigerator for at least 1 hour.

1 cup diced pineapple

½ cup diced jicama or Asian pear

¼ cup diced red bell pepper

1 tablespoon minced shallots

½ of a small fresh serrano pepper, seeds and membranes removed, chopped

1½ teaspoons chopped fresh cilantro

½ teaspoon lime juice

½ teaspoon kosher salt

MAKE THE SALSA:

In a small bowl, combine pineapple, jicama or Asian pear, bell peppers, shallots, serrano peppers, cilantro, lime juice, and salt.

2 teaspoons extra-virgin olive oil, divided

PAN-FRY THE CRAB CAKES:

In a medium nonstick skillet, heat 1 teaspoon oil over medium heat. Place 3 to 4 crab cakes in the skillet and pan-fry for 2 minutes on each side, or until golden brown. Repeat with 1 teaspoon oil and remaining crab cakes. Serve with fruit salsa.

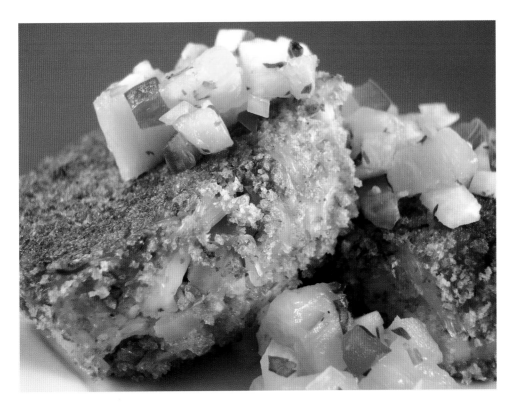

SWISS CHARD ROLLS

SERVES 4

Use colorful Swiss chard leaves for an updated take on stuffed cabbage. This whole-grain recipe is a great use of leftover millet.

⅔ cup water

⅔ cup low-sodium vegetable broth

⅔ cup millet, rinsed and drained

½ teaspoon kosher salt

PREPARE THE MILLET:
In a medium pot, combine water and vegetable broth and bring to a boil over high heat. Add millet and salt, reduce heat to low, cover, and simmer for 18 to 20 minutes, or until the liquid is almost absorbed. Remove from heat and keep covered for 5 minutes. Fluff with fork, allow to cool, and reserve.

1 teaspoon extra-virgin olive oil

½ cup diced yellow or white onions (about ½ of a small onion)

2 cloves garlic, minced

MAKE THE TOMATO SAUCE:
While the millet cools, heat oil in a medium skillet over medium heat. Add onions and cook for 2 minutes, then add garlic and cook for 1 minute.

1½ cups chopped fresh tomatoes

½ teaspoon dried oregano

3 sprigs fresh Italian parsley

2 tablespoons water

¼ teaspoon kosher salt

⅛ teaspoon freshly ground black pepper

Add tomatoes, oregano, parsley, water, salt, and black pepper. Reduce heat to low, cover, and simmer for 30 minutes.

1 tablespoon chopped fresh basil

Add basil during the last 2 minutes of cooking. Remove skillet from heat and discard parsley sprigs.

1 teaspoon extra-virgin olive oil

½ cup diced yellow or white onions (about ½ of a small onion)

2 cloves garlic, minced

MAKE THE MILLET FILLING:
In a large skillet, heat oil over medium heat. Add onions and cook for 2 minutes, then add garlic and cook for 1 minute.

2 cups chopped button or crimini mushrooms

2 tablespoons low-sodium vegetable broth

¼ cup diced carrots

¼ cup diced celery

¼ teaspoon dried marjoram

Add mushrooms and vegetable broth and cook for 4 minutes. Add carrots, celery, and marjoram, and cook for 2 minutes. Turn off the heat. Add reserved millet (or 2 cups of leftover cooked millet) to the pan and mix to incorporate. Allow the mixture to cool.

---

8 to 10 medium to large Swiss chard leaves

2 quarts water

2 tablespoons kosher salt

MAKE THE CHARD ROLLS:

Prepare the Swiss chard leaves by removing the thick stem from the center of each leaf using a v-shaped cut, making sure to leave the top of each leaf intact.

Prepare a large bowl of ice water.

In a medium pot, bring 2 quarts of water to a boil over high heat. Add salt and blanch chard leaves in boiling water for 3 minutes. Immediately place chard in the ice water to stop the cooking process. Set leaves on a towel and pat dry.

On a clean work surface, lay one chard leaf shiny-side down with the tip of the leaf pointing toward you. Overlap the two ends of the leaf where the stem was removed. Place ⅓ cup of millet filling on the leaf, about 2 inches from the tip. Fold the tip of the leaf over the filling, then fold the sides over top toward the center, and roll up tightly, like a burrito. Repeat with remaining leaves and filling.

Kosher salt to taste

When all chard rolls are complete, place them in the skillet with the tomato sauce. Sprinkle each roll with a pinch of salt to taste. Cover and simmer over medium-low heat for 5 minutes, or until heated through.

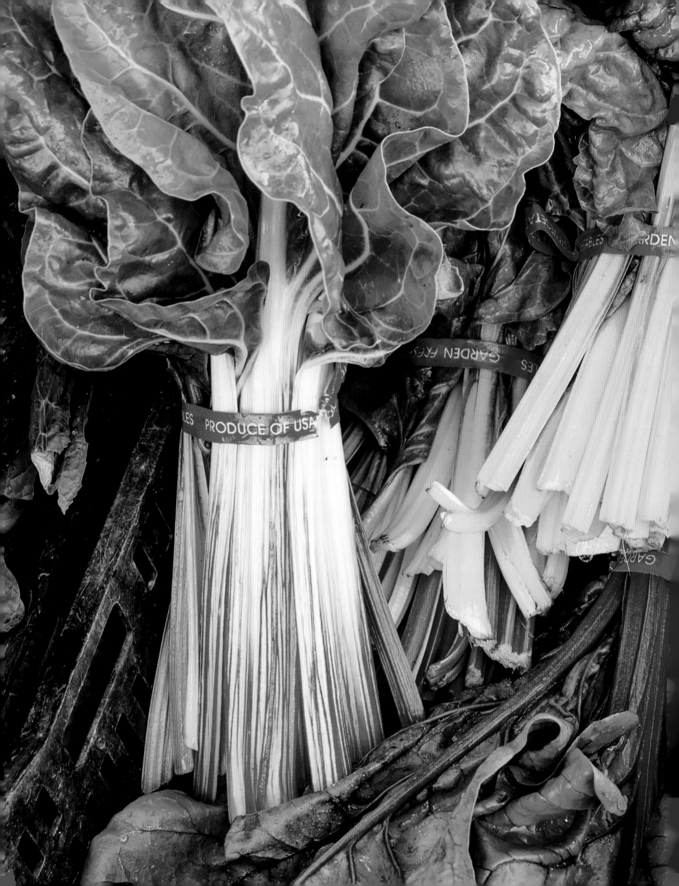

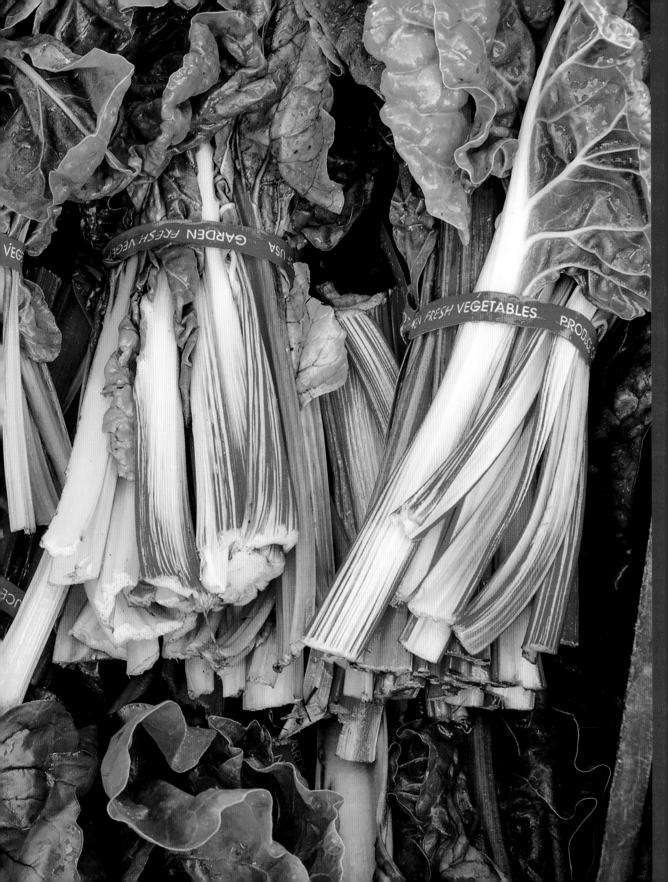

BANANA FIG BREAD

SERVES 6 TO 8

 (V) (DF)

Special equipment: 9-inch loaf pan, parchment paper (optional)

Ripe bananas and a moist swirl of figs give this quick bread a natural sweetness.

Olive oil cooking spray

Preheat oven to 350°F.

Spray a 9-inch loaf pan with cooking spray. If desired, add parchment paper to the bottom of the pan to prevent the bread from sticking.

½ cup dried figs

½ cup water

Heat water in a small pot over high heat until just boiling. Remove from heat and soak the dried figs in the water for 10 minutes or until softened. Remove softened figs from liquid and cut into chunks. Purée the figs in a food processor (preferable) or blender, gradually adding enough of the soaking liquid to reach a paste-like consistency.

1½ cups white whole-wheat flour

½ cup almond flour

1½ teaspoons baking soda

1 teaspoon ground cinnamon

½ teaspoon kosher salt

¼ teaspoon ground nutmeg

1 pinch ground cloves

In a medium bowl, mix together white whole-wheat flour, almond flour, baking soda, cinnamon, salt, nutmeg, and cloves.

---

4 very ripe bananas

2 eggs, beaten

¼ cup packed light brown sugar

¼ cup extra-virgin olive oil

½ teaspoon vanilla extract

In a large bowl, mash bananas with a fork. Mix in eggs, brown sugar, oil, and vanilla.

Add flour mixture to the banana mixture, and mix until just combined. Pour half of the batter into the pan. Spoon two-thirds of the fig paste over top of the batter. Pour remaining batter into the pan. Spoon the remaining one-third of the fig paste over top. Gently run a knife back and forth through the batter a few times to create a fig swirl.

Bake for 50 to 60 minutes, or until a toothpick inserted into the center comes out clean. Allow bread to cool before unmolding.

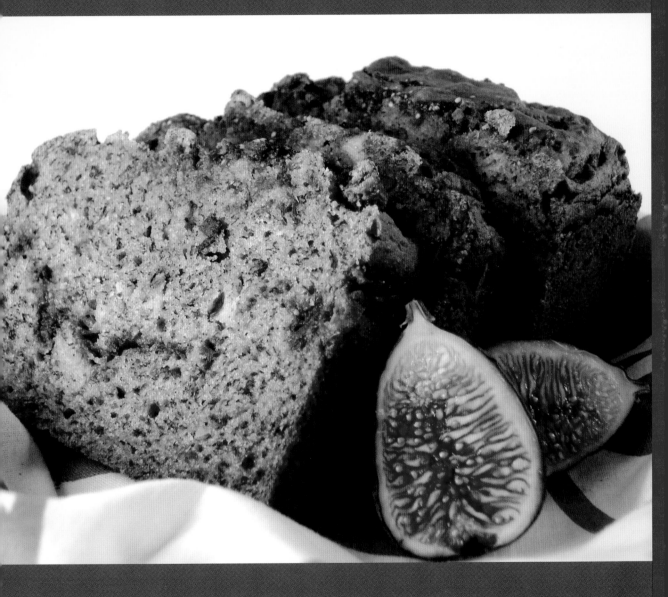

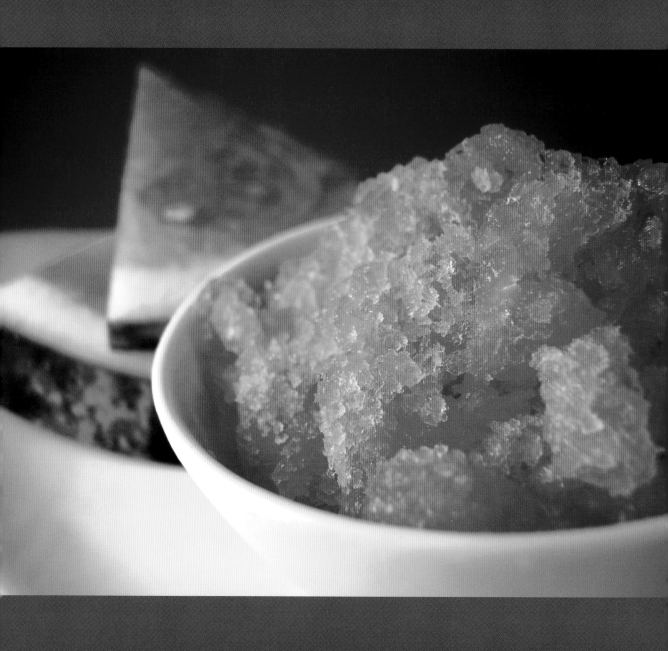

WATERMELON GRANITA

SERVES 4 TO 6

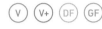

As one of the most cooling fruits, watermelon is beneficial for clearing heat and nourishing *yin*. With only four ingredients, this icy treat is the ideal refreshment for a hot summer day.

---

5 cups chopped watermelon, seeds and rind removed

In a blender, purée watermelon in batches.

---

2 teaspoons lemon juice

2 teaspoons agave nectar (optional)

1 pinch kosher salt

In a large, freezer-safe dish, mix watermelon purée with lemon juice, agave nectar, and salt. Place the mixture in the freezer. After 30 minutes, scrape the surface and sides with a fork, breaking up any large chunks. Continue scraping every 30 to 45 minutes for about 3 to 4 hours, or until the mixture is frozen and has a flaky texture.

Store in a covered container in the freezer until ready to serve.

The Indian Summer of life should be a little sunny and a little sad, like the season, and infinite in wealth and depth of tone, but never hustled.

– Henry Adams

Chapter 13
Indian Summer Recipes: building the foundation

As the transition between the bright growth of summer and the cool withdrawal of fall, Indian summer is the ideal time for centering the body and restoring balance. The warm, temperate climate of this season is best matched by eating foods that are neither too warming nor too cooling. For this reason, the Indian summer recipes emphasize the use of thermally neutral foods such as rice and potatoes.

Nourishing the body's center is the theme of Indian summer; this is accomplished by helping the body to digest foods as easily as possible. Foods should be cooked well and chewed thoroughly to encourage optimal digestion by the stomach and intestines. To curb the sweet cravings experienced by those with this seasonal body type, the following recipes use naturally sweet foods like corn, sweet potatoes, and beets instead of refined sugars. Animal proteins and dairy products are also helpful to boost energy and build body mass in the weakened Indian Summer body types. Vegetarians with this seasonal type can substitute the meat and fish found in these recipes with well-cooked legumes and soy products; however, these ingredients tend to be less beneficial for strengthening *qi*.

The recipes of Indian summer also reflect the grounding of the body to the Earth. Using foods that support the body's energetic center allows us to lay a foundation for the cooler seasons ahead. During this season, it is also important to pay respect to the Earth, plants, animals, and people that have helped to provide us with nourishing foods. By showing appreciation for our foods' origins, we further enhance our connection to the earth and our surrounding environment.

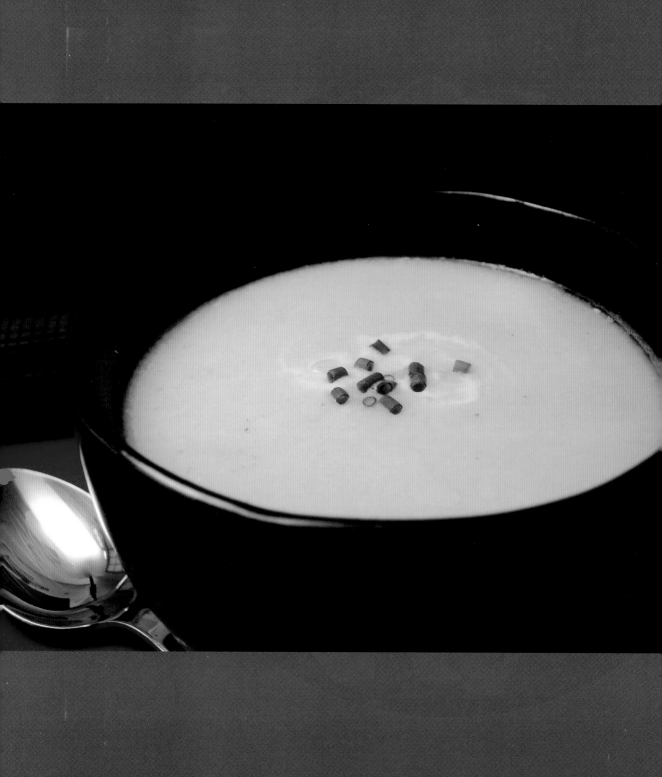

COCONUT CURRY CORN SOUP

SERVES 4

The naturally sweet flavors of fresh corn and coconut are helpful for strengthening *qi* within the body. In this recipe, they are combined with a hint of curry for a simple and nourishing soup.

4 cups water

8 ears fresh corn

2¼ teaspoons kosher salt

In a medium pot over high heat, bring water to a boil. Using a knife, cut off corn kernels to measure about 7 cups. After the water comes to a boil, add the corn and salt. Reduce heat to medium-low and simmer with lid slightly ajar for 15 minutes.

Drain corn and reserve the cooking liquid. Reserve ¾ cup of the corn kernels. Purée the remaining corn with 2½ cups of cooking liquid, adding more liquid if necessary to reach your desired consistency. If using an immersion blender, the soup can be directly blended in the cooking pot. If using a countertop blender, purée the soup in small batches, then pour it back into the cooking pot.

2 tablespoons coconut milk

¼ teaspoon curry powder

1 pinch ground white pepper

Add the reserved whole corn kernels to the blended soup, along with the coconut milk, curry powder, and white pepper. Cover and simmer over low heat for 5 minutes.

1 tablespoon chopped chives (optional)

Garnish with chives before serving, if desired.

WARM ROASTED BEET SALAD

SERVES 6

This beautiful crimson-red and golden beet salad can be added to greens or served on its own. With a sweet, earthy flavor, beets benefit the body by regulating and supplementing *qi*.

4 medium red and golden beets (about 2½ pounds)

PREPARE THE BEETS:

Preheat oven to 425°F.

Wrap each beet in aluminum foil. Place on a baking sheet and bake for 45 to 50 minutes, or until tender when pierced with a paring knife.

½ tablespoon red wine vinegar

½ tablespoon balsamic vinegar

½ teaspoon honey

⅛ teaspoon kosher salt

⅛ teaspoon freshly ground black pepper

3 tablespoons extra-virgin olive oil

MAKE THE DRESSING:

While the beets are roasting, whisk together red wine vinegar, balsamic vinegar, honey, salt, and black pepper in a small bowl. Add oil in a steady stream, whisking until emulsified.

1 teaspoon chopped fresh Italian parsley

¼ cup whole walnuts, toasted and chopped

Lettuce greens (optional)

ASSEMBLE THE SALAD:

When beets are cool enough to handle, peel them by rubbing the skins with a paper towel or with the aluminum foil in which they were wrapped. Cut beets into chunks.

To prevent red beets from bleeding onto the golden ones, first toss golden beets in the dressing and remove from bowl. Add red beets, parsley, and toasted walnuts to the remaining dressing and toss. Place the dressed golden beets over top. Serve with lettuce greens if desired.

VEGAN POTATO SALAD

SERVES 8

Instead of using mayonnaise, this potato salad incorporates a vegan tofu dressing for a creamy, low-fat alternative.

3 pounds red potatoes
(about 12 medium potatoes)

2 quarts water

1½ teaspoons kosher salt, divided

PREPARE THE POTATOES:
In a large pot, bring potatoes, water, and 1 teaspoon of salt to a boil over high heat. Reduce heat to medium-low and simmer with lid slightly ajar for 20 to 25 minutes, or until the potatoes are tender when pierced with a paring knife.

Drain potatoes and allow them to rest until cool enough to handle. Cut potatoes into 1½-inch pieces. Place potatoes in a medium bowl, season with remaining ½ teaspoon of salt, and toss together.

5 ounces firm tofu

1 tablespoon extra-virgin olive oil

1 teaspoon lemon juice

1 teaspoon Dijon mustard

½ teaspoon water

1 teaspoon kosher salt

MAKE THE VEGANNAISE DRESSING:
Blend together tofu, oil, lemon juice, mustard, water, and salt in a blender or food processor until very smooth.

½ cup peas (blanched if fresh, or thawed if frozen)

¼ cup shredded carrots

2 teaspoons chopped fresh Italian parsley

1 teaspoon kosher salt

⅛ teaspoon freshly ground black pepper

ASSEMBLE THE SALAD:
Add peas, carrots, parsley, salt, and black pepper to the potatoes. Add dressing and toss. Serve warm or cold.

ZESTY CORN FRITTERS

MAKES ABOUT 8 FRITTERS

This dish is a healthy alternative to deep-fried corn fritters. Using *masa harina*, a Mexican corn flour, enhances the naturally sweet flavor of the fresh corn.

---

5 ears fresh corn

1 egg, beaten

Using a box grater, grate about 4 ears of corn into a medium bowl to measure 1⅓ cups, collecting all pulp and juice. Using a knife, cut off whole corn kernels from about ½ of an ear to measure a heaping ¼ cup, and add it to the grated corn. Mix beaten egg into the corn mixture.

½ cup *masa harina*

⅛ teaspoon ground cumin

⅛ teaspoon smoked paprika

¾ teaspoon kosher salt

1 pinch freshly ground black pepper

In a small bowl, mix together *masa harina*, cumin, paprika, salt, and black pepper.

⅓ cup diced red bell pepper

1 teaspoon chopped fresh cilantro

Fold the *masa harina* mixture into the corn mixture, and then stir in the bell peppers and cilantro until well incorporated.

---

1 teaspoon extra-virgin olive oil

In a medium nonstick skillet, heat oil over medium-high heat. Drop heaping spoonfuls of the batter into the skillet to form fritters about 2 to 3 inches in diameter. Pan-fry for 2 to 3 minutes per side, or until golden brown. Repeat with remaining batter.

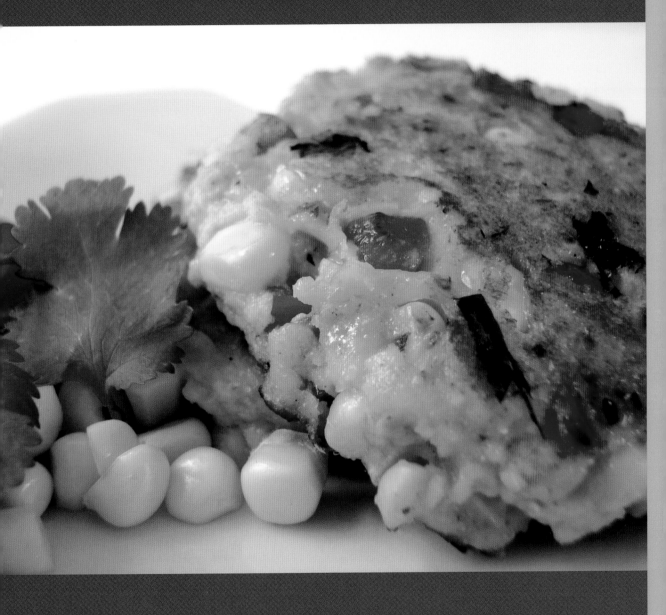

SPINACH NIÇOISE SALAD

SERVES 4

Seared fresh tuna and baby spinach add a twist to a classic French salad.

2 tablespoons lemon juice

½ teaspoon minced shallots

¼ teaspoon Dijon mustard

⅛ teaspoon mashed garlic

⅛ teaspoon anchovy paste

⅛ teaspoon kosher salt

⅛ teaspoon black pepper

4 tablespoons extra-virgin olive oil

MAKE THE DRESSING:

In a small bowl, whisk together lemon juice, shallots, mustard, garlic, anchovy paste, salt, and black pepper. Add the oil in a steady stream, whisking until emulsified.

---

2 eggs

ASSEMBLE THE SALAD:

Place eggs in a small pot and add just enough water to cover. Bring to a boil over high heat, uncovered. Remove pot from heat and cover for 14 minutes. Promptly drain eggs and place them in ice water until cool. Peel the eggs and cut them into quarters.

---

2 quarts water

2 tablespoons kosher salt

2½ cups halved green beans (about ½ pound)

Prepare a medium bowl of ice water.

In a medium pot, bring 2 quarts of water to a boil over high heat. Use this water to cook both the green beans and the potatoes. Add salt and blanch the green beans in the boiling water for 3 to 4 minutes. Remove the green beans and immediately place them in the ice water to stop the cooking process.

Drain the green beans and pat dry. In a medium bowl, toss the green beans with 1 teaspoon of the dressing.

---

12 fingerling potatoes (about 1¼ pounds)

⅛ teaspoon kosher salt

In the same pot of boiling water, add the potatoes and simmer uncovered for 10 to 20 minutes, or until tender when pierced with a paring knife. Drain the potatoes and toss with salt and 1 tablespoon of the dressing. Allow to cool.

1 teaspoon extra-virgin olive oil

8 ounces sushi-grade tuna

⅛ teaspoon kosher salt

⅛ teaspoon freshly ground
black pepper

In a medium skillet, heat oil over medium-high heat. Season the tuna with salt and black pepper. Sear the tuna for 1 minute on each side until golden brown, or cook to your desired doneness. Cut tuna into ¼-inch slices.

12 ounces baby spinach
(about 12 cups)

½ pint grape tomatoes

¼ cup Niçoise olives, drained

⅛ teaspoon kosher salt

⅛ teaspoon freshly ground
black pepper

In a medium bowl, combine spinach, tomatoes, and olives, and toss with 2 tablespoons of dressing. Season with salt and black pepper, then transfer to a serving platter.

Separately arrange eggs, green beans, potatoes, and tuna over the salad. Remaining dressing can be served on the side or lightly drizzled over the salad.

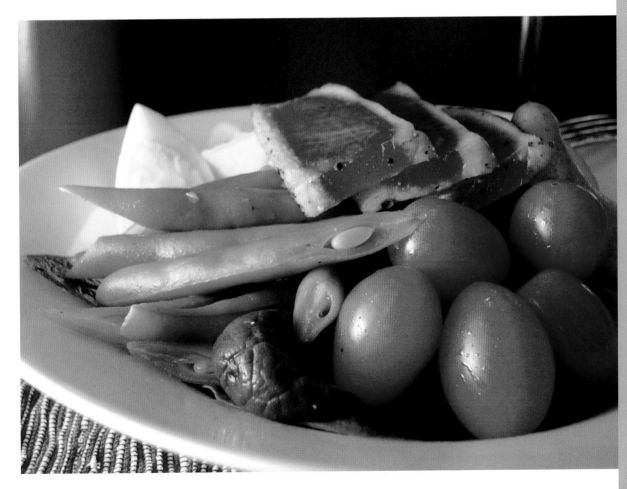

BAKED FALAFEL WITH AVOCADO TZATZIKI SAUCE

SERVES 4 (MAKES ABOUT 16 FALAFEL BALLS)

Baking the falafel at a high heat gives it a crisp, crunchy exterior without the need for deep-frying. Serve with whole-wheat pita bread, lettuce, tomatoes, avocado, cucumber, and kalamata olives for a Mediterranean-inspired meal.

1 cup plain Greek yogurt

2 teaspoons chopped fresh dill

1 cup chopped English cucumber, seeds removed

¼ of an avocado

1 clove garlic, minced

½ teaspoon lemon juice

½ teaspoon kosher salt

⅛ teaspoon freshly ground black pepper

1¾ cups (or one 15-ounce can) cooked garbanzo beans, drained

1 whole-wheat pita bread, torn into small pieces

¾ cup packed fresh Italian parsley

½ cup packed fresh cilantro

3 tablespoons chopped white or yellow onions

3 cloves garlic

1¼ teaspoons ground cumin

¾ teaspoon ground coriander

1 teaspoon kosher salt

MAKE THE TZATZIKI SAUCE:

Prepare Tzatziki sauce at least 1 hour prior to serving. In a blender (preferable) or food processor, blend yogurt, dill, cucumber, avocado, garlic, lemon juice, salt, and black pepper. Refrigerate until ready to serve.

MAKE THE FALAFEL:

Preheat oven to 400°F.

If working with a food processor, blend together garbanzo beans, pita, parsley, cilantro, onions, garlic, cumin, coriander, and salt, until the mixture is a uniform consistency, but slightly chunky.

If working without a food processor, place garbanzo beans in a medium bowl. Finely chop pita, parsley, cilantro, onions, and garlic, and add them to the bowl. Add cumin, coriander, and salt, and mash together until the mixture is a uniform consistency, but slightly chunky.

3 teaspoons white sesame seeds

Mix in sesame seeds by hand. Form the mixture into small balls, about 1 heaping tablespoon each, and place on a lightly oiled baking sheet. Bake for 10 minutes, then flip the falafel over and bake for 10 minutes. Serve with Tzatziki sauce.

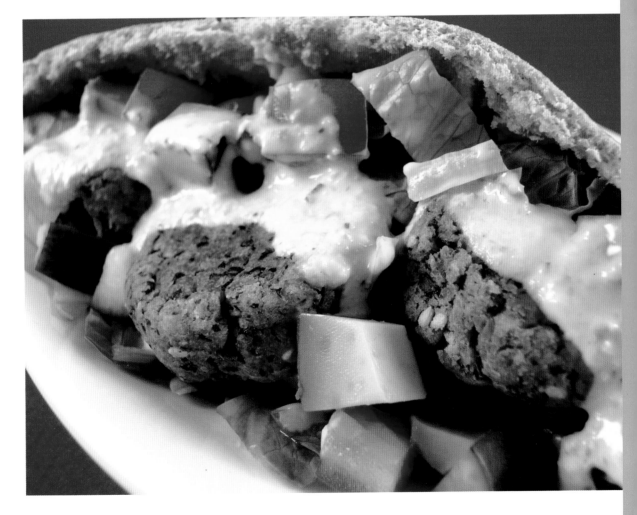

SWEET AND GOLDEN POTATO GRATIN

SERVES 12

Using both Yukon Gold and sweet potatoes, this recipe is a good source of complex carbohydrates and is beneficial for enhancing *qi*. It omits the heavy cream and large amounts of cheese found in traditional gratin recipes.

1½ cups whole milk

½ cup low-sodium vegetable broth

1 clove garlic, minced

¼ teaspoon dried thyme

1 pinch ground nutmeg

1 tablespoon chopped fresh Italian parsley

Preheat oven to 400°F.

In a medium pot over medium-low heat, simmer milk, vegetable broth, garlic, thyme, and nutmeg for 10 to 15 minutes.

Remove from heat and add parsley.

1½ pounds sweet potatoes (about 2 medium potatoes), cut into ⅛-inch slices

1½ pounds Yukon Gold potatoes (about 3 to 4 medium potatoes), cut into ⅛-inch slices

1 teaspoon kosher salt

⅛ teaspoon freshly ground black pepper

In a large bowl, toss sweet potato and Yukon Gold potato slices with salt and black pepper.

½ cup grated Parmigiano Reggiano cheese

½ cup grated Gruyere cheese

In a small bowl, mix together Parmagiano Reggiano and Gruyere cheeses.

2 teaspoons extra-virgin olive oil	Lightly oil the bottom and sides of a 2-quart (13 x 9 x 2") baking dish. Layer half of the potato mixture into the bottom of the dish and sprinkle half of the cheese mixture over top. Then layer the remaining potato mixture and remaining cheese mixture. Pour milk mixture over top. Cover with foil and bake for 30 minutes. Uncover and bake for 25 minutes, or until top of gratin is golden brown.
½ tablespoon chopped fresh Italian parsley (optional)	Cool for 10 minutes before serving. Garnish with parsley if desired.

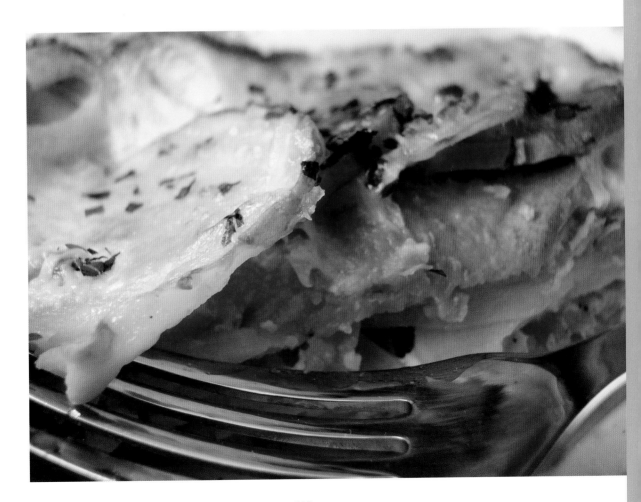

COCONUT CRUSTED FISH

SERVES 4

The sweet, tropical fruit salsa in this recipe tastes best when paired with a mild white fish.

2 mangoes, peeled, seeds removed, and cut into ½-inch chunks

¼ cup diced red bell pepper

1 tablespoon minced shallots

½ of a fresh jalapeño pepper, seeds and membranes removed, minced

2 tablespoons chopped fresh cilantro

⅛ teaspoon kosher salt

1½ tablespoons lime juice

MAKE THE MANGO SALSA:
In a small bowl, toss together mangoes, bell peppers, shallots, jalapeño peppers, cilantro, salt, and lime juice. Allow salsa to sit for 30 minutes so flavors can meld together.

¼ cup dried bread crumbs (or 1 to 2 slices whole-wheat bread, if making from fresh)

¼ cup unsweetened, shredded, dried coconut

2 tablespoons white whole-wheat flour

1 egg

PREPARE THE FISH:
Preheat oven to 425°F.

If making your own bread crumbs, pulse enough bread slices in a food processor (preferable) or blender to measure ½ cup fresh bread crumbs. In a small skillet, toast the bread crumbs over medium heat for 5 minutes until light golden brown, stirring continuously. Let cool. The toasted bread crumbs should measure about ¼ cup.

Mix ¼ cup toasted or store-bought bread crumbs and coconut in a bowl. Place flour in a second bowl and beat egg in a third bowl.

4 fish fillets (such as mahi mahi, snapper, or halibut, about 4 to 6 ounces each)

½ teaspoon kosher salt

1 pinch freshly ground black pepper

Season fish with salt and black pepper, and then dredge in the flour, shaking off any excess. Dip fish into the beaten egg, then coat with the bread crumb and coconut mixture.

1 teaspoon extra-virgin olive oil

In an oven-proof skillet or a regular skillet, heat oil over medium heat. Cook fish until crust is golden brown, about 1 minute on each side.

If using an oven-proof skillet, place skillet directly in the oven. If using a regular skillet, transfer fish to a baking sheet and place in the oven. Bake the fish for 12 to 15 minutes, or until cooked through. (Generally, the cooking time for fish is 8 to 10 minutes per inch of thickness.)

Top with mango salsa before serving.

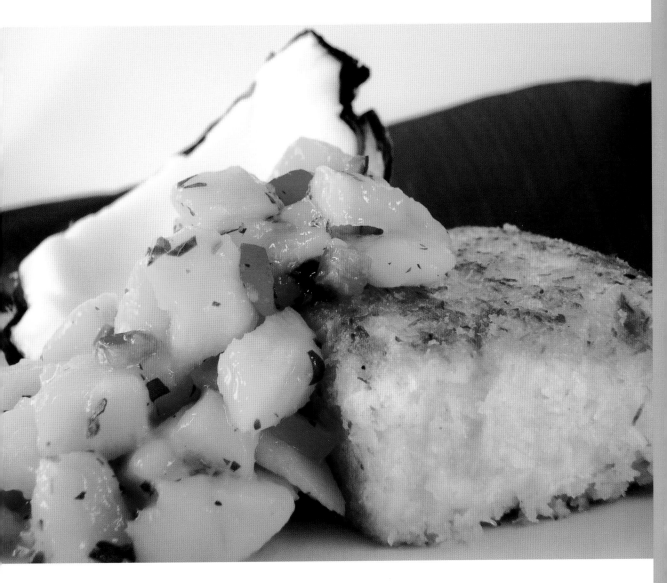

KOREAN CRISPY RICE BOWL

SERVES 2 TO 4

Special equipment: heat-proof stone bowls (optional)

Note: this recipe uses cooked brown rice, which should be prepared beforehand.

---

2 quarts water

1 tablespoon kosher salt

½ cup julienned carrots (about 1 medium carrot)

½ cup mung bean sprouts

½ cup julienned zucchini (about ½ of a small zucchini)

---

1 teaspoon extra-virgin olive oil

1 cup sliced fresh shiitake mushroom caps (about 2 large mushrooms)

1 clove garlic, minced

3 ounces spinach (about 3 cups)

---

1 teaspoon extra-virgin olive oil

2 eggs

---

2 teaspoons extra-virgin olive oil, divided

1½ cups cooked short-grain brown rice, divided

This recipe takes its cue from the classic Korean dish, *bibimbap*, which means "mixed rice" or "mixed meal." Traditionally, this balanced meal of grains, protein, and vegetables is cooked and served in a hot stone bowl.

Prepare a medium bowl of ice water.

In a medium pot, bring 2 quarts of water to a boil over high heat. Add salt and blanch carrots in the boiling water until they are just tender. Remove the carrots and immediately place them in the ice water to stop the cooking process. Drain and pat dry.

Repeat the blanching process with the bean sprouts and zucchini, keeping each group of vegetables separate.

In a small skillet, heat oil over medium heat. Add mushrooms and cook for 2 to 3 minutes, then add garlic and cook for 1 minute. Remove mushrooms and garlic, then add spinach in the same skillet and cook over low heat for 1 to 2 minutes, or until wilted.

Wipe skillet clean and heat oil over medium heat. Pan-fry eggs for 4 to 6 minutes until whites are cooked and yolks begin to set, or until desired doneness.

Use two heat-proof stone bowls, a cast iron skillet, or a nonstick skillet to crisp the rice. If using stone bowls, rub the cooking surface of each bowl with 1 teaspoon oil and add ¾ cup cooked rice to the bottom of each bowl. If using a skillet, coat with 2 teaspoons oil and evenly spread 1½ cups cooked rice on the bottom of the skillet.

Place the stone bowls or skillet on the stove over medium heat for about 8 to 10 minutes, or until the rice starts to sizzle. Occasionally press down on the rice with the back of a spoon so that the rice becomes golden brown and crispy.

Keep the stone bowls or skillet on the stove over medium heat. If using stone bowls, divide the carrots, bean sprouts, zucchini, mushrooms, and spinach between the two bowls and arrange them over top of the rice. If using a skillet, place all of the vegetables over top of the rice in the single skillet. Place the fried eggs over top of the vegetables, cover, and cook for 2 to 3 minutes. Serve hot in the stone bowls or skillet.

⅛ teaspoon sesame oil (optional)

Gochu jang (Korean chili pepper paste) (optional)

If desired, drizzle a small amount of sesame oil over the vegetables and serve with *gochu jang*, a traditional accompaniment to this dish. Use both condiments sparingly as they can be overpowering.

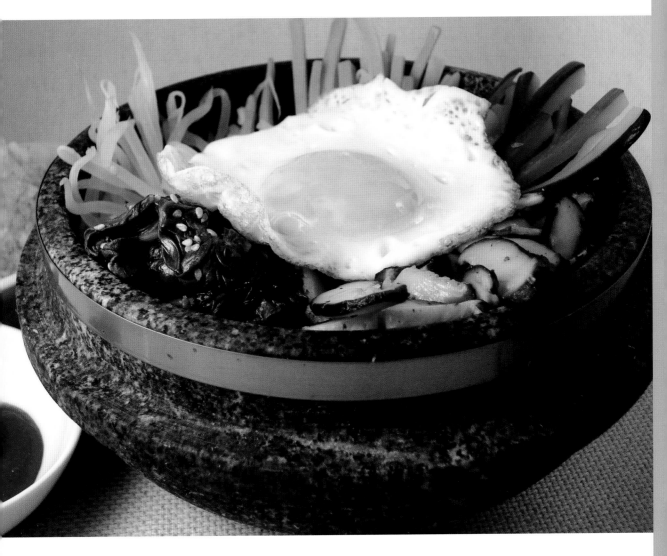

SWEET POTATO BROWN RICE RISOTTO

SERVES 4 TO 6

Note: this recipe uses cooked brown rice, which should be prepared beforehand.

Rice benefits the body by strengthening *qi* and soothing the stomach. This recipe uses whole-grain brown rice instead of the traditional Arborio rice for additional nutrients and fiber. Leftover risotto can be made into *arancini* by forming into balls, coating with bread crumbs and lightly pan-frying over medium heat.

1 pound sweet potatoes or yams, cut into 1-inch chunks (about 2 small potatoes)

⅛ teaspoon kosher salt

⅛ teaspoon freshly ground black pepper

1 tablespoon extra-virgin olive oil

Preheat oven to 375°F.

Place sweet potatoes on a baking sheet and toss with salt, black pepper, and oil. Bake for 15 to 20 minutes, or until sweet potatoes are tender, tossing occasionally.

4 cups low-sodium vegetable broth

In a small pot over medium heat, bring vegetable broth to a simmer. Reduce heat to low and cover.

1 tablespoon extra-virgin olive oil

1½ cups diced yellow onions (about 1 medium onion)

1 clove garlic, minced

In a large, heavy pot, heat oil over medium-low heat. Add onions and cook for 8 minutes or until soft, stirring occasionally. Add garlic and cook for 2 minutes.

3 cups cooked short-grain brown rice

1 pinch ground nutmeg

1 teaspoon kosher salt

⅛ teaspoon freshly ground black pepper

Add cooked brown rice, nutmeg, salt, and black pepper, and stir for 1 minute. Add 1 cup of hot broth and simmer over medium-low heat until broth is absorbed, stirring frequently. Continue to simmer for about 30 minutes while adding broth in ½ cup to 1 cup increments. Allow the risotto to absorb the broth before stirring in the next addition. Continue simmering and stir occasionally until risotto is creamy.

2 tablespoons grated Parmigiano Reggiano cheese

1 tablespoon shaved Parmigiano Reggiano cheese (optional)

1 teaspoon chopped fresh Italian parsley (optional)

Fold roasted sweet potatoes into the risotto. Remove from heat and stir in the grated cheese. Garnish with cheese shavings and chopped parsley, if desired.

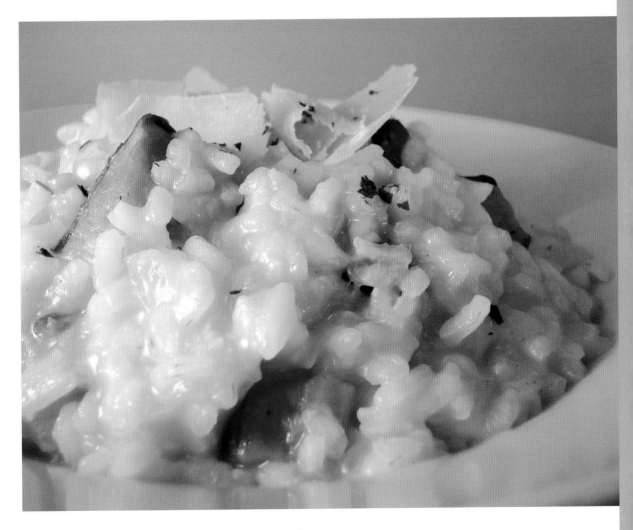

BEEF TAMALE PIE

SERVES 6

In this savory recipe inspired by Mexican tamales, the sweetness of the polenta topping complements the hearty spiced beef and vegetable filling.

½ pound lean ground beef

¾ cup diced yellow onions (about ½ of a medium onion)

MAKE THE FILLING:
In a large, heavy pot, brown ground beef over medium-high heat for 2 minutes. Add onions and cook for 2 minutes.

---

2 cloves garlic, minced

1 teaspoon ground cumin

½ teaspoon ground coriander

1 pinch chipotle chili pepper powder

1 teaspoon kosher salt

⅛ teaspoon freshly ground black pepper

Add garlic, cumin, coriander, chili pepper powder, salt, and black pepper, and cook for 1 minute.

1¾ cups (or one 15-ounce can) cooked black beans

1¾ cups (or one 15-ounce can) cooked pinto beans

1¾ cups (or one 15-ounce can) crushed tomatoes

½ cup (or one-quarter of a 15-ounce can) whole corn kernels, drained

½ cup diced carrots

½ cup diced fresh tomatoes

Drain black and pinto beans, reserving ¾ cup of the bean liquid. Add the black beans, pinto beans, reserved bean liquid, crushed tomatoes, corn, carrots, and fresh tomatoes to the pot. Reduce heat to medium-low, cover, and simmer for 10 minutes, or until the mixture thickens, stirring occasionally.

---

2 tablespoons chopped fresh cilantro

Remove from heat and mix in the cilantro. Pour the filling into a 2-quart (13 x 9 x 2") baking dish.

6 cups water

2 teaspoons kosher salt

2 cups polenta

MAKE THE POLENTA TOPPING AND ASSEMBLE:

Preheat a convection oven to 400°F.

In a medium pot, bring water to a boil over high heat. Add salt and gradually stir in the polenta. Reduce heat to medium and simmer for 20 minutes, until the mixture thickens and the cornmeal is tender, stirring frequently. Be careful of the hot polenta splattering as it bubbles.

Quickly spread polenta over the beef filling. Bake for 20 minutes, or until top is golden brown.

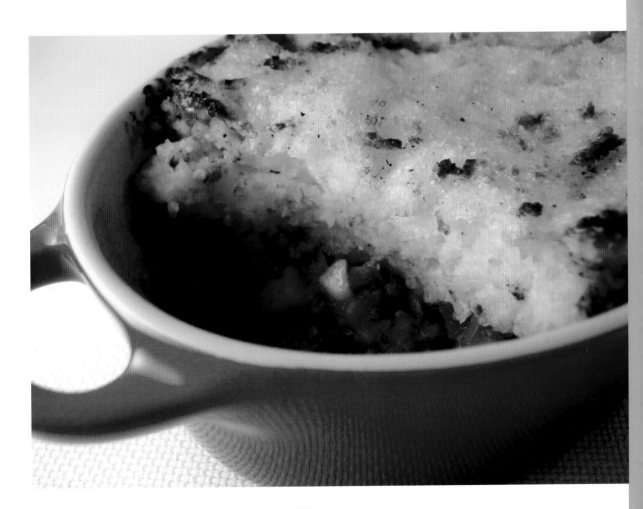

PULLED PORK WITH HONEY GLAZE AND TANGY SLAW

SERVES 6

Slow-roasting the pork for several hours turns a tough and inexpensive cut of meat into a tender and succulent dish. The natural sweetness of the honey has a harmonizing effect on the body and complements the salty and sour flavors in this recipe.

Note: overnight preparation is recommended for this recipe.

---

1 quart water

¾ cup kosher salt

6 tablespoons honey

3 pounds pork shoulder (Boston butt)

PREPARE THE PORK:

In a large bowl, make a brine solution by stirring together the water, salt, and honey until mostly dissolved. Place pork in brine, cover, and refrigerate overnight.

Remove pork from refrigerator 30 minutes prior to cooking, drain, and pat dry.

Preheat oven to 300°F.

Place pork in a medium roasting pan and cover with aluminum foil. Bake covered for 4 hours; baste the pork periodically with its own juices during the last 2 hours. After the pork is tender enough to pull apart easily with a fork, uncover and cook for 20 minutes to caramelize the edges.

---

2 tablespoons honey

1 teaspoon soy sauce

In a small bowl, stir together honey and soy sauce. Glaze the pork with this sauce and bake for 10 minutes. Remove pork from the pan, cover, and set aside to rest for 15 to 20 minutes. Shred pork into large pieces.

---

4 cups shredded green cabbage (about 1 small head)

2 cups shredded red cabbage (about ½ of a small head)

1 carrot, shredded

1 apple, shredded

MAKE THE SLAW:

While the pork rests, combine green cabbage, red cabbage, carrots, and apples in a medium bowl.

2 tablespoons apple cider vinegar

2 teaspoons honey

1 teaspoon soy sauce

1½ teaspoons kosher salt

⅛ teaspoon freshly ground black pepper

2½ tablespoons extra-virgin olive oil

In a small bowl, whisk together vinegar, honey, soy sauce, salt, and black pepper. Add the oil in a steady stream, whisking until emulsified.

¾ teaspoon black sesame seeds

Add dressing to the slaw and toss. Garnish with black sesame seeds and serve with the pulled pork.

GRILLED TERIYAKI SALMON WITH MIXED GRAIN PILAF

SERVES 4

In this simple yet elegant recipe, salmon is glazed with a sweet and salty teriyaki sauce and paired with a nutty, whole-grain pilaf.

Note: overnight preparation is recommended for this recipe.

½ cup wheat berries, rinsed and drained

½ cup short-grain brown rice, rinsed and drained

---

1 tablespoon extra-virgin olive oil

1 cup diced yellow onions (about 1 small onion)

1 clove garlic, minced

¼ cup wild rice, rinsed and drained

½ teaspoon kosher salt

⅛ teaspoon freshly ground black pepper

1¼ cups low-sodium vegetable broth

1¼ cups water

---

1 tablespoon chopped fresh Italian parsley

MAKE THE PILAF:

In a medium bowl, soak the wheat berries and brown rice overnight in enough room temperature water to cover.

In a medium pot, heat oil over medium heat. Add onions and cook for 4 minutes, then add garlic and cook for 1 minute, stirring frequently.

Drain the wheat berries and brown rice, and add them to the pot along with the wild rice, salt, and black pepper. Cook for 1 minute, stirring continuously.

Add broth and water, and bring to a boil over high heat. Reduce heat to medium-low, cover, and simmer for 45 to 60 minutes, or until liquid is absorbed.

Remove from heat, add parsley, and gently fluff with a fork. Do not over-stir or the pilaf will become mushy.

½ cup soy sauce

1½ tablespoons honey

1 teaspoon rice vinegar

1 teaspoon chopped fresh green onions

½ teaspoon finely minced or grated ginger

¼ teaspoon sesame oil

4 salmon fillets, about 4 to 6 ounces each

PREPARE THE SALMON:

In a shallow bowl, make the teriyaki sauce by combining the soy sauce, honey, vinegar, green onions, ginger, and sesame oil. Add salmon and marinate for 30 minutes.

⅛ teaspoon kosher salt

⅛ teaspoon freshly ground black pepper

4 teaspoons extra-virgin olive oil, divided

Remove the fish from the teriyaki marinade, scrape off any excess, and reserve remaining marinade. Season fish with salt and black pepper. Rub each fish fillet with 1 teaspoon oil to prevent it from sticking to the grill and burning. Using an outdoor grill or an indoor grill pan, grill fish over medium heat for about 5 minutes on each side, or until salmon is opaque in the center. (Generally, the cooking time for fish is 8 to 10 minutes per inch of thickness.)

Strain the reserved marinade into a small sauce pan and bring to a boil over high heat. Reduce heat to medium-low and cook for 4 to 5 minutes, or until sauce is slightly thickened.

---

1 tablespoon chopped fresh green onions (optional)

Pour teriyaki sauce over fish. Garnish with green onions before serving, if desired.

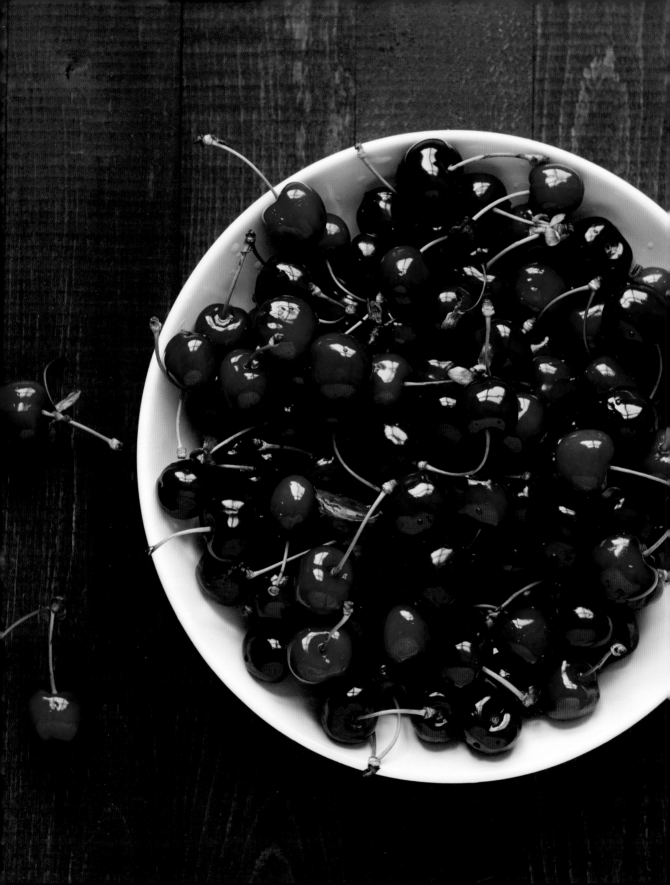

BAKED FRUIT CRUMBLE

SERVES 6

This light and healthy dessert pleases the palate with a combination of sweet and tart flavors. The whole-grain oat and almond topping complements whatever fresh fruit is in season.

---

2 apples, cut into chunks

5 cups fresh fruit (such as berries, plums, or cherries), pitted

3 tablespoons honey

1 teaspoon grated lemon zest

1 tablespoon lemon juice

Preheat oven to 400°F.

In a 2-quart (13 x 9 x 2") baking dish, mix together apples, fresh fruit, honey, lemon zest, and lemon juice.

---

2 cups rolled oats, divided

¼ cup sliced almonds

1 teaspoon ground cinnamon

1 pinch ground nutmeg

1 pinch kosher salt

3 tablespoons honey

2 tablespoons butter, melted

In a food processor (preferable) or blender, pulse ½ cup rolled oats until they reach a coarse meal consistency. In a medium bowl, mix together the ground oats, remaining 1½ cups rolled oats, almonds, cinnamon, nutmeg, and salt.

Add honey and melted butter, and mix until incorporated. Pour oat topping over fruit mixture.

Cover with aluminum foil and bake for 15 minutes. Uncover and bake for 15 minutes, or until topping is golden brown and fruit is bubbling. Allow to cool for 20 minutes before serving.

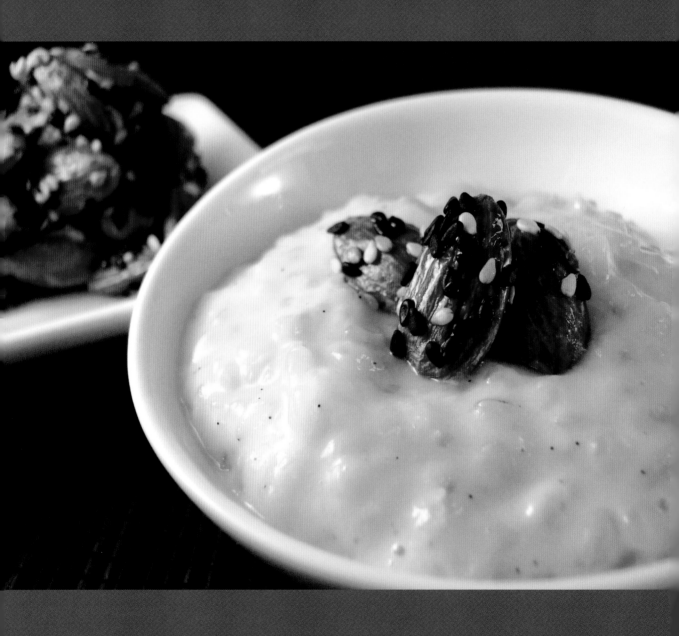

RICE PUDDING WITH *YIN-YANG* ALMONDS

Note: this recipe uses cooked brown rice, which should be prepared beforehand.

---

1 cup raw almonds

2 teaspoons honey

1 teaspoon black sesame seeds

1 teaspoon white sesame seeds

⅛ teaspoon kosher salt

---

2 cups cooked short-grain brown rice

4 cups whole milk

1 cinnamon stick

1 vanilla bean

---

2 tablespoons honey

SERVES 4 TO 6

In this recipe, the crunch of the almonds provides a contrast to the creaminess of the rice pudding. The black and white sesame honey almonds can also be eaten on their own as a healthy snack.

ROAST THE ALMONDS:

Preheat oven to 300°F.

In a small bowl, mix together almonds, honey, black and white sesame seeds, and salt until well incorporated. Spread mixture onto a lightly oiled baking sheet in a thin layer and bake for 20 minutes, tossing occasionally.

MAKE THE PUDDING:

In a medium pot, heat the cooked brown rice, milk, and cinnamon over medium heat. Cut the vanilla bean lengthwise, scrape out the seeds with a paring knife, and add both the seeds and the bean pod to the pot. Simmer for 45 to 60 minutes, stirring occasionally to prevent the mixture from sticking and burning. When the rice pudding is thickened and creamy in texture, remove from heat.

Discard vanilla bean pod and cinnamon stick, and then stir in honey. Serve warm or cold. Garnish with sesame honey almonds.

*Autumn is a second spring when
every leaf is a flower.*
– Albert Camus

Chapter 14
Fall Recipes: drying and bolstering

As the harvest season, fall is represented by a spirit of communal celebration and the giving of thanks. It is a time of change; the weather becomes cool, the skies start to gray, and the trees display their last bursts of color before winter arrives. The fall recipes in this chapter help to warm and invigorate the body, protecting it from external damp and cold.

Drying and aromatic spices play a prominent role in this season's dishes; cinnamon, cloves, cardamom, and nutmeg help to stimulate the body's internal fire. Slower cooking methods like baking, braising, and stewing enhance the flavor of these warming spices and emulate fall's slower pace. The fall recipes emphasize whole grains such as rye, buckwheat, amaranth, and basmati rice, which are especially beneficial for the swollen joints and edema that are common among this body type. Seasonal foods also include kohlrabi, turnips, quince, and the familiar fall staple, pumpkin.

As the cycle of seasons shifts from *yang* to *yin*, fall encourages us to turn inward. Focus centers on the home, and the season's bountiful gifts are shared with family and friends. By emphasizing the fall themes of harvest and storage, we can strengthen our reserves and prepare for the coming winter.

BUTTERNUT SQUASH AND ADZUKI BEAN SOUP

SERVES 4 TO 6

This velvety soup combines sweet squash and adzuki beans with a hint of spice, and is perfect for cool, crisp fall evenings. Commonly used in Asian cooking, adzuki beans have a diuretic effect on the body and are beneficial for reducing edema.

---

6 cups peeled, seeded, and cubed butternut or winter squash (about 1 medium squash)

2 tablespoons extra-virgin olive oil

½ teaspoon kosher salt

⅛ teaspoon freshly ground black pepper

Preheat oven to 375°F.

On a baking sheet, toss together squash, oil, salt, and black pepper, and bake for 15 to 20 minutes. Increase oven temperature to 450°F, toss squash, and bake for 10 minutes to caramelize the edges.

½ cup low-sodium vegetable broth

In a blender (preferable) or food processor, purée 2 cups of the roasted squash pieces with the vegetable broth. Reserve purée and remaining squash pieces.

½ teaspoon extra-virgin olive oil

1 cup diced yellow onions (about 1 small onion)

1 clove garlic, minced

½ teaspoon curry powder

¼ teaspoon ground cumin

In a large pot, heat oil over medium heat. Add onions and cook for 3 minutes, stirring occasionally. Add garlic and cook for 1 minute. Add curry powder and cumin and cook for 1 minute.

---

2 cups low-sodium vegetable broth

¼ cup water

1¾ cups (or one 15-ounce can) cooked adzuki beans, drained

1 teaspoon soy sauce

¾ teaspoon kosher salt

⅛ teaspoon freshly ground black pepper

Add reserved squash purée, reserved roasted squash pieces, vegetable broth, water, adzuki beans, soy sauce, salt, and black pepper. Bring to a boil over high heat. Reduce heat to low, cover, and simmer for 20 minutes.

CHICKEN PAPAYA SOUP

SERVES 4

Sweet papaya and fresh ginger add a unique flavor to this Asian-style chicken soup, a twist on a nourishing and healing tradition.

(DF)

2 teaspoons extra-virgin olive oil

4 chicken thighs, bone-in and skin removed (about 1 to 1½ pounds)

In a large pot, heat oil over medium-high heat. Brown chicken for 2 minutes on each side. Remove chicken from pot and reserve.

---

1 cup sliced yellow onions (about 1 small onion)

1 inch ginger, peeled and sliced

1 teaspoon minced ginger

Reduce heat to medium. Add the onions, sliced ginger, and minced ginger, and cook for 3 minutes, stirring frequently.

---

2 cups low-sodium chicken broth

2 cups water

Deglaze the pot by adding the chicken broth and water and scraping the caramelized bits from the bottom of the pot with a wooden spoon until dissolved.

---

2 celery stalks, cut into chunks

½ teaspoon kosher salt

⅛ teaspoon freshly ground black pepper

Add the reserved chicken, celery, salt, and black pepper, and bring to a boil over high heat. Reduce heat to low, cover, and simmer for 45 minutes or until the chicken is tender. If desired, shred the chicken and discard the bones.

---

1 teaspoon soy sauce

1½ cups barely ripe papaya, peeled, seeded, and cut into 1-inch chunks

Add the soy sauce and papaya. Cook for 5 to 10 minutes, or until papaya is tender but not mushy.

---

1 tablespoon chopped fresh green onions (optional)

Garnish with green onions before serving, if desired.

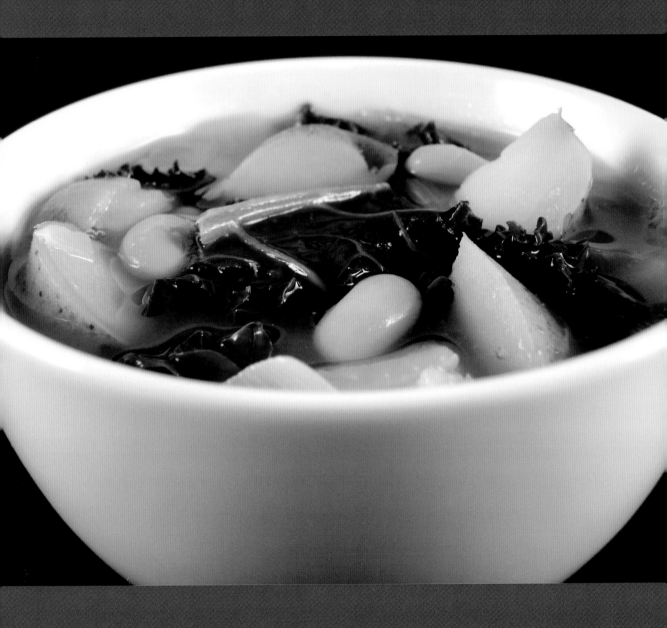

KALE AND WHITE BEAN SOUP

SERVES 4

The lightness of this soup is ideal for the transition between the warm days of Indian summer and the cool nights of fall. Use a ham shank or hock to infuse the broth with a deep, smoky flavor.

½ teaspoon extra-virgin olive oil

1 cup diced yellow onions (about 1 small onion)

In a large pot, heat oil over medium heat. Add onions and cook for 3 minutes until softened.

---

3 cloves garlic, minced

8 ounces smoked ham shank or ham hock

Add garlic and ham shank or ham hock, and cook for 2 minutes, stirring occasionally to prevent garlic from burning.

---

2 cups low-sodium chicken broth

2 cups water

Add chicken broth and water and bring to a boil over high heat. Reduce heat to low, cover, and simmer for 10 minutes.

---

3 medium red potatoes, cut into 1-inch chunks

1¾ cups (or one 15-ounce can) cooked cannellini beans, drained

1 teaspoon chopped fresh rosemary leaves

1 teaspoon kosher salt

⅛ teaspoon freshly ground black pepper

Add potatoes, cannellini beans, rosemary, salt, and black pepper. Cover and simmer for 10 minutes.

---

1 bunch of kale, large stems removed and leaves chopped (about 3 cups)

Add kale, cover, and simmer for 5 minutes.

AMARANTH STUFFED MUSHROOMS

SERVES 4 TO 6

Traditionally eaten in India, Mexico, and Peru, amaranth is high in protein and calcium, and helps to drain excess fluids from the body. With a crunchy texture and nutty flavor, it can also be used as a nutritious filling for stuffed mushrooms.

½ cup low-sodium vegetable broth

½ cup water

½ cup amaranth, rinsed and drained

In a medium pot, bring vegetable broth and water to a boil over high heat. Stir in the amaranth, reduce heat to low, and simmer with lid slightly ajar for 20 minutes, or until liquid is absorbed, stirring occasionally.

½ cup dried bread crumbs, divided (or 2 to 3 slices whole-wheat bread if making from fresh)

½ teaspoon extra-virgin olive oil

If making your own bread crumbs, pulse enough bread slices in a food processor (preferable) or blender to measure 1 cup fresh bread crumbs. In a small skillet, toast the bread crumbs over medium heat for 5 minutes until light golden brown, stirring continuously. Let cool. The toasted breadcrumbs should measure about ½ cup.

Reserve ¼ cup of toasted or store-bought bread crumbs for the stuffing mixture. In a small bowl, mix the remaining ¼ cup of bread crumbs with the oil, and reserve for topping.

10 large mushrooms (such as button, brown, or crimini)

1 teaspoon extra-virgin olive oil

1½ tablespoons minced shallots

3 cloves garlic, minced

2 tablespoons minced kale

Preheat oven to 400°F.

Remove the stems from the mushrooms and keep both the stems and the caps.

To prepare the stuffing mixture, chop the stems into small pieces. In a small skillet, heat oil over medium-low heat. Add chopped mushroom stems, shallots, garlic, and kale, and cook for 2 minutes.

1 tablespoon minced fresh Italian parsley	Remove from heat and stir in the cooked amaranth, ¼ cup reserved bread crumbs, parsley, salt, and black pepper.
½ teaspoon kosher salt	
⅛ teaspoon freshly ground black pepper	

Olive oil cooking spray	Lightly spray a baking sheet with cooking spray. Place mushroom caps cavity-side down on the baking sheet and lightly spray the mushrooms with cooking spray. Turn mushrooms over and season with salt. Fill each mushroom with about 1 tablespoon of the stuffing mixture. Sprinkle reserved ¼ cup bread crumb and oil mixture over top of the stuffed mushrooms.
⅛ teaspoon kosher salt	

Bake for 10 to 15 minutes, or until the topping is golden brown and the mushrooms are just tender. Be careful not to over-bake or the mushrooms will become dry and rubbery.

1 tablespoon minced fresh Italian parsley (optional)	Garnish with parsley before serving if desired.

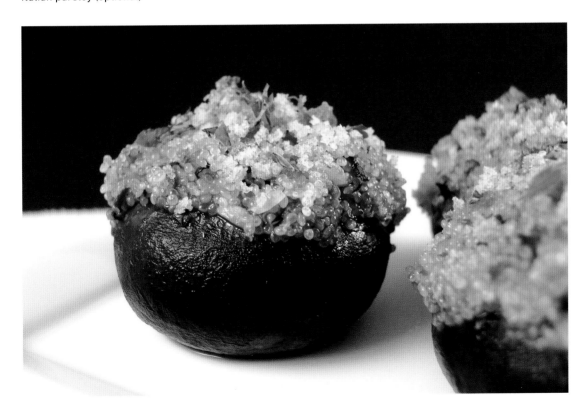

WARM RYE BERRY AND BEAN SALAD

SERVES 4

Note: overnight preparation is recommended for this recipe.

Tender white beans, tart dried cherries, and whole grains offer a contrast of textures and flavors in this recipe. Cherries warm the body and strengthen *qi*, while rye berries reduce edema and excess fluids.

---

1 cup rye berries, rinsed and drained

3 cups water

½ teaspoon kosher salt

¼ cup dried cherries

½ cup water

---

1 teaspoon extra-virgin olive oil

¼ cup minced shallots

¼ cup diced celery

1 cup (or about ½ of a 15-ounce can) cooked cannellini beans, drained

---

2 tablespoons chopped fresh green onions

1 tablespoon chopped fresh Italian parsley

PREPARE THE SALAD:

In a medium pot, soak rye berries in room temperature water overnight.

Add the salt to the rye berries and soaking water and bring to a boil over high heat. Reduce heat to low, cover, and simmer for 1½ hours, or until berries are cooked through. Some berries may split open during cooking.

In a small pot, bring water to a boil over high heat. Remove from heat and soak the dried cherries in the water for 3 minutes, or until soft. Drain and discard the soaking liquid, then roughly chop the cherries and reserve.

In a large skillet, heat oil over medium heat. Add shallots and cook for 1 minute. Add celery and cook for 2 minutes, then add cannellini beans and cook for 3 minutes.

Remove mixture from heat and stir in the cooked rye berries, reserved cherries, green onions, and parsley.

½ tablespoon water

½ teaspoon grated lemon zest

1 tablespoon lemon juice

½ teaspoon kosher salt

⅛ teaspoon freshly ground black pepper

2 tablespoons extra-virgin olive oil

MAKE THE DRESSING:

In a small bowl, combine water, lemon zest, lemon juice, salt, and black pepper. Add oil in a steady stream and whisk together until emulsified. Add dressing to the rye berry mixture and toss until well incorporated.

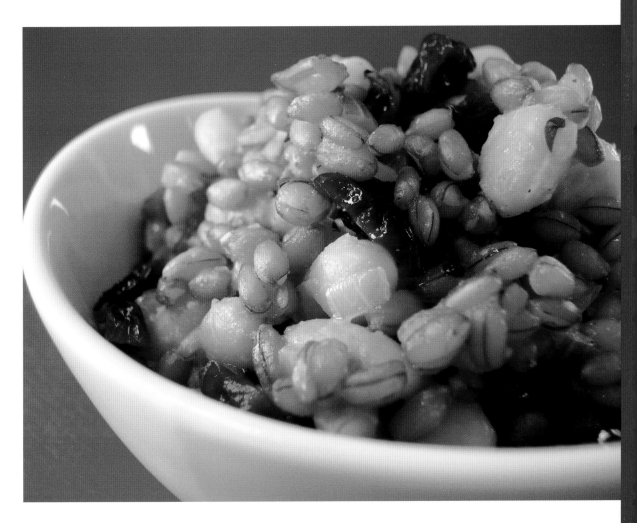

HEARTY TURKEY CHILI

SERVES 6 TO 8

This California-style chili is packed with flavorful vegetables, beans, and spices. If desired, you can substitute the turkey with any other ground meat, or omit it entirely for a meatless version.

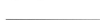

---

1 fresh pasilla pepper

Roast the pasilla pepper briefly over the flame of a gas burner or under the broiler, turning occasionally, so that the skin becomes blackened on all sides. Place the pepper in a paper bag and close. Let sit for 5 minutes or until the skin is soft. Peel off the blackened skin, cut into ½-inch pieces, and reserve.

---

2 teaspoons extra-virgin olive oil

1½ cups diced yellow onions (about 1 medium onion)

1 pound ground turkey

In a large pot, heat oil over medium heat. Add onions and cook for 1 minute. Add the ground turkey and brown for 3 minutes, stirring occasionally.

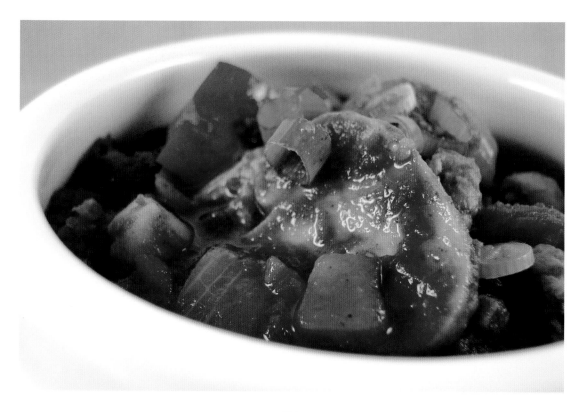

2 cups sliced mushrooms (such as button, brown, or crimini)	Add mushrooms and cook for 4 minutes. Stir in garlic and tomato paste and cook for 1 minute.
3 cloves garlic, minced	
2 tablespoons tomato paste	

1¾ cups (or one 15-ounce can) tomato sauce	Add tomato sauce, stewed tomatoes, beans, broth or water, jalapeño peppers, bay leaves, chili powder, paprika, cumin, oregano, Worcestershire sauce, coriander, red pepper flakes, cayenne pepper, salt, and black pepper. Bring to a boil over high heat. Reduce heat to low, cover, and simmer for 30 minutes.
1¾ cups (or one 14.5-ounce can) stewed tomatoes	
3½ cups (or two 15-ounce cans) cooked beans (such as black, kidney, or garbanzo), drained	
1½ cups low-sodium chicken broth or water	
1 fresh jalapeño pepper, seeds and membranes removed, minced	
2 dried bay leaves	
2 tablespoons chili powder	
1 teaspoon smoked paprika	
1 teaspoon ground cumin	
1 teaspoon dried oregano	
1 teaspoon Worcestershire sauce	
¼ teaspoon ground coriander	
¼ teaspoon crushed red pepper flakes	
1 pinch ground cayenne pepper	
1 teaspoon kosher salt	
⅛ teaspoon freshly ground black pepper	

1¾ cups (or one 15-ounce can) whole corn kernels, drained	Add reserved roasted pasilla peppers, corn, and red and green bell peppers, and simmer for 5 minutes.
½ of a red bell pepper, chopped	
½ of a green bell pepper, chopped	

¼ cup chopped fresh green onions	Remove bay leaves and garnish with green onions.

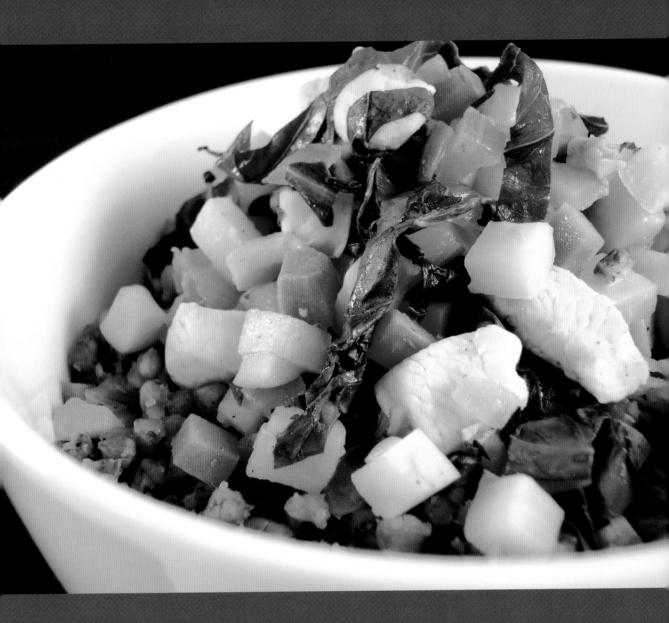

CHICKEN KASHA BOWL

SERVES 4

Kasha, or toasted buckwheat groats, serves as an aromatic base for this quick and simple stir-fry. This recipe uses both the bulb and the leaves of kohlrabi, a vegetable in the cabbage family that has a sweet, broccoli-like flavor.

2 teaspoons extra-virgin olive oil

1 cup medium-cut (cracked) kasha, rinsed and drained

PREPARE THE KASHA:

In a medium pot, heat oil over medium heat. Add kasha and toast for 2 minutes, stirring occasionally to prevent from burning.

1 cup low-sodium vegetable broth

⅛ teaspoon kosher salt

Add vegetable broth and salt and bring to a boil over high heat. Reduce heat to low, cover, and simmer for 10 minutes, or until the liquid is absorbed.

2 teaspoons extra-virgin olive oil

¾ cup diced yellow onions (about ½ of a medium onion)

2 cloves garlic, minced

MAKE THE STIR-FRY:

In a large skillet, heat oil over medium-high heat. Add onions and cook for 1 minute, then add garlic and cook for 1 minute.

1 cup diced mushrooms (such as button, brown, or crimini)

½ cup diced carrots

½ cup diced celery

Add mushrooms, carrots, and celery, and cook for 2 minutes, stirring occasionally.

1 pound boneless, skinless chicken breasts, cut into ½-inch pieces

1 kohlrabi, bulb peeled and diced, stems discarded, and leaves chopped

Add chicken and cook for 2 to 3 minutes, or until cooked through. Add kohlrabi bulb and leaves, and cook for 2 minutes.

½ teaspoon dried thyme

¼ teaspoon dried sage

¾ teaspoon kosher salt

⅛ teaspoon freshly ground black pepper

Add thyme, sage, salt, and black pepper, and cook for 1 minute.

Spoon the stir-fry mixture over top of the kasha before serving.

SOBA NOODLE STIR-FRY

SERVES 4

Common in Japanese cooking, soba noodles are made from buckwheat and can be served hot or cold. In this recipe, they are served hot along with a warming stir-fry of ginger, garlic, and onions to help the body ward off the cold, damp weather of the season.

½ teaspoon soy sauce

¼ teaspoon minced ginger

⅛ teaspoon kosher salt

⅛ teaspoon freshly ground black pepper

8 ounces boneless, skinless chicken breasts, cut into medium-sized pieces

In a medium bowl, mix together soy sauce, ginger, salt, and black pepper.

Add chicken and marinate in refrigerator for 30 minutes.

---

8 ounces dried soba noodles

Prepare soba noodles according to package directions. Drain cooked noodles and rinse them under cold water until the water runs clear. Place the noodles in a bowl of cold water to cover, then reserve.

---

2 teaspoons extra-virgin olive oil

⅓ cup sliced yellow onions (about ¼ of a medium onion)

In a large skillet, heat oil over medium heat. Add onions and cook for 1 minute. Add marinated chicken and cook for 3 minutes.

---

1 cup sliced fresh shiitake mushroom caps (about 2 large mushrooms)

1 clove garlic, minced

½ teaspoon minced ginger

Add mushrooms and cook for 2 minutes, then add garlic and ginger and cook for 1 minute, stirring occasionally.

---

2 baby bok choy, quartered lengthwise

1 celery stalk, sliced diagonally into ½-inch pieces

2 tablespoons low-sodium vegetable broth or water

Add bok choy, celery, and broth or water. Cover and cook for 2 to 3 minutes.

1 tablespoon chopped fresh green onions

1 tablespoon chopped fresh cilantro

1 teaspoon soy sauce

¼ teaspoon kosher salt

⅛ teaspoon freshly ground black pepper

Drain the reserved noodles.

Add the noodles, green onions, cilantro, soy sauce, salt, and black pepper to the skillet. Toss and cook for 1 minute.

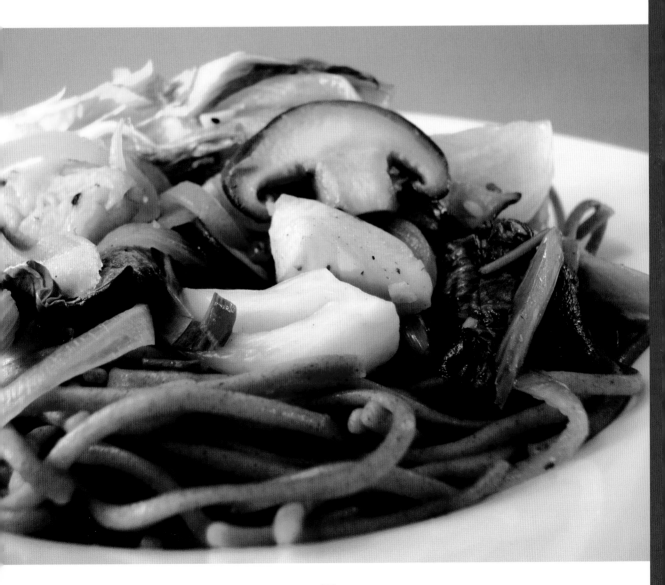

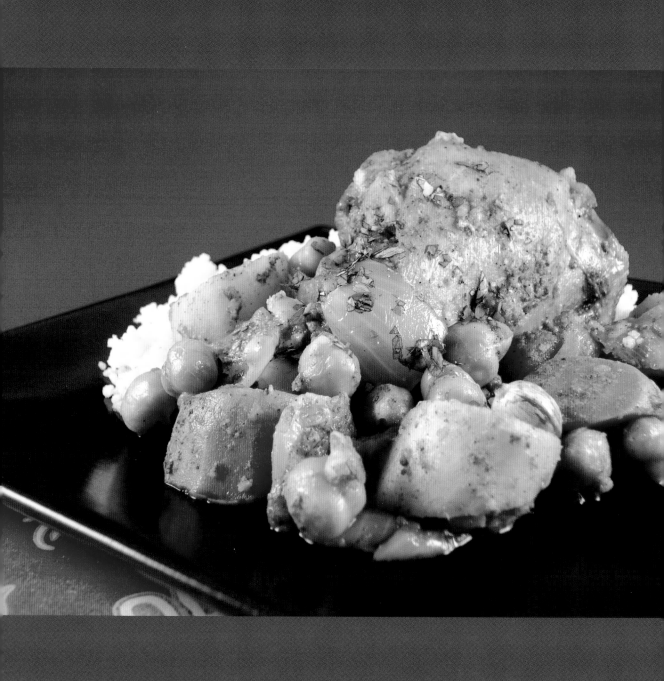

MOROCCAN CHICKEN TAGINE

SERVES 4

Special equipment (optional): tagine pot

A tagine is a slow-cooked stew that is traditionally prepared in a cone-shaped pot. This dish pairs well with couscous, a small, pellet-shaped pasta made from semolina.

---

2 teaspoons extra-virgin olive oil

4 chicken leg pieces (drumsticks or thighs), bone-in and skin removed

In a tagine pot or large skillet, heat oil over medium heat. Brown chicken for 2 minutes on each side. Remove chicken and reserve.

---

1 cup diced yellow onions (about 1 small onion)

2 cloves garlic, minced

Add onions and cook for 3 minutes, then add garlic and cook for 1 minute, stirring occasionally.

---

1 cinnamon stick

1 teaspoon ground cinnamon

3 dried cardamom pods

½ teaspoon ground ginger

¼ teaspoon ground nutmeg

⅛ teaspoon ground cloves

Add cinnamon stick, ground cinnamon, cardamom, ginger, nutmeg, and cloves. Toast the spices for 30 seconds, stirring continuously to prevent them from burning.

---

1 parsnip, cut into 1-inch chunks

1 carrot, cut into 1-inch chunks

1 cup (or about ½ of a 15-ounce can) cooked garbanzo beans, drained

½ cup water

1 teaspoon kosher salt

⅛ teaspoon freshly ground black pepper

Add reserved chicken, parsnips, carrots, garbanzo beans, water, salt, and black pepper, and bring to a boil over high heat. Reduce heat to low, cover, and simmer for 45 to 60 minutes, or until the chicken is tender.

¼ teaspoon *harissa* (North African red pepper sauce)

1 tablespoon chopped fresh Italian parsley (optional)

Mix in *harissa* and simmer uncovered for 2 minutes. Garnish with parsley before serving if desired.

MINI STUFFED PUMPKINS

SERVES 4

Use miniature pumpkins or squash for a visually appealing and edible presentation of this hearty wild-rice stuffing.

1 teaspoon extra-virgin olive oil	In a medium pot, heat oil over medium heat. Cook onions for 4 minutes or until softened. Add garlic and cook for 1 minute, stirring occasionally.
1 cup diced yellow onions (about 1 small onion)	
1 clove garlic, minced	
1 cup short-grain brown rice, rinsed and drained	Stir in the brown rice and wild rice and cook for 1 minute.
½ cup wild rice, rinsed and drained	
2 cups low-sodium vegetable broth	Add vegetable broth, water, mushrooms, rosemary, salt, and black pepper, and bring to a boil over high heat. Reduce heat to low, cover, and simmer for 45 to 55 minutes, or until the liquid is almost absorbed.
1 cup water	
⅛ cup dried mushrooms (such as porcini or shiitake)	
1 teaspoon chopped fresh rosemary leaves	
¾ teaspoon kosher salt	
⅛ teaspoon freshly ground black pepper	
4 miniature pumpkins	While the rice is cooking, preheat oven to 350°F.
¼ teaspoon kosher salt	Cut off the tops of the pumpkins and scrape out the seeds. Separately place pumpkin tops and bottoms on a lightly oiled baking sheet. Season the cavities of the pumpkin bottoms with salt. Bake for 35 minutes.

½ cup chopped kale, large
stems removed

Finish the stuffing by gently stirring the kale into the rice mixture
over low heat. Cook for 4 to 5 minutes. Do not over-stir or the rice will
become mushy.

When pumpkins are done baking, remove pumpkin tops from the
baking sheet and set them aside. Spoon the stuffing mixture into the
pumpkin bottoms. Leftover stuffing can be stored in the refrigerator
for 3 to 5 days.

Place the stuffed pumpkins back into the oven and bake for 20 to
30 minutes, or until the pumpkins are tender and easily pierced with
a paring knife. Serve with pumpkin tops if desired.

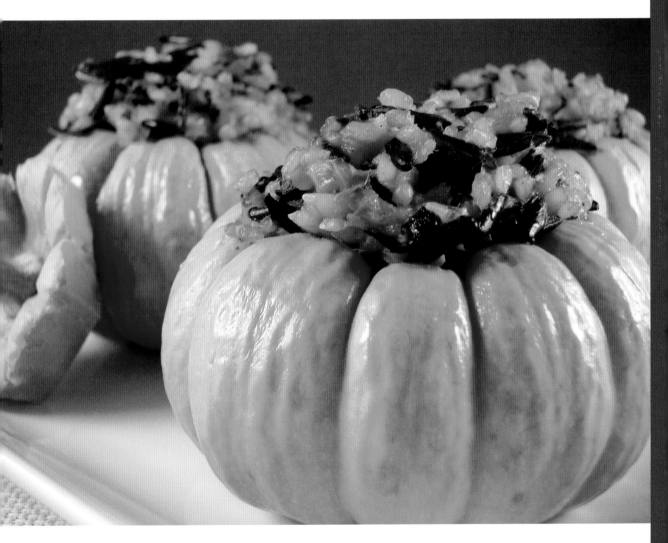

JAMAICAN PORK, BEANS, AND RICE

SERVES 3 TO 4

(DF) (GF)

Note: overnight preparation is recommended for this recipe.

The versatile jerk spice rub in this recipe can be used for pork, chicken, or fish. Adding a side of red beans and whole-grain rice tempers the spiciness of the meat.

½ cup chopped fresh green onions

½ of a fresh scotch bonnet or habañero pepper, seeds and membranes removed

2 cloves garlic

¼ cup packed fresh Italian parsley

1 tablespoon fresh thyme leaves

1 tablespoon lime juice

1 tablespoon lightly packed light brown sugar

1 teaspoon ground allspice

¼ teaspoon ground nutmeg

¼ teaspoon ground cinnamon

⅛ teaspoon ground cloves

½ teaspoon kosher salt

1 pound pork loin

PREPARE THE PORK:

In a food processor (preferable) or blender, blend together green onions, scotch bonnet or habañero peppers, garlic, parsley, thyme, lime juice, brown sugar, allspice, nutmeg, cinnamon, cloves, and salt until mixture becomes a smooth paste.

Place pork in a shallow bowl. Coat with marinade, cover, and refrigerate for 8 hours or overnight.

½ teaspoon extra-virgin olive oil

Remove pork from refrigerator 30 minutes prior to cooking.

Preheat oven to 350°F.

In an oven-proof skillet or a regular skillet, heat oil over medium-high heat. Sear pork for 1 to 2 minutes on each side.

If using an oven-proof skillet, place skillet directly in the oven. If using a regular skillet, transfer pork to a lightly oiled baking sheet and place in the oven. Cover and bake for 15 minutes, or until a meat thermometer inserted into the thickest part of the meat reads 150°F. Remove pork from the oven and allow it to rest covered for 10 minutes. Cut into ¼-inch slices before serving.

½ teaspoon extra-virgin olive oil

½ cup diced yellow onions
(about ½ of a small onion)

1 clove garlic, minced

MAKE THE RICE:

In a medium pot, heat oil over medium heat. Add onions and cook for 3 minutes. Add garlic and cook for 1 minute, stirring occasionally.

½ teaspoon ground allspice

1 cup long-grain brown rice
(such as basmati or jasmine),
rinsed and drained

Add allspice and brown rice and stir for 1 minute.

1 cup water

1 cup low-sodium vegetable broth

3 sprigs fresh thyme

¾ teaspoon kosher salt

1 pinch freshly ground black
pepper

Add water, vegetable broth, thyme, salt, and black pepper, and bring to a boil over high heat. Reduce heat to low, cover, and simmer for 30 minutes.

1¾ cups (or one 15-ounce can)
cooked kidney beans, drained

Gently mix in kidney beans and cook for 15 minutes.

¼ cup chopped fresh green
onions

Add the green onions and fluff the mixture with a fork; do not over-stir or the rice will become mushy. Remove thyme sprigs before serving.

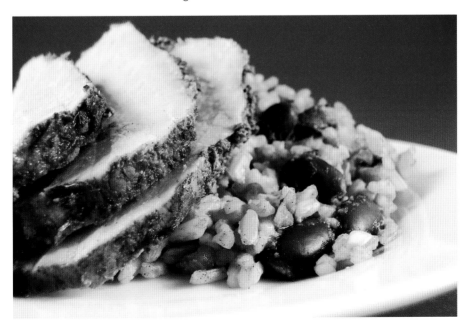

BAKED TANDOORI CHICKEN AND INDIAN-SPICED CAULIFLOWER

SERVES 4 TO 6

Note: overnight preparation is recommended for this recipe.

In this recipe, zesty spices add flavor and pizzazz to everyday ingredients. They are also beneficial for stimulating digestion and warming the body.

1 teaspoon ground ginger

1 teaspoon ground cumin

1 teaspoon ground coriander

1 teaspoon paprika

1 teaspoon ground turmeric

½ teaspoon ground cayenne pepper

1 teaspoon lemon juice

1 teaspoon minced fresh ginger

1 clove garlic, minced

1½ teaspoons kosher salt

6 chicken leg pieces (drumsticks or thighs), bone-in and skin removed

PREPARE THE CHICKEN:

In a shallow medium bowl, mix together ground ginger, cumin, coriander, paprika, turmeric, cayenne pepper, lemon juice, fresh ginger, garlic, and salt.

Add chicken and marinate covered in the refrigerator for 8 hours or overnight.

Remove chicken from refrigerator 30 minutes prior to cooking.

Preheat oven to 500°F.

Place chicken on a lightly oiled baking sheet and cover loosely with foil. Bake covered for 20 minutes, then remove foil and bake for 5 minutes, or until chicken is browned and cooked through.

1 tablespoon extra-virgin olive oil

1 teaspoon yellow mustard seeds

½ teaspoon cumin seeds

½ teaspoon ground cumin

¼ teaspoon ground coriander

1 pinch ground cayenne pepper

2 dried bay leaves

MAKE THE CAULIFLOWER:

In a large pot, heat oil over medium heat. Add mustard seeds, cumin seeds, ground cumin, coriander, cayenne pepper, and bay leaves, and toast for 1 minute, stirring continuously to prevent spices from burning.

1 cup sliced yellow onions (about 1 small onion)	Add onions and water and cook for 2 minutes. Add garlic, ginger, and jalapeño peppers, and cook for 1 minute.
2 tablespoons water	
2 cloves garlic, minced	
1 teaspoon minced fresh ginger	
1 teaspoon minced fresh jalapeño pepper, seeds and membranes removed	

1 cup chopped turnips	Add turnips and vegetable broth. Reduce heat to low, cover, and simmer for 5 minutes.
½ cup low-sodium vegetable broth	

2¼ cups chopped russet potatoes (about 1 large potato)	Add potatoes, cauliflower, turmeric, garam masala, red pepper flakes, salt, and black pepper. Cover and cook for 15 minutes, or until turnips are tender.
5 cups cauliflower florets (about 1 head of cauliflower)	
¼ teaspoon ground turmeric	
¼ teaspoon garam masala	
⅛ teaspoon crushed red pepper flakes	
1½ teaspoons kosher salt	
⅛ teaspoon freshly ground black pepper	

2 tomatoes, chopped	Remove from heat and mix in tomatoes and cilantro. Remove bay leaves before serving.
1 tablespoon packed chopped fresh cilantro	

LENTIL CURRY

SERVES 4

Herbs and spices are infused into this seasonal duo of lentils and cauliflower for a hearty vegan meal. Brown basmati rice serves as an ideal accompaniment to this dish.

2 teaspoons extra-virgin olive oil

1½ cups diced yellow onions (about 1 medium onion)

In a medium pot, heat oil over medium heat. Add onions and cook for 1 minute.

3½ teaspoons curry powder

1 teaspoon kosher salt

1 dried bay leaf

1 cup dried green lentils, rinsed and drained

2 cups low-sodium vegetable broth

½ cup water

Add curry powder, salt, bay leaf, lentils, vegetable broth, and water, and bring to a boil over high heat. Reduce heat to low, cover, and simmer for 30 to 40 minutes, or until the lentils are just tender.

2 cups cauliflower florets

Add cauliflower, cover, and simmer for 10 minutes.

1 teaspoon extra-virgin olive oil

2 teaspoons minced fresh jalapeño or serrano pepper, seeds and membranes removed

2 teaspoons cumin seeds

2 cloves garlic, minced

1 teaspoon minced ginger

While the cauliflower is cooking, heat oil in a small skillet over medium-high heat. Add jalapeño or serrano peppers, cumin seeds, garlic, and ginger, and toast for 1 minute, stirring continuously to prevent spices from burning.

Add toasted spices to the lentils and cauliflower, and cook uncovered for 5 minutes so that the flavors meld together.

1 teaspoon lemon juice

3 teaspoons chopped fresh cilantro, divided

Remove the bay leaf and stir in the lemon juice and 2 teaspoons of cilantro. Garnish with remaining 1 teaspoon of cilantro before serving.

PUMPKIN AMARANTH MUFFINS

MAKES 9 TO 12 MUFFINS

Special equipment: muffin pan, cupcake liners (optional)

With a hint of spice, these seasonal muffins are perfect for a sweet snack or a breakfast treat.

Olive oil cooking spray (optional)

Preheat oven to 375°F.

Spray muffin pan with a small amount of cooking spray, or use cupcake liners and omit oil.

1 cup (or about ⅓ of a 15-ounce can) pumpkin purée

½ cup extra-virgin olive oil

2 eggs

1 teaspoon grated orange zest

¼ cup plus 1 tablespoon orange juice

½ cup lightly packed light brown sugar

1 teaspoon vanilla extract

In a medium bowl, mix together pumpkin purée, oil, eggs, orange zest, orange juice, brown sugar, and vanilla.

1⅓ cups white whole-wheat flour

⅔ cup amaranth flour

1 teaspoon baking soda

1½ teaspoons ground cinnamon

½ teaspoon ground nutmeg

½ teaspoon ground ginger

⅛ teaspoon ground cloves

⅛ teaspoon kosher salt

In a large bowl, mix together white whole-wheat flour, amaranth flour, baking soda, cinnamon, nutmeg, ginger, cloves, and salt.

Add pumpkin mixture to flour mixture and stir until just combined.

½ cup chopped raw walnuts, divided

Reserve two tablespoons of walnuts for the topping. Stir the remaining walnuts into the batter and spoon it into the prepared muffin pan. Sprinkle the reserved walnuts over top.

Bake for 20 to 25 minutes, or until a toothpick inserted into the center of a muffin comes out clean. Let muffins cool for 5 minutes, then remove from pan.

269

PEAR, QUINCE, AND APPLE TART

SERVES 6 TO 8 (MAKES ONE 8-INCH TART)

Special equipment:
8-inch tart pan

Quince is a pear-shaped fruit that is seasonally available in the fall. Its tart flavor complements the sweetness from the pear, apple, and chewy almond crust in this simple, elegant dessert.

Olive oil cooking spray

MAKE THE CRUST:
Lightly coat an 8-inch tart pan with cooking spray.

1½ cups blanched or raw almonds

1 pinch kosher salt

In a food processor, pulse almonds and salt until they reach a coarse consistency.

Heaping ¼ cup chopped dried and pitted dates

Add dates to the ground almonds and pulse until the mixture is uniform. The crust mixture should stick together when you squeeze it into a ball; if necessary, gradually add more dates and pulse again. Firmly press the crust mixture into the tart pan in an even layer.

1 apple (such as Golden Delicious or Granny Smith), peeled, cored, and halved

1 Bosc pear, peeled, cored, and halved

1 quince, peeled, cored, and halved

⅛ teaspoon lemon juice

MAKE THE FILLING:
In a small bowl, coat one-half of each fruit with lemon juice to prevent the fruit from turning brown, and reserve. Cut the other halves of the fruit into ½-inch pieces for the filling.

¼ cup water

½ teaspoon lemon juice

½ tablespoon packed light brown sugar

¼ teaspoon ground cinnamon

1 pinch ground cloves

1 pinch ground nutmeg

¼ teaspoon vanilla extract

In a small skillet over medium heat, add apple, pear, and quince pieces with water, lemon juice, brown sugar, cinnamon, cloves, nutmeg, and vanilla, and bring to a simmer. Reduce heat to low, cover, and cook for 20 minutes.

In a food processor or blender, purée the fruit mixture until it reaches a sauce-like consistency with some small pieces remaining. Spread the fruit sauce over the crust in a thin layer.

Preheat oven to 350°F.

Cut the reserved halves of the fruit into ¼-inch slices. Arrange the slices in an overlapping circle over top of the fruit sauce.

½ teaspoon ground cinnamon ½ teaspoon packed light brown sugar	Mix together cinnamon and brown sugar and sprinkle over top of the fruit. Cover the tart with aluminum foil and bake for 20 minutes. Uncover and bake for 10 to 15 minutes, or until the fruit is tender and the crust is golden brown. Allow the tart to cool before unmolding.
2 tablespoons apricot jam (optional)	If desired, briefly heat up apricot jam until liquid and brush it over top of the sliced fruit as a glaze.

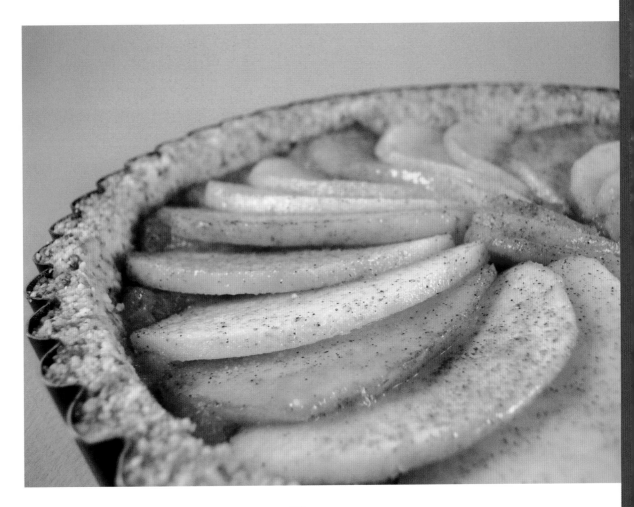

The color of springtime is in the flower.
The color of winter is in the imagination.
– Ward Elliot Hour

Chapter 15
Winter Recipes: warming and nourishing

As the cycle of seasons slowly comes to its end, the Earth withdraws into a cold, deep *yin*. The stark, barren landscape of winter displays a quiet peace; this is a time of rest and reflection. Taking shelter from the bitter elements, we retreat into the warmth of our homes and are comforted by the aroma of slow-cooked soups, stews, and roasts.

Winter's harsh environment does not support the delicate, tender greens that are available in warmer seasons. Instead, sustenance comes from hardy root vegetables grown within the earth. The following recipes make use of seasonal vegetables like turnips, fennel, and parsnips, as well as foods that are rich in complex carbohydrates like winter squash and chestnuts. To nourish and protect the body from the external cold, these hearty dishes also incorporate animal protein sources like lamb, chicken, and shrimp. In addition, members of the onion family and spices like pepper, rosemary, thyme, and cloves are used to boost flavor and provide warmth.

With its short days, long nights, and gray skies, winter sets a tone of introspective meditation. The season encourages us to reflect on the events of the past year and gain insight from our experiences. However harsh winter's decline may be, it is never permanent. As with any cycle, the end also serves as a transition to a new beginning. Winter offers us the opportunity to slow down and conserve, as we once again await the arrival of spring and look forward to a new year ahead.

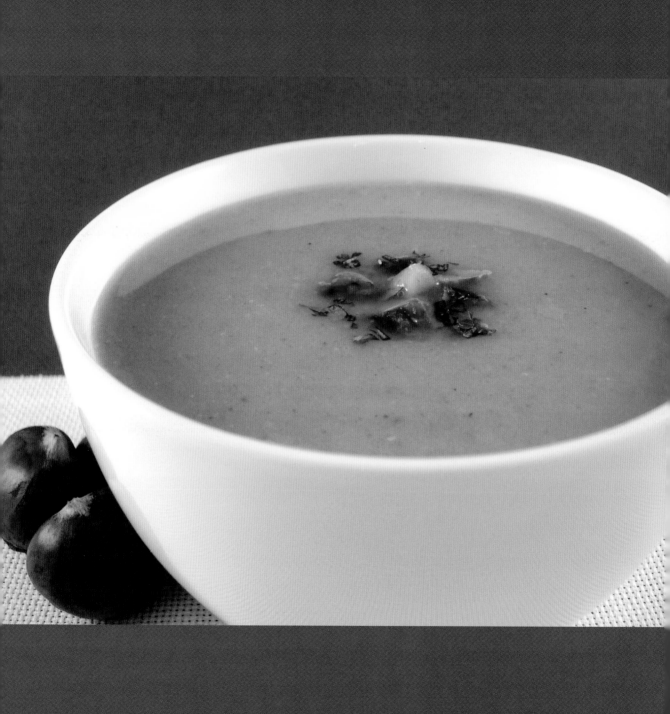

CREAMY CHESTNUT SOUP

SERVES 4 TO 6

This rich, velvety soup is a great starter to any winter meal. Although roasting fresh chestnuts takes a bit of time, the result is well worth the effort. For a vegan alternative, substitute the chicken broth in this recipe with vegetable broth.

---

3 cups raw chestnuts or 1½ cups cooked, peeled, and chopped chestnuts

If roasting the chestnuts yourself, preheat oven to 450°F. Score an "X" on the outside of each chestnut with a knife. Place the chestnuts on a baking sheet and roast for 20 to 30 minutes, or until the chestnut meat is tender and the shells begin to split open. Allow chestnuts to cool, then crack and peel, being sure to remove the inner skin.

Chop the cooked chestnuts to yield 1½ cups. Reserve 1 to 2 tablespoons of chestnuts for garnish, if desired.

---

1 teaspoon extra-virgin olive oil

½ cup chopped white onions (about ½ of a small onion)

½ cup chopped leeks, white parts, rinsed thoroughly (about 1 medium leek)

1 clove garlic, minced

In a medium pot, heat oil over medium heat. Add onions and cook for 2 minutes. Add leeks and garlic and cook for 2 minutes.

---

2 cups low-sodium chicken broth or vegetable broth

1½ cups water

¾ cup peeled and chopped red potatoes (about 1 medium potato)

1 dried bay leaf

3 sprigs fresh Italian parsley

1 sprig fresh thyme

1¼ teaspoons kosher salt

⅛ teaspoon freshly ground black pepper

Add roasted chestnuts, broth, water, potatoes, bay leaf, parsley, thyme, salt, and black pepper, and bring to a boil over high heat. Reduce heat to low, cover, and simmer for 20 minutes.

Remove from heat and discard bay leaf, parsley, and thyme. Purée the soup. If using an immersion blender, the soup can be directly blended in the cooking pot. If using a countertop blender, purée the soup in small batches and combine before serving. Add additional broth or water if necessary to achieve desired consistency.

---

1 tablespoon chopped fresh Italian parsley (optional)

Garnish with reserved chopped chestnuts and Italian parsley, if desired.

CHINESE CHICKEN PORRIDGE

SERVES 4

Creamy rice porridge has been eaten for centuries in Asian cultures and is also known as *jook* or congee. Traditionally, this porridge is made with white rice, though you can also use whole-grain brown rice, as suggested here. Considered to have warming and healing properties, this slow-cooked soup is a nice alternative to the traditional chicken noodle and is perfect for cold winter mornings.

(DF)

Note: this recipe uses cooked brown rice, which should be prepared beforehand.

---

4 cups water

8 ounces boneless, skinless chicken breasts

½ teaspoon kosher salt

In a large pot, bring water to a boil over high heat. Add chicken and salt, reduce heat to low, cover, and poach the chicken for 10 to 15 minutes. Remove chicken from liquid, let cool, and reserve in the refrigerator. Strain 2 cups of the poaching liquid for cooking the congee and discard the remaining liquid.

---

2 cups low-sodium chicken broth

2 cups cooked short-grain brown rice

½ inch ginger, peeled and sliced

½ teaspoon kosher salt

½ teaspoon soy sauce

In the same pot, add the 2 cups of poaching liquid, chicken broth, cooked rice, ginger, and salt, and bring to a boil over high heat. Reduce heat to low, cover, and simmer for 2 ½ hours, stirring occasionally.

Shred the reserved chicken into bite-sized pieces. Add the chicken and soy sauce to the porridge, and cook uncovered for 45 to 60 minutes. Stir regularly and scrape the bottom of the pot to prevent the rice from sticking.

---

2 tablespoons chopped fresh green onions, divided

1 tablespoon chopped fresh cilantro, divided

¼ cup roasted, salted peanuts (optional)

Remove from heat and stir in 1 tablespoon of green onions and ½ tablespoon of cilantro. Garnish with remaining 1 tablespoon of green onions and ½ tablespoon of cilantro before serving. Garnish with peanuts if desired.

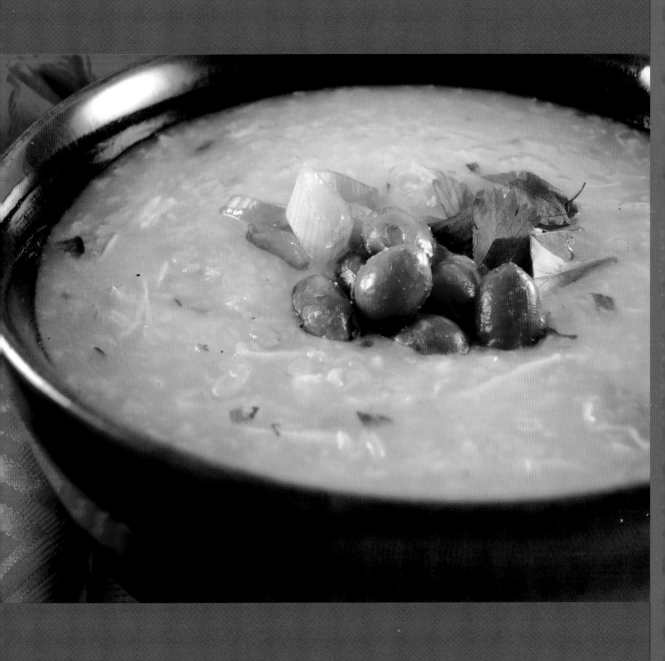

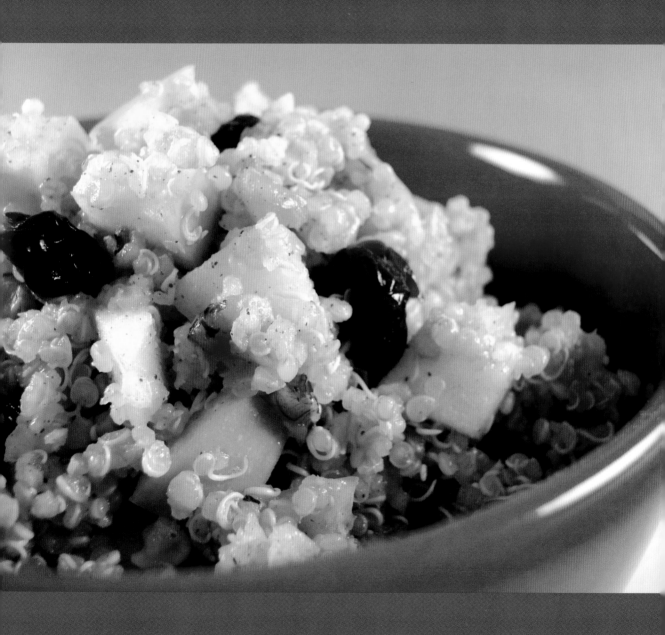

WARM QUINOA AND APPLE SALAD

SERVES 4

Originally cultivated in South America, quinoa is a seed with a high protein content and a slightly crunchy texture. It serves as the base for this warm winter salad of tart cherries, crisp apples, and toasted walnuts.

---

2 cups water

¼ teaspoon kosher salt

1 cup quinoa, rinsed and drained

PREPARE THE SALAD:

In a medium pot, bring the water to a boil over high heat. Add salt and quinoa, reduce heat to low, cover, and simmer for 15 minutes, or until liquid is almost absorbed.

¼ cup dried cherries

¼ cup water

While the quinoa is cooking, heat the water in a small pot over high heat until just boiling. Remove from heat and soak the cherries for 5 minutes. Drain and discard soaking liquid, then cut cherries in half.

---

1 green apple, diced

1 teaspoon lemon juice

In a medium bowl, toss the cherries with the apples and lemon juice.

½ teaspoon grated lemon zest

2 tablespoons lemon juice

½ teaspoon ground cinnamon

1 pinch ground nutmeg

½ teaspoon kosher salt

1 pinch freshly ground black pepper

¼ cup extra-virgin olive oil

MAKE THE DRESSING:

In a small bowl, whisk together lemon zest, lemon juice, cinnamon, nutmeg, salt, and black pepper. Add the oil in a steady stream, whisking until emulsified.

½ cup chopped toasted walnuts

ASSEMBLE THE SALAD:

Add quinoa, dressing, and walnuts to the cherry and apple mixture, and toss together. Serve warm or at room temperature.

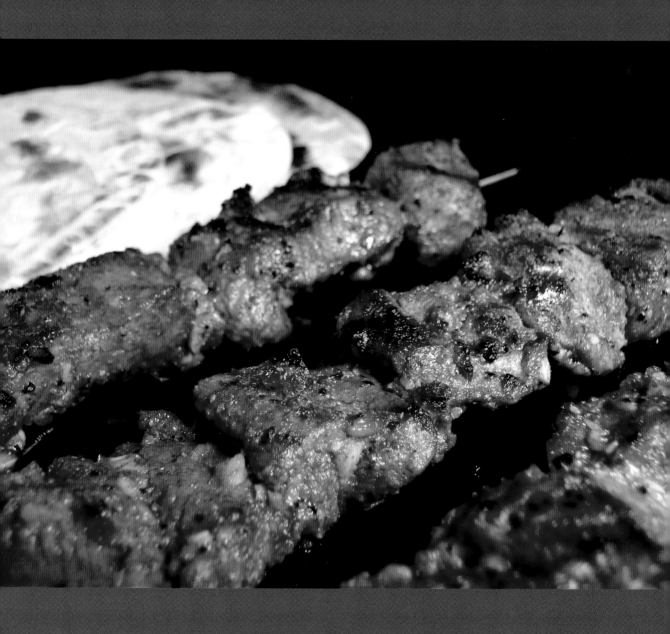

MOROCCAN SPICED LAMB SKEWERS

SERVES 4

Special equipment: four wooden or metal skewers

Note: overnight preparation is recommended for this recipe.

Throw these warming skewers on the grill and serve them as a quick appetizer, or pair them with flatbread, couscous, or caramelized onions for an easy meal. The vibrant spice blend also works nicely on chicken or beef.

2 tablespoons extra-virgin olive oil

½ tablespoon grated lemon zest

2 tablespoons lemon juice

3 cloves garlic, minced

1 teaspoon ground cumin

1 teaspoon paprika

½ teaspoon ground coriander

¼ teaspoon ground cinnamon

1½ teaspoons kosher salt

1 teaspoon freshly ground black pepper

1 pound lamb (loin or leg), de-boned and cut into 1½-inch pieces

In a medium bowl, mix together oil, lemon zest, lemon juice, garlic, cumin, paprika, coriander, cinnamon, salt, and black pepper to make a paste.

Add the lamb pieces, coat, cover, and marinate in the refrigerator for 8 hours or overnight.

Cooking spray or vegetable oil

Remove lamb from refrigerator 30 minutes prior to cooking.

If using wooden skewers, soak them in enough water to cover for 10 minutes to prevent them from burning on the grill. Thread the marinated lamb pieces onto the skewers.

Spray outdoor grill or indoor grill pan with cooking spray, or wipe with oil. Grill skewers over medium heat for 2 to 3 minutes on each side, or until lamb is cooked to your desired doneness.

GARLIC SHRIMP WITH ROSEMARY QUINOA

SERVES 4

This recipe combines the warming effect of garlic and rosemary with the *yang*-nourishing properties of shrimp and quinoa.

(GF)

2 cups water

¼ teaspoon kosher salt

1 sprig fresh rosemary

1 cup quinoa, rinsed and drained

---

1 teaspoon extra-virgin olive oil

1 teaspoon chopped fresh rosemary leaves

¼ teaspoon kosher salt

1 pinch freshly ground black pepper

---

2 teaspoons extra-virgin olive oil

½ cup diced yellow onions (about ½ of a small onion)

5 cloves garlic, minced

---

1 pound shrimp (about 28 extra-large shrimp), peeled and de-veined

¼ teaspoon kosher salt

⅛ teaspoon freshly ground black pepper

1 teaspoon butter

MAKE THE QUINOA:

In a medium pot, bring water to a boil over high heat. Add salt, rosemary sprig, and quinoa. Reduce heat to low, cover, and simmer for 15 minutes, or until liquid is almost absorbed. Remove from heat and remove rosemary sprig.

In a medium skillet, heat oil over medium-low heat. Add chopped rosemary and cook for 1 minute. Add cooked quinoa, salt, and black pepper, and cook for 1 minute.

PREPARE THE SHRIMP:

In a medium skillet, heat oil over medium heat. Add onions and cook for 1 minute, then add garlic and cook for 1 minute.

Add the shrimp and cook for 1 to 2 minutes on each side, or until just cooked through. Remove from heat. Add salt, black pepper, and butter to coat.

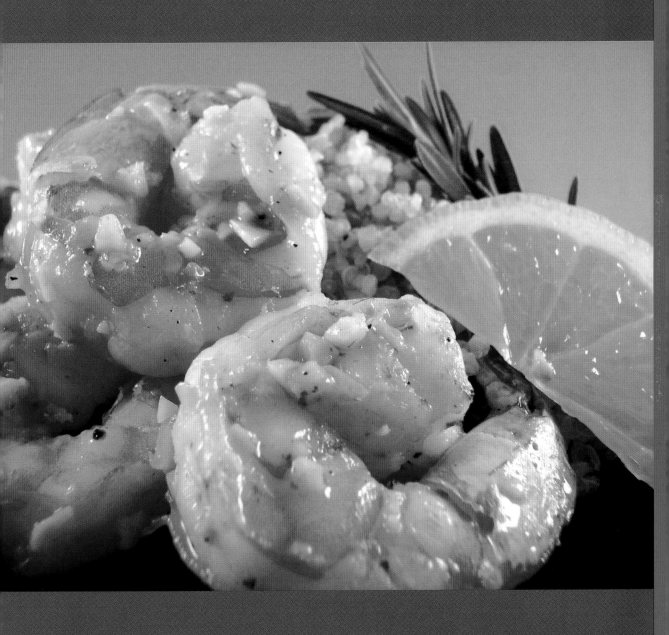

BEEF AND CHERRY STIR-FRY

SERVES 4 TO 6

In this recipe, dried cherries add a sweet and tart flavor to thinly sliced beef, peppers, and onions. The warming thermal nature of these ingredients helps the body to defend against the cold of the season. Serve this dish over rice, or with warmed tortillas for an Asian-style fajita.

½ teaspoon extra-virgin olive oil

1 tablespoon chopped shallots

1 teaspoon minced ginger

1 clove garlic, minced

1 fresh serrano pepper, seeds and membranes removed, minced

PREPARE THE BEEF:
In a small skillet, heat oil over medium heat. Add shallots, ginger, garlic, and serrano peppers, and cook for 1 minute.

½ cup water

⅓ cup dried cherries

Reduce heat to low, add the water and dried cherries, cover, and cook for 10 minutes.

⅓ cup water

1 pinch kosher salt

½ teaspoon soy sauce

1 pound beef sirloin, cut into ¼-inch strips

In a blender (preferable) or food processor, purée the cooked cherry mixture with the water, salt, and soy sauce.

In a medium bowl, coat the beef strips with 4 tablespoons of the cherry purée and marinate for 30 minutes. Reserve the remaining cherry purée.

½ cup dried cherries

½ cup water

MAKE THE STIR-FRY:
While the beef is marinating, heat the water in a small pot over high heat until just boiling. Remove from heat and soak the dried cherries in the water for 15 minutes, then drain and discard the water.

2 teaspoons extra-virgin olive oil

1 cup sliced yellow onions (about 1 small onion)

1 teaspoon minced ginger

1 clove garlic, minced

In a large skillet, heat oil over medium-high heat. Add the onions and cook for 2 minutes. Add the ginger and garlic and cook for 1 minute.

1 red bell pepper, cut into ¼-inch strips

1 green bell pepper, cut into ¼-inch strips

1½ teaspoons soy sauce

1 teaspoon kosher salt

⅛ teaspoon freshly ground black pepper

¼ cup chopped fresh green onions

Add marinated beef and cook for 3 minutes, or until the meat is browned. Add red and green bell peppers and cook for 1 minute. Add reserved cherry purée, soaked cherries, soy sauce, salt, and black pepper, and cook for 1 minute.

Remove from heat and add green onions.

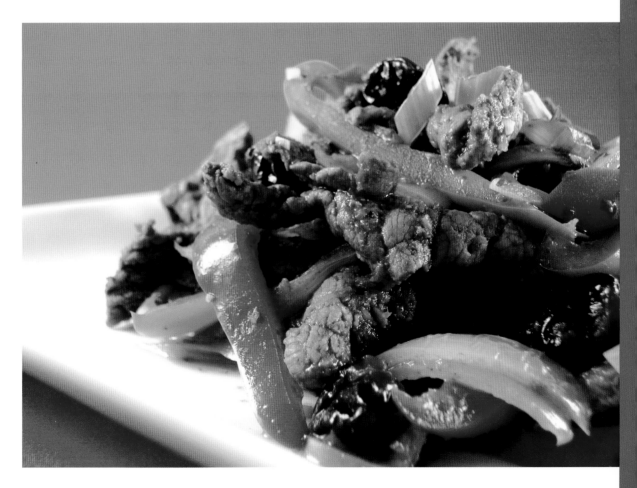

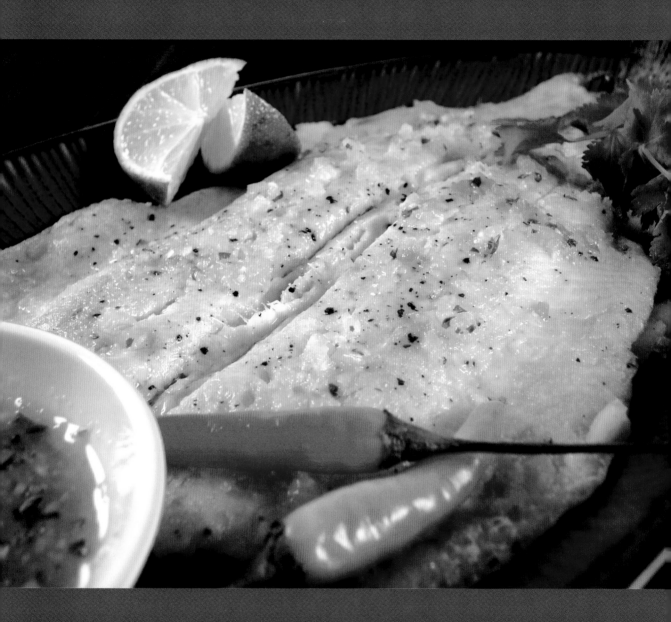

TROUT WITH SWEET CHILI SAUCE

SERVES 3 TO 4

Whole, butterflied trout fillets are pan-fried in this Thai-inspired recipe. Using agave nectar in the sauce adds a mild sweet flavor that balances the spicy chilies and tangy lime juice.

2 tablespoons minced shallots

1 clove garlic, minced

1 fresh Thai chili pepper, seeds and membranes removed, minced

¼ teaspoon minced ginger

⅛ teaspoon kosher salt

2 tablespoons water

1 teaspoon lime juice

2 teaspoons agave nectar

2 teaspoons water

½ teaspoon chopped fresh cilantro

2 teaspoons extra-virgin olive oil, divided

2 trout, about 10 to 12 ounces each, butterflied and heads removed

½ teaspoon kosher salt

⅛ teaspoon freshly ground black pepper

MAKE THE CHILI SAUCE:

In a large skillet over medium-low heat, add shallots, garlic, chili peppers, ginger, salt, and water and cook for 2 minutes.

In a blender (preferable) or food processor, blend together the cooked shallot mixture, lime juice, agave nectar, water, and cilantro.

PREPARE THE TROUT:

Wipe the skillet clean and heat 1 teaspoon oil over medium-high heat. Season both sides of the trout with salt and black pepper. Pan-fry one trout flesh-side down for 3 minutes. Carefully flip trout over and pan-fry it skin-side down for 3 minutes, or until cooked through. Remove trout from skillet. Repeat with remaining 1 teaspoon oil and remaining trout.

Serve the chili sauce over top of the trout or on the side.

HEARTY VEGETABLE CASSOULET

SERVES 4

Even without the sausage or other meats found in traditional versions of this French dish, this vegetable stew is quite warming. Slowly cooking the stew in the oven allows its flavors to meld together with the crust of herbs and bread crumbs.

---

1 tablespoon extra-virgin olive oil

1½ cups chopped yellow onions (about 1 medium onion)

12 medium mushrooms (such as button, brown, or crimini), halved

3 cloves garlic, minced

Preheat oven to 350°F.

In a large, oven-proof pot, heat oil over medium heat. Add onions and cook for 2 minutes. Add mushrooms and cook for 1 minute, then add garlic and cook for 1 minute.

½ cup low-sodium vegetable broth

Deglaze the pot by adding the vegetable broth and scraping the caramelized bits from the bottom of the pot with a wooden spoon until dissolved.

---

2 medium carrots, cut into 1-inch chunks

1 celery stalk, cut into 1-inch chunks

2 small turnips, cut into 1-inch chunks

2 dried bay leaves

1 teaspoon fresh thyme leaves

1¼ teaspoons kosher salt

⅛ teaspoon freshly ground black pepper

Add carrots, celery, turnips, bay leaves, thyme, salt, and black pepper, and cook for 5 minutes.

1¾ cups (or one 15-ounce can) cooked white beans, drained

1½ cups low-sodium vegetable broth

Add beans and vegetable broth and bring to a boil over high heat. Remove from heat.

¾ cup dried bread crumbs
(or 3 to 4 slices whole-wheat
bread if making from fresh)

¼ teaspoon chopped fresh
thyme leaves

2 teaspoons chopped fresh
Italian parsley

2 teaspoons extra-virgin olive oil

1 pinch kosher salt

If making your own bread crumbs, pulse enough bread slices in a
food processor (preferable) or blender to measure 1½ cups fresh bread
crumbs.

In a small bowl, mix the 1½ cups fresh bread crumbs or ¾ cup store-
bought bread crumbs with thyme, parsley, oil, and salt. Sprinkle the
herbed bread crumbs over the vegetables to cover.

Place the oven-proof pot in the oven and bake uncovered for 60 to
75 minutes, or until the vegetables are tender. The bread crumbs
should be golden brown and most of the liquid should be absorbed.
Remove bay leaves before serving.

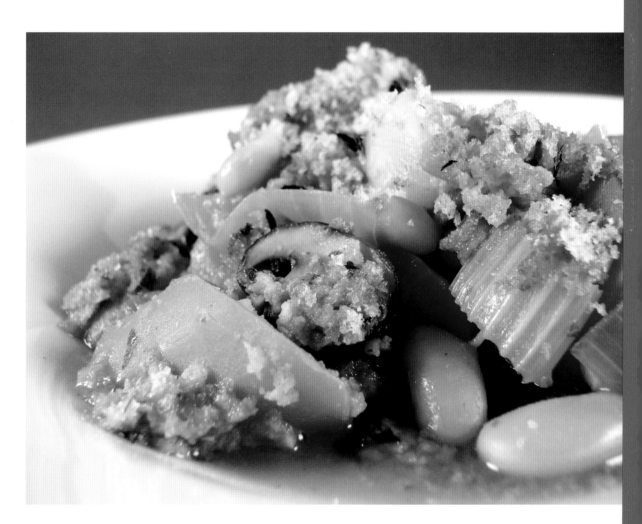

CHICKEN MOLE

SERVES 4 TO 6

This Mexican-inspired recipe blends together smoky chili peppers, sweet spice, and a hint of chocolate. Less time-consuming than traditional versions, this mole still offers a rich and complex flavor.

6 chicken leg pieces (drumsticks and/or thighs), bone-in and skin removed

¼ teaspoon dried oregano, preferably Mexican

½ teaspoon kosher salt

⅛ teaspoon freshly ground black pepper

½ teaspoon extra-virgin olive oil

MAKE THE CHICKEN MOLE:
Season the chicken with oregano, salt, and black pepper. In a large skillet, heat oil over medium heat. Brown the chicken for 2 minutes on each side. Remove the chicken from the skillet and reserve.

1 teaspoon extra-virgin olive oil

1 cup sliced yellow onions (about 1 small onion)

In the same skillet, heat oil over low heat. Add onions and caramelize for 15 minutes, stirring occasionally.

2 garlic cloves, minced

1 dried pasilla pepper, seeds and stems removed, broken into pieces

2 dried California or Anaheim peppers, seeds and stems removed, broken into pieces

¼ cup raisins

2 tablespoons raw almonds

1 tablespoon white sesame seeds

½ of a cinnamon stick, preferably Mexican

1 teaspoon dried oregano, preferably Mexican

⅛ teaspoon ground coriander

⅛ teaspoon ground cumin

Add garlic, pasilla peppers, California peppers, raisins, almonds, sesame seeds, cinnamon stick, oregano, coriander, and cumin, and cook for 2 minutes.

2¼ cups low-sodium chicken broth	Add chicken broth, tomatoes, salt, and black pepper. Cover and simmer for 20 minutes.
½ cup (or about ⅓ of a 15-ounce can) diced tomatoes	Remove from heat and purée the mixture in a blender (preferable) or food processor until smooth.
1½ teaspoons kosher salt	
⅛ teaspoon freshly ground black pepper	
1½ ounces semi-sweet chocolate, chopped	In the same skillet, pour in the mole sauce and add the chocolate. Stir until the chocolate is melted and well incorporated.
	Add reserved browned chicken, cover, and simmer over low heat for 30 minutes, or until chicken is cooked through.
½ teaspoon white sesame seeds (optional)	Garnish with sesame seeds before serving if desired.
4 cups low-sodium chicken broth	MAKE THE RICE:
1 cup (or about ½ of a 15-ounce can) diced tomatoes	While the mole is cooking, bring chicken broth and tomatoes to a boil in a medium pot over high heat.
2 cups long-grain brown rice, rinsed and drained	Reduce heat to low and add rice, salt, bay leaf, and celery stalk. Cover and simmer for 45 to 60 minutes, or until liquid is absorbed and rice is tender. Remove from heat and set aside covered for 5 minutes.
¾ teaspoon kosher salt	
1 dried bay leaf	Remove celery stalk and bay leaf and gently fluff rice with a fork. Do not over-stir or the rice will become mushy.
½ of a celery stalk, including the leaves	
1 tablespoon chopped fresh green onions (optional)	Garnish with green onions before serving if desired.

THAI WINTER SQUASH CURRY

SERVES 6 TO 8

This rich, stew-like curry can be served with rice for a hearty meal on a cold night. The warming effect of the onions and curry spices is balanced by the natural sweetness of the squash and the creaminess of the coconut milk. Use any variety of winter squash, such as acorn, kabocha, or butternut, as suggested here.

1 tablespoon extra-virgin olive oil

1 cup chopped yellow onions (about 1 small onion)

½ cup chopped leeks, white parts, rinsed thoroughly (about 1 medium leek)

In a medium pot, heat oil over medium heat. Add onions and cook for 1 minute, then add leeks and cook for 1 minute.

3 cloves garlic, minced

1 tablespoon minced ginger

1 fresh serrano pepper, seeds and membranes removed, minced

1 tablespoon curry powder

1 tablespoon soy sauce

Add garlic, ginger, serrano peppers, curry powder, and soy sauce, and cook for 1 minute.

4 cups peeled, seeded, and cubed butternut squash (about 1 small squash)

1 carrot, cut into 1-inch chunks

1 medium russet potato, cut into 1-inch chunks

2 cups low-sodium vegetable broth

1 cup water

1 teaspoon kosher salt

⅛ teaspoon freshly ground black pepper

Add butternut squash, carrots, potatoes, vegetable broth, water, salt, and black pepper, and bring to a boil over high heat. Reduce heat to low, cover, and simmer for 15 minutes, or until vegetables are tender, stirring occasionally.

10 ounces firm tofu, cubed

1⅔ cups (or one 14-ounce can) coconut milk

2 teaspoons agave nectar (optional)

2 tablespoons packed fresh cilantro leaves

Add tofu, coconut milk, and agave nectar if desired, and cook for 5 minutes.

Remove from heat and add cilantro.

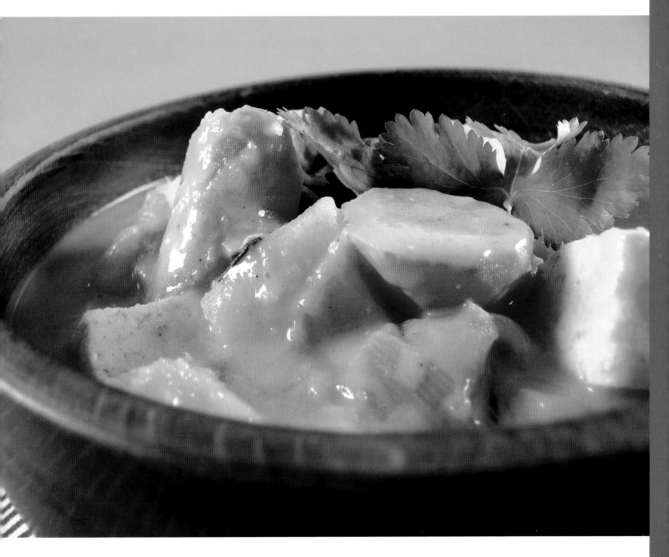

JAMBALAYA

SERVES 4 TO 5

Try this Creole-style jambalaya for a filling, one-pot dish of chicken, shrimp, and sausage mixed with rice, tomatoes, and a variety of spices. Slowly simmering the dish allows the flavors to meld together and enhances its warming thermal nature.

1½ teaspoons paprika

1¼ teaspoons dried minced onions

¾ teaspoon dried oregano

¾ teaspoon dried thyme

¾ teaspoon garlic powder

¼ teaspoon ground cayenne pepper

⅛ teaspoon freshly ground black pepper

In a small bowl, mix together paprika, dried onions, oregano, thyme, garlic powder, cayenne pepper, and black pepper.

8 ounces shrimp (about 16 large shrimp), peeled, de-veined, and cut into ½-inch pieces

8 ounces boneless, skinless chicken breasts, cut into ½-inch pieces

⅛ teaspoon kosher salt

In a small bowl, toss together shrimp and 1 teaspoon of the spice mixture. In another small bowl, toss together chicken, salt, and 1 teaspoon of the spice mixture. Reserve the remaining spice mixture.

Set shrimp and chicken aside to marinate for 30 minutes.

1 teaspoon extra-virgin olive oil

In a large, heavy pot, heat oil over medium-high heat. Add the marinated chicken and brown for 2 minutes. Remove the chicken from the pot and reserve.

½ teaspoon extra-virgin olive oil

6 ounces sausage (about 1 to 2 sausages), cut into ¼-inch slices

In the same pot, heat oil over medium-high heat. Add the sausage and brown for 2 minutes. Remove the sausage from the pot and reserve.

1 teaspoon extra-virgin olive oil	In the same pot, heat oil over medium heat. Add the onions and cook for 1 minute. Add garlic and cook for 1 minute. Stir in rice to coat and cook for 1 minute.
½ cup diced yellow onions (about ½ of a small onion)	
2 cloves garlic, minced	
1 cup long-grain brown rice, rinsed and drained	

½ teaspoon crushed red pepper flakes	Add reserved spice mixture, red pepper flakes, bay leaf, salt, and black pepper, and cook for 1 minute.
1 dried bay leaf	
1¼ teaspoons kosher salt	
⅛ teaspoon freshly ground black pepper	

2½ cups low-sodium chicken broth	Add chicken broth, tomatoes, and red and green bell peppers, and bring to a boil over high heat. Reduce heat to low, cover, and simmer for 40 minutes, or until rice is al dente.
1¾ cups (or one 15-ounce can) diced tomatoes	Stir in the reserved browned chicken and sausage and cook for 7 minutes. Add the marinated shrimp and cook for 5 minutes.
½ cup diced red bell pepper (about ½ of a pepper)	
½ cup diced green bell pepper (about ½ of a pepper)	

1 tablespoon chopped fresh green onions (optional)	Remove bay leaf before serving. Garnish with green onions if desired.

BUTTERNUT SQUASH LASAGNA

SERVES 8

Incorporating sweet butternut squash and tender spinach, this vegetarian recipe is a lighter alternative to traditional lasagnas, which tend to be heavy and greasy.

---

4 quarts peeled, seeded, and cubed butternut squash (about 2 medium squash or 4½ pounds)

2 teaspoons chopped fresh rosemary leaves

4 cloves garlic, minced

2 tablespoons extra-virgin olive oil

2 teaspoons kosher salt

¼ teaspoon freshly ground black pepper

MAKE THE FILLING COMPONENTS:
Preheat oven to 425°F.

In a large bowl, toss together butternut squash, rosemary, garlic, oil, salt, and black pepper. Divide mixture between two baking sheets and bake for 20 minutes, or until the squash is tender and lightly browned, tossing occasionally.

Remove the squash from the oven and reduce the oven temperature to 375°F.

1¾ cups low-sodium vegetable broth

½ cup water

1 teaspoon kosher salt

1½ tablespoons chopped fresh Italian parsley

Reserve one-third of the roasted butternut squash chunks.

In a blender (preferable) or food processor, blend the remaining two-thirds of the roasted butternut squash with vegetable broth, water, salt, and parsley in batches. Add additional water if necessary and blend again to achieve a thick, but smooth, consistency.

---

2 teaspoons extra-virgin olive oil

1 cup diced yellow onions (about 1 small onion)

4 cloves garlic, minced

8 cups washed, drained, and roughly chopped spinach (about 3 bunches)

1¼ teaspoons kosher salt

In a large skillet, heat oil over medium heat. Add onions and cook for 1 minute, then add garlic and cook for 1 minute. Add spinach and salt and cook for 4 to 5 minutes, or until the spinach is tender. Drain and discard cooking liquid.

---

12 whole-wheat lasagna noodles

Cook lasagna noodles according to package directions and drain.

1 cup grated mozzarella cheese 5 tablespoons grated Parmigiano Reggiano cheese	In a small bowl, mix together mozzarella and Parmigiano Reggiano cheeses. Reserve half of the cheese mixture for the topping. Divide the remaining cheese mixture into three portions for the three lasagna layers.
1½ cups pasta sauce ½ teaspoon crushed red pepper flakes	In a medium bowl, mix together pasta sauce and red pepper flakes.
Olive oil cooking spray	ASSEMBLE AND BAKE THE LASAGNA:

In a lightly oiled 2-quart (13 x 9 x 2") baking dish, evenly spread 1 cup of the butternut squash purée on the bottom of the dish. Place three cooked lasagna noodles side by side over the purée. Spread 1 cup of the squash purée over the noodles, then add one-third of the reserved butternut squash chunks, one-third of the spinach mixture, ½ cup of the pasta sauce mixture, and one-third of the cheese mixture over top.

Repeat for two more layers, starting with the lasagna noodles and ending with the cheese mixture.

Top with the three remaining lasagna noodles. Spread 1 cup of squash purée over top of the noodles, then sprinkle the reserved half of the cheese mixture over top.

Lightly spray a sheet of aluminum foil with cooking spray to prevent the cheese from sticking to it. Cover lasagna with the foil and bake for 30 minutes. Uncover and bake for 10 minutes, then broil for 1 to 2 minutes, or until the cheese is golden brown. Let cool for 10 minutes before serving.

BRAISED LAMB WITH ROASTED VEGETABLES

SERVES 3 TO 4

The classic combination of meat and potatoes is brightened up with the addition of oven-roasted carrots, parsnips, onions, and fennel in this hearty winter dish. As one of the most warming foods, lamb is beneficial for nourishing *yang* and strengthening *qi* in the body.

---

3 lamb shanks, membranes trimmed

¾ teaspoon kosher salt

⅛ teaspoon freshly ground black pepper

2 teaspoons extra-virgin olive oil

PREPARE THE LAMB:
Season the lamb with salt and black pepper. In a large pot, heat oil over medium heat. Add lamb and brown for 3 minutes on each side. Remove lamb from the pot and set aside.

½ teaspoon extra-virgin olive oil

1 cup diced yellow onions (about 1 small onion)

½ cup diced carrots (about 1 medium carrot)

1 celery stalk, diced

In the same pot, add oil, onions, carrots, and celery, and cook for 3 minutes.

---

2 cloves garlic, minced

2 teaspoons tomato paste

Add garlic and cook for 1 minute. Stir in tomato paste and cook for 1 minute.

2½ cups low-sodium beef broth

1 teaspoon fresh rosemary leaves

4 sprigs fresh thyme

1 dried bay leaf

1 teaspoon kosher salt

¼ teaspoon freshly ground black pepper

Add browned lamb, beef broth, rosemary, thyme, bay leaf, salt, and black pepper, and bring to a boil over high heat. Reduce heat to low, cover, and simmer for 2½ to 3 hours, or until lamb is tender.

Remove thyme sprigs and bay leaf before serving.

1 small yellow onion, cut into medium chunks

2 medium carrots, cut into medium chunks

2 medium Yukon Gold potatoes, cut into medium chunks

1 parsnip, cut into medium chunks

1 fennel bulb, cut into large pieces

1 teaspoon chopped fresh rosemary leaves

1 teaspoon chopped fresh thyme leaves

1 clove garlic, minced

1 tablespoon extra-virgin olive oil

¾ teaspoon kosher salt

⅛ teaspoon freshly ground black pepper

ROAST THE VEGETABLES:

About 1 hour before the lamb is done cooking, preheat oven to 400°F.

In a large bowl, toss together onions, carrots, potatoes, parsnips, fennel, rosemary, thyme, garlic, oil, salt, and black pepper.

Place vegetables on a lightly oiled baking sheet and roast for 45 to 50 minutes, or until vegetables are tender and browned.

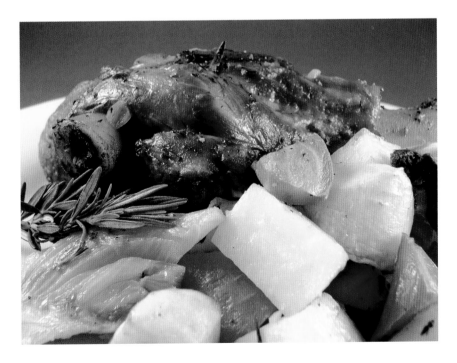

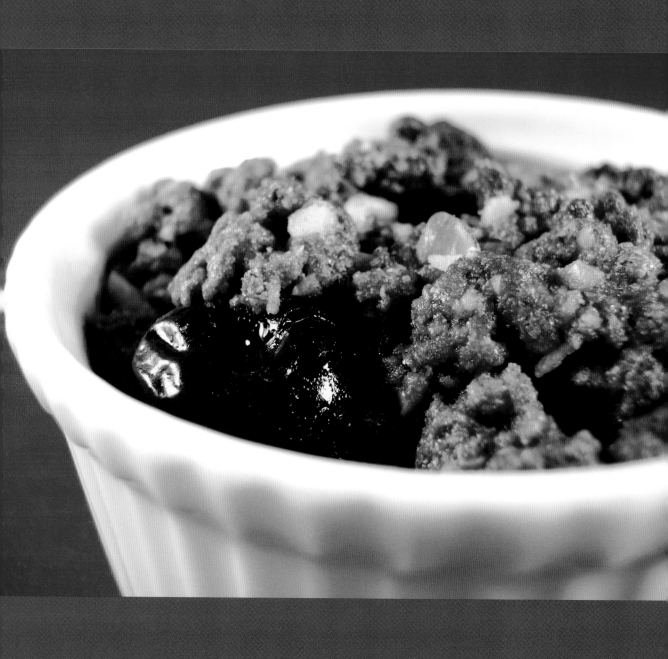

CHOCOLATE CHERRY CRISP

SERVES 4

Special equipment: four 4-ounce ramekins or one small baking dish

For a warm and comforting dessert, try this simple combination of plump, juicy cherries with a crunchy walnut, cinnamon, and cocoa topping.

---

3 cups fresh or frozen cherries, thawed and pitted

¼ cup dried cherries

1 teaspoon grated orange zest

1 tablespoon orange juice

1 tablespoon lightly packed light brown sugar

Preheat oven to 350°F.

In a small bowl, mix together fresh or thawed cherries, dried cherries, orange zest, orange juice, and brown sugar. Divide mixture among four ramekins or pour into one small baking dish.

¾ cup white whole-wheat flour

¼ cup lightly packed light brown sugar

½ cup chopped raw walnuts

2 teaspoons unsweetened cocoa powder

½ teaspoon ground cinnamon

1 pinch kosher salt

In a medium bowl, mix together flour, brown sugar, walnuts, cocoa powder, cinnamon, and salt.

---

2 ounces cold, unsalted butter, cut into small cubes

4 to 6 teaspoons ice water

Gently incorporate butter into the dry ingredients. Be sure not to over-mix; the topping mixture should have small, coarse lumps remaining. Add 1 teaspoon of ice water at a time to the topping mixture and lightly toss together. Use only enough water for the mixture to just come together; it should be crumbly, but not dough-like.

Sprinkle the topping mixture over the cherry mixture. Place the ramekins or baking dish on a baking sheet and bake for 20 to 30 minutes, or until the topping is browned and crisp, and the juices are bubbly. Let cool for 5 minutes before serving.

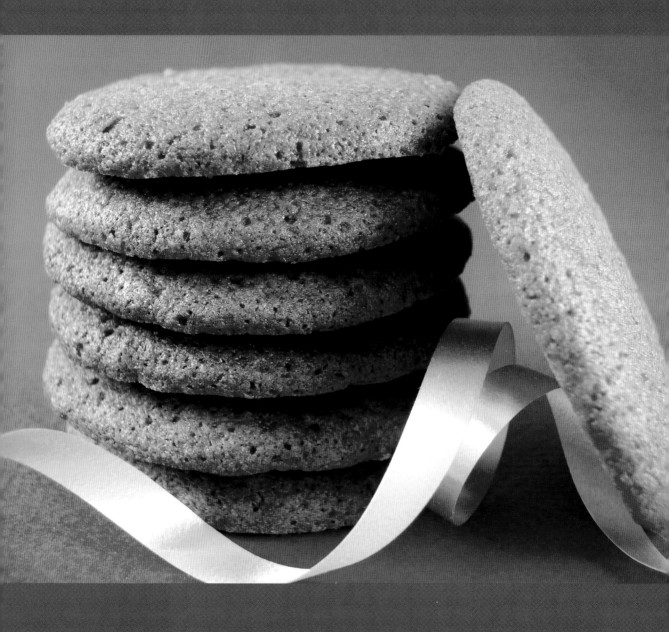

GINGERSNAP COOKIES

MAKES ABOUT 3 DOZEN COOKIES

A welcome gift or treat for any occasion, these seasonal cookies incorporate fresh ginger and ground black pepper for a spicy kick.

(V)

Special equipment: parchment paper (optional)

Cooking spray (optional)

Preheat oven to 375°F.

Spray two baking sheets with a small amount of cooking spray, or line them with parchment paper and omit spray.

---

3 ounces unsalted butter, softened

½ cup lightly packed light brown sugar

1 tablespoon finely minced or grated fresh ginger

1 tablespoon ground ginger

1 teaspoon ground cinnamon

⅛ teaspoon ground nutmeg

⅛ teaspoon freshly ground black pepper

1 pinch ground cloves

In a large bowl, cream together butter, brown sugar, fresh ginger, ground ginger, cinnamon, nutmeg, black pepper, and cloves with a mixer on low speed, until incorporated.

---

1 cup white whole-wheat flour

½ teaspoon baking soda

1 pinch kosher salt

In a small bowl, mix together flour, baking soda, and salt.

Mix the flour mixture into the butter mixture until just combined.

---

3 tablespoons dark molasses

1 egg, lightly beaten

Add molasses and egg and mix until just incorporated.

Drop rounded teaspoons of cookie dough onto the baking sheets and flatten them slightly with the palm of your hand. Bake for 8 minutes, rotate the pans from top to bottom and front to back, and bake for 7 minutes, or until golden brown.

SEASONAL BODY TYPES
CHARACTERISTICS AND HEALING PRINCIPLES

	SPRING	SUMMER	INDIAN SUMMER	FALL	WINTER
Amount of yin and yang	Yin — Yang Decreasing yin and increasing yang	Yin — Yang Least yin and most yang	Yin — Yang Balance of yin and yang	Yin — Yang Increasing yin and decreasing yang	Yin — Yang Most yin and least yang
Body thermal nature	Warm	Hot	Neutral	Cool	Cold
Theme	Birth	Growth	Foundation	Harvest	Withdrawal
Element	Wood	Fire	Earth	Metal	Water
Traditional Chinese Medicine diagnoses	*Qi* stasis, Blood stasis	*Yin* deficiency, Heat excess, Damp/Heat excess	*Qi* deficiency, Blood deficiency	Damp/Cold excess	*Yang* deficiency, Cold excess
Common physical symptoms	Muscle tension, migratory pain, headaches, constipation, pre-menstrual symptoms, frequent sighing, eye conditions	Hot palms and soles, flushed complexion, frequent thirst, night sweats, skin inflammation/rash, high blood pressure, diabetes, heartburn, insomnia, arthritis or edema worse in hot, humid weather	Fatigue, dizziness, weakened immune system, asthma, environmental allergies, easy bruising, weak digestion, constipation, loose stool, dry eyes or skin, sweet food cravings	Cold and clammy hands and feet, sinus congestion with white sputum, arthritis or edema worse in cold, damp weather, foggy-headedness, overweight, feeling of heaviness in the body, sticky stool	Aversion to cold, pale complexion, dark circles under the eyes, low vitality, slow movement, excessive sleep, lack of appetite, clear and copious urine, infertility
Common personality characteristics	Determined, hard-working, moody, irritable, uptight	Outgoing, passionate, adventurous, talkative, hot-tempered, easily angered	Compassionate, reliable, mild-mannered, passive, anxious, worried	Cautious, deliberate, has trouble concentrating or making decisions, gloomy	Sensitive, intuitive, thoughtful, introverted, shy, insecure, fearful
Common tongue characteristics	Purple, reddish-purple, or lavender color, and/or purple spots	Red color, yellow coating, cracks, or red spots	Scalloped edges or teeth marks	Wet surface and a sticky/pasty white coating	White coating that is not sticky/pasty

	SPRING	SUMMER	INDIAN SUMMER	FALL	WINTER
Healing principles	Move and cleanse	Cool and refresh	Build and strengthen	Dry and bolster	Warm and nourish
Mindfulness recommendations	Practicing forgiveness, expressing emotions, seeing things in new ways, releasing the need to control	Meditating, practicing progressive relaxation, quieting the mind, developing patience and restraint	Doing walking meditations, developing self-awareness, practicing affirmations, building confidence, caring for oneself	Expressing gratitude, learning to lighten up and release, healing from loss	Processing emotions, setting goals, taking risks, overcoming fears
Activity recommendations	Stretching and increasing flexibility, releasing tension, improving circulation, receiving bodywork/massage, practicing expressive arts	Practicing slow and mindful exercise, emphasizing fluid movement, getting ample rest and relaxation	Improving postural alignment and balance, strengthening the core, practicing deep abdominal breathing, being outdoors, hiking	Exercising aerobically, working up a sweat, participating in group activities, volunteering in the community, playing club sports	Creating warmth in the body, elevating heart rate, lighting competitive fire, participating in races and adventure sports
Food recommendations	Emphasize light foods, leafy greens, herbs and spices, garlic, onions. Minimize fatty foods, refined oils	Emphasize cooling fruits, vegetables, legumes, seafood, seaweeds, low-fat foods. Minimize heavy foods, meats, spicy foods, stimulants	Emphasize naturally sweet foods, foods with a neutral thermal nature, whole grains, meats, dairy, foods with high-quality *qi*, easily digestible foods. Minimize raw foods, refined sugars	Emphasize warming spices, whole and drying grains, foods that promote diuresis and drain excess fluids. Minimize fatty foods, dairy, cold foods, iced drinks	Emphasize hearty meats, root vegetables, warming spices, energy-dense foods. Minimize raw foods, cold foods, iced drinks
Therapeutic flavors	Sour	Bitter	Sweet	Pungent	Salty
Food preparation recommendations	Lightly cooked, stir-fries	Steamed, blanched, poached, minimally cooked, raw if tolerable	Well-cooked	Baked dishes, casseroles	Slow-cooked, simmered, braised, soups, stews, roasts

Glossary

acquired *qi* – the life force energy that is acquired from one's environment, including the air one breathes and the food one eats.

acupuncture – a type of Traditional Chinese Medicine therapy in which very thin needles are inserted into the skin at different points along energetic channels in order to manipulate *qi*.

Ayurvedic medicine – a holistic medical system from India which is based on the balancing of humors and elements known as *doshas*.

biofeedback – a mind-body technique used to increase awareness of physiological processes (e.g. breathing, heart rate, muscle tension, and skin temperature) and improve one's health and performance through the control and manipulation of those processes.

cold – a term used in Traditional Chinese Medicine to describe a health pattern or *yin* condition which results from an excess of cold energy in the body. It manifests as physical symptoms such as a feeling of cold, a pale complexion, weakness, slow movement, and low energy, and is treated with warming foods and activities that nourish *yang*.

congenital *qi* or ***yuan qi*** – the life force energy that is inherited from one's parents.

constitution – a characterization of one's body structure, physical makeup, emotional temperament, and personality, which can be associated with different health patterns and one's susceptibility to disease.

constitutionology – the study of individual body types and constitutions and their correlation to health states and the development of disease.

dan tian – the energy center and storage location for *qi* within the body, located a few centimeters below the navel.

dampness – a term used in Traditional Chinese Medicine to describe a health pattern in which excess fluids, moisture, and mucus accumulate in the body, leading to symptoms of edema, swelling, sinus congestion, arthritis, yeast infections, sluggishness, and feelings of heaviness.

deficiency – a term used in Traditional Chinese Medicine to describe a health pattern in which the body lacks *qi* or other substances; it is commonly characterized by general weakness, fatigue, a soft voice, and withdrawal.

excess – a term used in Traditional Chinese Medicine to describe a health pattern in which the body has an abundance of heat or congestion; it is commonly characterized by a robust constitution, hyperactivity, a loud and powerful voice, and extroversion.

Fall body type – an individual who displays symptoms of excess dampness and cold, such as cold and clammy hands and feet, sinus congestion, arthritis or edema which feels worse in cold weather, and feelings of heaviness or fogginess. Fall body types are deliberate and careful, and can also have trouble making decisions or have a gloomy outlook. Healing principles for Fall body types include eating warming and drying foods, burning off excess fluids through aerobic exercise, and lightening up, both physically and emotionally.

feng shui – the art of arranging one's environment, home, and workspace to promote the harmonious flow of *qi* and enhance one's health and well-being.

Five Element theory – a systematic framework used in Traditional Chinese Medicine to classify health in terms of five elements (wood, fire, earth, metal, and water) and the natural processes which transform those elements.

five flavors – a collection of terms used in Traditional Chinese Medicine to describe a food's medicinal properties, which may or may not correlate with the food's actual taste when eaten. Bitter foods have a drying and draining effect on the body, pungent foods promote circulation and dispersion, sweet foods build and strengthen the body, sour foods are cleansing and astringent, and salty foods moisten and promote downward movement.

five seasons – a collection of terms used in Traditional Chinese Medicine to describe the different phases and periods of the year in relation to the cycles of *yin* and *yang*. Spring and summer are *yang* seasons, fall and winter are *yin* seasons, and Indian summer represents the balance and transition between *yin* and *yang*.

guided imagery – a mind-body technique that directs the mind to visualize and imagine a sensory experience in order to promote relaxation, stress reduction, and healing.

heat – a term used in Traditional Chinese Medicine to describe a health pattern or *yang* condition which results from an excess of hot energy in the body. It manifests as physical symptoms such as a feeling of warmth, a red complexion, thirst, high blood pressure, skin rashes, and inflammation, and is balanced with cooling foods and activities that nourish *yin*.

homeostasis – the ability or tendency of a body to regulate physiological processes in order to maintain an internal equilibrium.

holism – the consideration of the sum and integration of individual components, rather than each component separately. Holistic medicine views an individual's health as the combination of mind, body, and spirit within the context of one's environment.

humoral medicine – a medical system with origins from ancient Greece which views health in terms of the balance of opposing elements or humors (blood, phlegm, yellow bile, and black bile).

Indian summer – the transitional period between the summer and fall seasons, in which the climate includes long days of sunshine and mild weather.

Indian Summer body type – an individual who displays symptoms of *qi* deficiency, such as fatigue, a low immune system, weak digestion, and environmental allergies. Indian Summer body types are mild-mannered and reliable, and can also be anxious and prone to worrying. Healing principles for Indian Summer body types include eating neutral staples and grains that build *qi*, strengthening the physical core and emotional resolve, and grounding the body.

intention – the focus of one's attention or thoughts toward a determined result.

meditation – a mind-body technique that develops awareness, trains the mind, and induces a relaxed state of consciousness through the focus of one's thoughts and attention.

meridian – an energetic channel or pathway in the body through which *qi* flows and circulates.

mindful exercise – the practice of being aware of one's environment and physiological processes (e.g. breath, heart rate, muscle contractions, and feelings of pain) during exercise.

mindfulness – the practice of paying attention and focusing awareness on the present moment.

organic foods – foods or food products that are grown or raised in an environment free of pesticides, synthetic chemicals, antibiotics, and growth hormones.

phytonutrients or **phytochemicals** – natural plant compounds that have a protective effect on the body and have antioxidant, anti-inflammatory, and other health-promoting properties.

plant-based diet – a diet which emphasizes foods that originate from plant sources such as whole grains, vegetables, fruits, legumes, and nuts.

psychoneuroimmunology (PNI) – the study of how psychological processes affect the central nervous and immune systems, and their relation to health and disease.

qi or **chi** – the universal energy and vital force present in all forms of life.

qi gong or **chi gung** – an exercise and healing art that encourages the cultivation and flow of *qi* within the body.

seasonal body type – a health pattern in which one lives in discordance with nature's seasonal cycles. A seasonal body type chronically displays symptoms from one season and climate throughout the year, in contrast with a neutral, balanced body which transitions along with the seasons.

seasonal diet – a diet which emphasizes foods that are predominantly available and harvested within a specific season and geographic region.

seasonality – a term used to describe the season in which a food is naturally available, grown, and harvested within a geographic region.

Spring body type – an individual who displays symptoms of *qi* stagnation, such as muscle tightness, tension headaches, migratory pain, and frequent sighing. Spring body types are determined and hard-working, and can also be moody and impatient. Healing principles for Spring body types include eating leafy greens, cleansing physical and emotional spaces, and increasing the circulation of *qi* within the body.

stagnation – a term used in Traditional Chinese Medicine to describe a health pattern in which the flow of *qi* within energetic meridians is blocked or stuck, leading to symptoms of tension, headaches, muscle stiffness, pain, frustration, and anger.

Summer body type – an individual who displays symptoms of excess heat, such as hot palms and soles, a flushed complexion, skin inflammations, rashes, high blood pressure, and insomnia. Summer body types are outgoing and adventurous, and can also be hot-tempered and easily angered. Healing principles for Summer body types include eating cooling raw fruits and vegetables, practicing physical and emotional restraint, nourishing *yin*, and relaxing the body.

sustainable foods – foods or food products that are grown or raised using ecologically friendly practices, in a manner which preserves natural resources and minimizes damage to the environment and human health.

tai chi or **tai ji quan** – an exercise and meditative health practice originally developed as a martial art and used to enhance *qi* within the body.

taijitu – the black and white symbol representing the balance and relationship between *yin* and *yang*.

tao – the "way" or the "one." The central organizing principle of the universe according to Taoist beliefs.

Taoism – a philosophical and cultural tradition that emphasizes the relationship between nature, humanity, and the divine, and uses nature as the model for an ideal life.

thermal nature – an intrinsic, abstract quality which describes a food's effect on the body when eaten. Foods with a warming thermal nature like most meats, energy-dense foods, and root vegetables create warmth in the body. Foods with a cooling thermal nature like most fruits, quick-growing vegetables, and raw foods refresh and cool down the body. Foods with a neutral thermal nature like most grains, starches, and legumes have no effect on the energetic temperature of the body.

Traditional Chinese Medicine (TCM) – an alternative medical system that describes health in terms of the balance of natural elements and phenomena, and includes holistic therapies such as acupuncture, herbal medicine, dietary therapy, massage, and bodywork.

whole foods diet – a diet which emphasizes unprocessed or minimally processed foods, eaten in their whole, natural, and unrefined forms with their original fiber, minerals, and nutrients intact.

Winter body type – an individual who displays symptoms of excess cold, such as an aversion to cold, a pale complexion, slow movement, a lack of appetite, and low vitality. Winter body types are intuitive and empathetic, and can also be fearful and insecure. Healing principles for Winter body types include eating warming and hearty foods, overcoming fears, boosting *yang*, and warming the body.

yang – a natural force and energy which is represented by light, warmth, masculinity, fire, external direction, activity, and change.

yin and *yang* – two complementary and opposing forces which are used to describe the nature of disease, the energetic properties of foods, and other universal phenomena. Optimal health is achieved when *yin* and *yang* are in balance.

yin – a natural force and energy which is represented by darkness, cold, femininity, water, internal direction, stability, and stillness.

Recommended Reading

Beinfield, Harriet, and Efrem Korngold. *Between Heaven and Earth: A Guide to Chinese Medicine.* New York: Ballantine Books, 1991.

Campbell, T. Colin, and Thomas M. Campbell II. *The China Study: Startling Implications for Diet, Weight Loss and Long Term Health.* Dallas: BenBella Books, 2006.

Flaws, Bob. *The Tao of Healthy Eating: Dietary Wisdom According to Chinese Medicine.* Boulder, CO: Blue Poppy Press, 1998.

Haas, Elson M. *Staying Healthy With the Seasons.* New York: Celestial Arts, 2003.

Kabat-Zinn, Jon. *Wherever You Go, There You Are: Mindfulness Meditation in Everyday Life.* New York: Hyperion, 1994.

Fallon, Sally, and Mary Enig. *Nourishing Traditions: The Cookbook that Challenges Politically Correct Nutrition and the Diet Dictocrats.* Washington, D.C.: NewTrends Publishing, 2001.

Kaptchuk, Ted J. *The Web That Has No Weaver.* New York: McGraw-Hill, 2000.

Kastner, Joerg. *Chinese Nutrition Therapy: Dietetics in Traditional Chinese Medicine (TCM).* Stuttgart, Germany: Thieme, 2004.

Kingsolver, Barbara, with Steven L. Hopp and Camille Kingsolver. *Animal, Vegetable, Miracle: A Year of Food Life.* New York: HarperCollins Publishers, 2007.

Leggett, Daverick. *Recipes for Self-Healing.* Totnes, England: Meridian Press, 1999.

Miller, Daphne. *The Jungle Effect: A Doctor Discovers the Healthiest Diets from Around the World – Why They Work and How to Bring Them Home.* New York: HarperCollins Publishers, 2008.

Pitchford, Paul. *Healing With Whole Foods: Asian Traditions and Modern Nutrition.* Berkeley: North Atlantic Books, 2002.

Pollan, Michael. *In Defense of Food: An Eater's Manifesto.* New York: The Penguin Press, 2008.

Pollan, Michael. *The Omnivore's Dilemma: A Natural History of Four Meals.* New York: The Penguin Press, 2006.

Prout, Linda. *Live in the Balance: The Ground-Breaking East-West Nutrition Program.* New York: Marlowe and Company, 2000.

Thich, Nhat Hanh. *Peace Is Every Step: The Path of Mindfulness in Everyday Life.* New York: Bantam Books, 1992.

Thich, Nhat Hanh. *The Miracle of Mindfulness.* Boston: Beacon Press, 1999.

Willcox, Bradley J., D. Craig Willcox, and Makoto Suzuki. *The Okinawa Program: How the World's Longest-Lived People Achieve Everlasting Health – And How You Can Too.* New York: Three Rivers Press, 2001.

Resources

Visit our website for seasonal body type information, recipes, and healing principles: www.whatsyourseason.com

Complementary and Alternative Medicine

American Association of Naturopathic Physicians
818 18th Street, NW, Suite 250, Washington, DC 20006
866-538-2267
www.naturopathic.org

American Association of Acupuncture and Oriental Medicine (AAAOM)
P.O. Box 96503 #44114, Washington, DC 20090
866-455-7999
www.aaaomonline.org

American Chiropractic Association
1701 Clarendon Boulevard, Suite 200, Arlington, VA 22209
703-276-8800
www.acatoday.org

American Massage Therapy Association (AMTA)
500 Davis Street, Suite 900, Evanston, IL 60201
877-905-0577
www.amtamassage.org

National Center for Complementary and Alternative Medicine (NCCAM)
9000 Rockville Pike, Bethesda, MD 20892
888-644-6226
www.nccih.nih.gov

National Center for Homeopathy
7918 Jones Branch Drive, Suite 300, McLean, VA 22102
703-506-7667
www.homeopathycenter.org

National Certification Commission for Acupuncture and Oriental Medicine (NCCAOM)
76 South Laura Street, Suite 1290, Jacksonville, FL 32202
904-598-1005
www.nccaom.org

Preventive Medicine Research Institute
900 Bridgeway, Sausalito, CA 94965
www.pmri.org

Mindfulness and Meditation

Center for Mindfulness
55 Lake Avenue North, Worcester, MA 01655
508-856-2656
www.umassmed.edu/cfm

Guided Mindfulness Meditation Practices with Jon Kabat-Zinn
508-856-2656
www.mindfulnesscds.com

Plum Village Mindfulness Practice Centre founded by Thich Nhat Hanh
Le Pey 24240, Thenac, France
www.plumvillage.org

Mind-Body Exercise and Energy Healing Therapies

Emotional Freedom Technique
www.thetappingsolution.com/what-is-eft-tapping

Feldenkrais Guild of North America
401 Edgewater Place, Suite 600, Wakefield, MA 01880
781-876-8935
www.feldenkrais.com

International Association of Reiki Professionals
P.O. Box 104, Harrisville, NH 03450
www.iarp.org

National Qi Gong Association
P.O. Box 270065, St. Paul, MN 55127
888-815-1893
www.nqa.org

Yoga Journal
www.yogajournal.com

Organic Food and Farming

California Certified Organic Farmers (CCOF)
2155 Delaware Avenue,
Suite 150, Santa Cruz, CA 95060
831-423-2263
www.ccof.org

Organic Consumers Association
6771 South Silver Hill Drive,
Finland, MN 55603
218-226-4164
www.organicconsumers.org

Organic Farming Research Foundation
303 Potrero Street, Suite 29-203,
Santa Cruz, CA 95060
831-426-6606
www.ofrf.org

Seasonal Food Guides

Eat the Seasons – North America
www.eattheseasons.com

National Resources Defense Council Guide to Seasonal Produce
40 West 20th Street,
New York, NY 10011
212-727-2700
www.simplesteps.org/eat-local

GRACE Communications Foundation – Sustainable Table Seasonal Food Guide
215 Lexington Avenue,
New York, NY 10016
212-726-9161
www.sustainabletable.org/
seasonalfoodguide

Local Foods and Farmers' Markets

LocalHarvest
P.O. Box 1292, Santa Cruz,
CA 95061
831-515-5602
www.localharvest.org

USDA National Farmers Market Directory
202-720-8356
www.ams.usda.gov/
local-food-directories/
farmersmarkets

Sustainable Agriculture

Biodynamic Association
1661 North Water Street,
Suite 307, Milwaukee, WI 53202
262-649-9212
www.biodynamics.com

Ecological Farming Association
2901 Park Avenue,
Suite D-2, Soquel, CA 95073
831-763-2111
www.eco-farm.org

National Sustainable Agriculture Coalition
110 Maryland Avenue NE,
Suite 209, Washington, DC 20002
202-547-5754
www.sustainableagriculture.net

Sustainable Agriculture Research and Education (SARE)
USDA-NIFA, Stop 2223,
1400 Independence Avenue, SW,
Washington, DC 20250
www.sare.org

Sustainable Table
215 Lexington Avenue,
New York, NY 10016
212-726-9161
www.sustainabletable.org

The Land Institute
2440 East Water Well Road,
Salina, KS 67401
785-823-5376
www.landinstitute.org

Sustainable Seafood

Marine Stewardship Council
2110 North Pacific Street, Suite
102, Seattle, WA 98103
206-691-0188
www.msc.org

Monterey Bay Aquarium Seafood Watch
886 Cannery Row,
Monterey, CA 93940
www.seafoodwatch.org

Environmental Conservation and Food Sustainability

Center for Food Safety
660 Pennsylvania Avenue, SE, #302, Washington, DC 20003
202-547-9359
www.centerforfoodsafety.org

Environmental Defense Fund
1875 Connecticut Avenue, NW, Suite 600, Washington, DC 20009
800-684-3322
www.edf.org

Environmental Working Group
1436 U Street, NW, Suite 100, Washington, DC 20009
202-667-6982
www.ewg.org

National Resources Defense Council
40 West 20th Street, New York, NY 10011
212-727-2700
www.nrdc.org

Non-Genetically Modified Foods

Center for Food Safety Shoppers Guide to Avoiding GE Food
660 Pennsylvania Avenue, SE, #302, Washington, DC 20003
202-547-9359
www.truefoodshoppersguide.org

Institute for Responsible Technology Non-GMO Shopping Guide
P.O. Box 469, Fairfield, IA 52556
641-209-1765
www.nongmoshopping guide.com

Non-GMO Project
1200 Harris Avenue, Suite #305, Bellingham, WA 98225
877-358-9240
www.nongmoproject.org

Vegetarianism and Veganism

The Vegan Society
Donald Watson House, 21 Hylton Street, Birmingham B18 6HJ, United Kingdom
www.vegansociety.com

Vegetarian Resource Group
P.O. Box 1463, Baltimore, MD 21203
410-366-8343
www.vrg.org

Nutrition

USDA Food and Nutrition Information Center
National Agricultural Library, 10301 Baltimore Avenue, Room 108, Beltsville, MD 20705
www.fnic.nal.usda.gov

USDA Food and Nutrition Service
3101 Park Center Drive, Alexandria, VA 22302
www.fns.usda.gov

USDA National Nutrient Database for Standard Reference
Nutrient Data Laboratory, USDA-ARS, 10300 Baltimore Avenue, Building 005, Room 107, BARC-West, Beltsville, MD 20705
301-504-0630
ndb.nal.usda.gov

Other

Humane Farm Animal Care
P.O. Box 727, Herndon, VA 20172
703-435-3883
www.certifiedhumane.org

Slow Food USA
68 Summit Street, 2B, Brooklyn, NY 11231
718-260-8000
www.slowfoodusa.org

Weston A. Price Foundation (food, farming and healing arts traditions)
PMB 106-380, 4200 Wisconsin Avenue, NW, Washington, DC 20016
202-363-4394
www.westonaprice.org

References

Chapter 1

1. Hesketh, T., and W.X. Zhu. 1997. Traditional Chinese medicine: One country, two systems. *BMJ* 315(7100):115-17.

2. Xu, J., and Y. Yang. 2009. Traditional Chinese medicine in the Chinese health care system. *Health Policy* 90:133-39.

3. Eisenberg, D.M., R.B. Davis, S.L. Ettner, et al. 1998. Trends in alternative medicine use in the United States, 1990-1997. *JAMA* 280(18):1569-75.

4. O'Connor, B.B. 2014. Conceptions of the body in complementary and alternative medicine. In Kelner, M., B. Wellman, B. Pescosolido, et al., eds. *Complementary and Alternative Medicine: Challenge and Change.* Oxon: Routledge, 39-60.

5. Balch, P.A. 2002. *Prescription for Herbal Healing: An Easy-to-Use A-to-Z Reference to Hundreds of Common Disorders and Their Herbal Remedies.* New York: Avery, vii.

6. White, A.R., J. Filshie, and T.M. Cummings. 2001. Clinical trials of acupuncture: Consensus recommendations for optimal treatment, sham controls and blinding. *Complement Ther Med* 9:237-45.

7. Jiang, M., J. Yang, C. Zhang, et al. 2010. Clinical studies with traditional Chinese medicine in the past decade and future research and development. *Planta Med* 76(17):2048-64.

8. Birch, S., J.K. Hesselink, F.A.M. Jonkman, et al. 2004. Clinical research on acupuncture: Part 1. What have reviews of the efficacy and safety of acupuncture told us so far? *J Altern Complement Med* 10(3):468-80.

9. Acupuncture. 1997. *NIH Consens Statement* 15(5):1-34.

Chapter 2

1. Frazão, E. 1996. The American diet: A costly health problem. *FoodReview*, U.S. Department of Agriculture, Economic Research Service 19(1):2-6.

2. Food and Agriculture Organization of the United Nations. 2002. The Spectrum of Malnutrition Fact Sheet. http://www.fao.org/worldfoodsummit/english/fsheets/malnutrition.pdf

3. World Health Organization. 2006. Enriching lives: Overcoming under- and over-nutrition. *Global Programming Note 2006-2007.* Geneva: World Health Organization. http://www.who.int/nmh/donorinfo/nutrition/nutrition_helvetica.pdf

4. Popkin, B.M. 2001. The nutrition transition and obesity in the developing world. *J Nutr* 131(3):871S-73S.

5. Hossain, P., B. Kawar, and M. El Nahas. 2007. Obesity and diabetes in the developing world – A growing challenge. *N Engl J Med* 356(3):213-15.

6. Kennedy, E.T. 2005. The global face of nutrition: What can governments and industry do? *J Nutr* 135(4):913-15.

7. Morrill, A.C., and C.D. Chinn. 2004. The obesity epidemic in the United States. *J Public Health Policy* 25(3-4):353-66.

8. National Alliance for Nutrition and Activity. 2010. National health priorities: Reducing obesity, heart disease, cancer, diabetes, and other diet- and inactivity-related diseases, costs, and disabilities.

Atlanta, GA: Department of Health and Human Services, Centers for Disease Control and Prevention.

9. Frazão, E. 1999. High costs of poor eating patterns in the United States. In Frazão, E., ed. *America's Eating Habits: Changes and Consequences.* Washington, D.C.: U.S. Department of Agriculture, Economic Research Service, Agriculture Information Bulletin 750:5-32.

10. Wallin, M.S., and A.M. Rissanen. 1994. Food and mood: Relationship between food, serotonin and affective disorders. *Acta Psychiatr Scand* Suppl 377:36-40.

11. Parker, G., N.A. Gibson, H. Brotchie, et al. 2006. Omega-3 fatty acids and mood disorders. *Am J Psychiatry* 163:969-78.

12. Christensen, L. 1993. Effects of eating behavior on mood: A review of the literature. *Int J Eat Disord* 14(2):171-83.

13. Ludwig, D.S. 2011. Technology, diet, and the burden of chronic disease. *JAMA* 305(13):1352-53.

14. Drewnowski, A., and S.E. Specter. 2004. Poverty and obesity: The role of energy density and energy costs. *Am J Clin Nutr* 79:6-16.

15. Milburn, M.P. 2004. Indigenous nutrition: Using traditional food knowledge to solve contemporary health problems. *American Indian Quarterly* 28(3-4):411-34.

16. Miller, D. 2008. *The Jungle Effect: A Doctor Discovers the Healthiest Diets from Around the World – Why They Work and How to Bring Them Home.* New York: Harper-Collins Publishers, 36.

17. Rembialkowska, E. 2007. Quality of plant products from organic agriculture. *J Sci Food Agric* 87(15):2757-62.

18. Pitchford, P. 2002. *Healing With Whole Foods: Asian Traditions and Modern Nutrition.* 3rd ed. Berkeley: North Atlantic Books, 19-21.

19. Kastner, J. 2004. *Chinese Nutrition Therapy.* Stuttgart, Germany: Thieme, 44.

20. Pitchford, P. 2002. *Healing With Whole Foods: Asian Traditions and Modern Nutrition.* 3rd ed. Berkeley: North Atlantic Books, 254-56.

21. American Heart Association. 2015. Suggested servings from each food group. http://www.heart.org/HEARTORG/GettingHealthy/NutritionCenter/HealthyEating/Suggested-Servings-from-Each-Food-Group_UCM_318186_Article.jsp#.VmXu9rgrKHs

22. Hu, F.B. 2003. Plant-based foods and prevention of cardiovascular disease: An overview. *Am J Clin Nutr* 78(suppl):544S-51S.

23. Campbell, T.C., and T.M. Campbell II. 2006. *The China Study: Startling Implications for Diet, Weight Loss and Long Term Health.* Dallas: BenBella Books.

24. Willcox, D.C., B.J. Willcox, H. Todoriki, et al. 2006. Caloric restriction and human longevity: What can we learn from the Okinawans? *Biogerontology* 7(3):173-77.

25. Pollan, M. 2004. Our national eating disorder. *The New York Times Magazine,* 17 October.

26. Andrade, A.M., G.W. Greene, and K.J. Melanson. 2008. Eating slowly led to decreases in energy intake within meals in healthy women. *J Am Diet Assoc* 108(7):1186-91.

27. Pitchford, P. 2002. *Healing With Whole Foods: Asian Traditions and Modern Nutrition.* 3rd ed. Berkeley: North Atlantic Books, 447-48.

28. Rudkowska, I., and L. Pérusse. 2012. Individualized weight management: What can be learned from nutrigenomics and nutrigenetics? *Prog Mol Biol Transl Sci* 108:347-82.

29. Ordovas, J.M. 2008. Genotype–phenotype associations: Modulation by diet and obesity. *Obesity* 16(S3):S40-S46.

30. Qi, L. 2014. Gene–diet interaction and weight loss. *Curr Opin Lipidol* 25(1):27-34.

31. Lairon, D., C. Defoort, J.C. Martin, et al. 2009. Nutrigenetics: Links between genetic background and response to Mediterranean-type diets. *Public Health Nutr* 12(9A):1601-06.

Chapter 3

1. Greaves, M. 2000. *Cancer: The Evolutionary Legacy.* Oxford: Oxford University Press, 10-14.

2. Reiche, E.M.V., S.O.V. Nunes, and H.K. Morimoto. 2004. Stress, depression, the immune system, and cancer. *Lancet Oncol* 5:617-25.

3. Vitetta, L., B. Anton, F. Cortizo, et al. 2005. Mind-body medicine: Stress and its impact on overall health and longevity. *Ann NY Acad Sci* 1057:492-505.

4. Baum, A., and D.M. Posluszny. 1999. Health psychology: Mapping biobehavioral contributions to health and illness. *Annu Rev Psychol* 50:137-63.

5. Wansink, B. 2006. *Mindless Eating: Why We Eat More Than We Think.* New York: Bantam Books, 106-07.

6. Astin, J.A., S.L. Shapiro, D.M. Eisenberg, et al. 2003. Mind-body medicine: State of the science, implications for practice. *J Am Board Fam Pract* 16(2):131-47.

7. Pistoia, F., S. Sacco, and A. Carolei. 2013. Behavioral therapy for chronic migraine. *Curr Pain Headache Rep* 17(1):304.

8. Selye, H. 1976. *Stress in Health and Disease.* Boston: Butterworth.

9. Cohen, S., and T.B. Herbert. 1996. Health psychology: Psychological factors and physical disease from the perspective of human psychoneuroimmunology. *Annu Rev Pscyhol* 47:113-42.

10. Ader, R., and N. Cohen. 1995. Psychoneuroimmunology: Interactions between the nervous system and the immune system. *Lancet* 345(8942):99-103.

11. Temoshok, L. 1987. Personality, coping style, emotion, and cancer: Towards an integrative model. *Cancer Surv* 6:545-67.

12. Chida, Y., and A. Steptoe. 2009. The association of anger and hostility with future coronary heart disease: A meta-analytic review of prospective evidence. *J Am Coll Cardiol* 53(11):936-46.

13. Carney, R.M., and K.E. Freedland. 2003. Depression, mortality, and medical morbidity in patients with coronary heart disease. *Biol Psychiatry* 54:241-47.

14. Giltay, E.J., M.H. Kamphuis, S. Kalmijn, et al. 2006. Dispositional optimism and the risk of cardiovascular death: The Zutphen elderly study. *Arch Intern Med* 166:431-36.

15. Marin, M.F., C. Lord, J. Andrews, et al. 2011. Chronic stress, cognitive functioning and mental health. *Neurobiol Learn Mem* 96(4):583-95.

16. Daubenmier, J., J. Kristeller, F.M. Hecht, et al. 2011. Mindfulness intervention for stress eating to reduce cortisol and abdominal fat among overweight and obese women: An exploratory randomized controlled study. *J Obes* 2011:1-13.

17. Rimmele, U., B.C. Zellweger, B. Marti, et al. 2007. Trained men show lower cortisol, heart rate and psychological responses to psychosocial stress compared with untrained men. *Psychoneuroendocrinology* 32(6):627-35.

18. Nabkasorn, C., N. Miyai, A. Sootmongkol, et al. Effects of physical exercise on depression, neuroendocrine stress hormones and physiological fitness in adolescent females with depressive symptoms. *Eur J Public Health* 16(2):179-84.

19. Kahn, A. 2006. *The Encyclopedia of Stress and Stress-Related Diseases.* 2nd ed. New York: Facts On File, 73-74.

20. Rakel, D. 2012. *Integrative Medicine.* 3rd ed. Philadelphia: Elsevier, 815-16.

21. Hart, J. 2008. Guided imagery. *Altern Complement Ther* 14(6):295-99.

22. van Tilburg, M.A.L., D.K. Chitkara, O.S. Palsson, et al. 2009. Audio-recorded guided imagery treatment reduces functional abdominal pain in children: A pilot study. *Pediatrics* 124(5):e890-97.

23. Eller, L.S. 1999. Guided imagery interventions for symptom management. *Annu Rev Nurs Res* 17(1):57-84.

24. Bonilla, E. 2008. Evidence about the power of intention. *Invest Clin* 49(4):595-615 (in Spanish).

25. Schlitz, M., D. Radin, B. Malle, et al. 2003. Distant healing intention: Definitions and evolving guidelines for laboratory studies. *Altern Ther Health Med* 9(3 Suppl):A31-43.

26. Achterberg, J., K. Cooke, T. Richards, et al. 2005. Evidence for correlations between distant intentionality and brain function in recipients: A functional magnetic resonance imaging analysis. *J Altern Complement Med* 11(6):965-71.

27. Waber, R.L., B. Shiv, Z. Carmon, et al. 2008. Commercial features of placebo and therapeutic efficacy. *JAMA* 299(9):1016-17.

28. Benedetti, F., H.S. Mayberg, T.D. Wager, et al. 2005. Neurobiological mechanisms of the placebo effect. *J Neurosci* 25(45):10390-402.

29. Koller, M., W. Lorenz, K. Wagner, et al. 2000. Expectations and quality of life of cancer patients undergoing radiotherapy. *J R Soc Med* 93(12):621-28.

30. Wood, A.M., J.J. Froh, and A.W.A. Geraghty. 2010. Gratitude and well-being: A review and theoretical integration. *Clin Psychol Rev* 30(7): 890-905.

31. Emmons, R.A., and M.E. McCullough. 2003. Counting blessings versus burdens: An experimental investigation of gratitude and subjective well-being in daily life. *J Pers Soc Psychol* 84(2):377-89.

32. Kabat-Zinn, J. 1994. *Wherever You Go, There You Are: Mindfulness Meditation in Everyday Life.* New York: Hyperion, 4.

33. Greeson, J. 2009. Mindfulness research update: 2008. *Complement Health Pract Rev* 14(1):10-18.

34. Lutz, A., L.L. Greischar, N.B. Rawlings, et al. 2004. Long-term meditators self-induce high-amplitude gamma synchrony during mental practice. *Proc Natl Acad Sci* 101(46):16369-73.

35. Masters, K.S., and B.M. Ogles. 1998. Associative and dissociative cognitive strategies in exercise and running: 20 years later, what do we know? *Sport Psychol* 12:253-70.

36. Gardner, F.L., and Z.E. Moore. 2007. *The Psychology of Enhancing Human Performance: The Mindfulness-Acceptance-Commitment (MAC) Approach.* New York: Springer, 34.

37. University of California Los Angeles Laboratory of Neuro Imaging. 2008. Brain Trivia. http://www.loni.usc.edu/about_loni/education/brain_trivia.php

Chapter 4

1. U.S. Department of Health and Human Services, Office of the Assistant Secretary for Planning and Evaluation. 2002. Physical activity fundamental to preventing disease. http://aspe.hhs.gov/health/reports/physicalactivity/

2. Chenoweth, D., and J. Leutzinger. 2006. The economic cost of physical inactivity and excess weight in American adults. *J Phys Act Health* 3:148-63.

3. Centers for Disease Control and Prevention. 2007. Prevalence of regular physical activity among adults – United States, 2001 and 2005. *MMWR* 56(46):1209-12.

4. Centers for Disease Control and Prevention. 2005. Trends in leisure-time physical inactivity by age, sex, and race/ethnicity – United States, 1994-2004. *MMWR* 54(39):991-94.

5. Booth, F.W., S.E. Gordon, C.J. Carlson, et al. 2000. Waging war on modern chronic diseases: Primary prevention through exercise biology. *J Appl Physiol* 88(2):774-87.

6. Blair, S.N. 1993. Evidence for success of exercise in weight loss and control. *Ann Intern Med* 119(7 Pt 2):702-06.

7. Donnelly, J.E., B. Smith, D.J. Jacobsen, et al. 2004. The role of exercise for weight loss and maintenance. *Best Pract Res Clin Gastroenterol* 18(6):1009-29.

8. Anderson, J.W., C.W. Kendall, and D.J.A. Jenkins. 2003. Importance of weight management in type 2 diabetes: Review with meta-analysis of clinical studies. *J Am Coll Nutr* 22(5):331-39.

9. Sullivan, P.W., E.H. Morrato, V. Ghushchyan, et al. 2005. Obesity, inactivity, and the prevalence of diabetes and diabetes-related cardiovascular comorbidities in the U.S., 2000-2002. *Diabetes Care* 28(7):1599-603.

10. Goodyear, L.J., and B.B. Kahn. 1998. Exercise, glucose transport, and insulin sensitivity. *Annu Rev Med* 49:235-61.

11. Myers, J. 2003. Exercise and cardiovascular health. *Circulation* 107(1):e2-e5.

12. Warburton, D.E.R., C.W. Nicol, and S.S.D. Bredin. 2006. Health benefits of physical activity: The evidence. *CMAJ* 174(6):801-09.

13. McTiernan, A., C. Ulrich, S. Slate, et al. 1998. Physical activity and cancer etiology: Associations and mechanisms. *Cancer Causes Control* 9(5):487-509.

14. Oliveria, S.A., and P.J. Christos. 1997. The epidemiology of physical activity and cancer. *Ann N Y Acad Sci* 833:79-90.

15. Wallace, B.A., and R.G. Cumming. 2000. Systematic review of randomized trials of the effect of exercise on bone mass in pre- and postmenopausal women. *Calcif Tissue Int* 67:10-18.

16. Kelley, G.A., K.S. Kelley, and Z.V. Tran. 2001. Resistance training and bone mineral density in women: A meta-analysis of controlled trials. *Am J Phys Med Rehabil* 80:65-77.

17. Granacher, U., T. Muehlbauer, L. Zahner, et al. 2011. Comparison of traditional and recent approaches in the promotion of balance and strength in older adults. *Sports Med* 41(5):377-400.

18. Granacher, U., T. Muehlbauer, A. Gollhofer, et al. 2011. An intergenerational approach in the promotion of balance and strength for fall prevention – a mini-review. *Gerontology* 57(4):304-15.

19. Wolf, S.L., H.X. Barnhart, N.G. Kutner, et al. 2003. Reducing frailty and falls in older persons: An investigation of tai chi and computerized balance training. *J Am Geriatr Soc* 51:1794-803.

20. Wolfson, L., R. Whipple, C. Derby, et al. 1996. Balance and strength training in older adults: Intervention gains and tai chi maintenance. *J Am Geriatr Soc* 44:498-506.

21. Dussa, K.R. 2012. Rehabilitation and return to sports after conservative and surgical treatment of upper extremity injuries. In Doral, M.N., ed. *Sports Injuries: Prevention, Diagnosis, Treatment and Rehabilitation.* New York: Springer, 201-08.

22. Emery, C.A. 2005. Injury prevention and future research. In Caine, D.J., and N. Maffulli, eds. *Epidemiology of Pediatric Sports Injuries.* Basel: Karger Publishers, 48:179-200.

23. Hillman, C.H., K.I. Erickson, and A.F. Kramer. 2008. Be smart, exercise your heart: Exercise effects on brain and cognition. *Nat Rev Neurosci* 9(1):58-65.

24. Kramer, A.F., S.J. Colcombe, E. McAuley, et al. 2005. Fitness, aging and neurocognitive function. *Neurobiol Aging* 26S(1):S124-27.

25. Fox, K.R. 1999. The influence of physical activity on mental well-being. *Public Health Nutr* 2(3a):411-18.

26. Schoenfeld, T.J., P. Rada, P.R. Pieruzzini, et al. 2013. Physical exercise prevents stress-induced activation of granule neurons and enhances local inhibitory mechanisms in the dentate gyrus. *J Neurosci* 33(18):7770-77.

27. Greenwood, B.N., and M. Fleshner. 2008. Exercise, learned helplessness, and the stress-resistant brain. *Neuromol Med* 10(2):81-98.

28. Olfson, M., and S.C. Marcus. 2009. National patterns in antidepressant medication treatment. *Arch Gen Psychiatry* 66(8):848-56.

29. Jahnke, R. 2006. Physiology of qigong, tai chi, and yoga. In Rakel, D.P., and N. Faass, eds. *Complementary Medicine in Clinical Practice*. Sudbury, MA: Jones and Bartlett, 133-43.

30. Larkey, L., R. Jahnke, J. Etnier, et al. 2009. Meditative movement as a category of exercise: Implications for research. *J Phys Act Health* 6(2):230-38.

31. Jahnke, R., L. Larkey, C. Rogers, et al. 2010. A comprehensive review of health benefits of qigong and tai chi. *Am J Health Promot* 24(6):e1-e25.

32. Field, T. 2011. Yoga clinical research review. *Complement Ther Clin Pract* 17(1):1-8.

33. Pineau, T.R., C.R. Glass, and K.A. Kaufman. 2014. Mindfulness in sport performance. In Ie A., C.T. Ngnoumen, and E.J. Langer, eds. *The Wiley Blackwell Handbook of Mindfulness*. Oxford: John Wiley & Sons, 1004-33.

34. Gavin, J. 2007. The body-mind cube: How to make any exercise program mindful. *IDEA Fitness Journal* 4(9):99.

Chapter 5

1. McGinnis, J.M. 2001. United States. In Koop, C.E., C.E. Pearson, and M.R. Schwarz, eds. *Critical Issues in Global Health*. San Francisco: Jossey-Bass, 80-90.

2. Chakravarti, A., and P. Little. 2003. Nature, nurture and human disease. *Nature* 421(6921):412-14.

3. U.S. Environmental Protection Agency. 2008. EPA's 2008 report on the environment. National Center for Environmental Assessment, Washington, D.C.: U.S. Environmental Protection Agency. EPA/600/R-07/045F.

4. Bearer, C.F. 1995. Environmental health hazards: How children are different from adults. *Future Child* 5(2):11-26.

5. Gavidia, T.G., J.P. de Garbino, and P.D. Sly. 2009. Children's environmental health: An under-recognised area in paediatric health care. *BMC Pediatrics* 9:10.

6. U.S. Environmental Protection Agency. 1992. Respiratory health effects of passive smoking: Lung cancer and other disorders. Washington, D.C.: U.S. Environmental Protection Agency. EPA/600/6-90/006F.

7. U.S. Department of Health and Human Services. 2006. The health consequences of involuntary exposure to tobacco smoke: A report of the Surgeon General. Atlanta, GA: U.S. Department of Health and Human Services, Centers for Disease Control and Prevention, Coordinating Center for Health Promotion, National Center for Chronic Disease Prevention and Health Promotion.

8. Lewtas, J. 2007. Air pollution combustion emissions: Characterization of causative agents and mechanisms associated with cancer, reproductive, and cardiovascular effects. *Mutat Res* 636(1):95-133.

9. Pope III, C.A., D.V. Bates, and M.E. Raizenne. 1995. Health effects of particulate air pollution: Time for reassessment? *Environ Health Perspect* 103(5):472-80.

10. Morris, R.D. 1995. Drinking water and cancer. *Environ Health Perspect* 103(Suppl 8):225-31.

11. Morris, R.D., A.M. Audet, I.F. Angelillo, et al. 1992. Chlorination, chlorination by-products, and cancer: A meta-analysis. *Am J Public Health* 82(7):955-63.

12. Gopal, K., S.S. Tripathy, J.L. Bersillon, et al. 2007. Chlorination byproducts, their toxicodynamics and removal from drinking water. *J Hazard Mater* 140(1):1-6.

13. Järup, L. 2003. Hazards of heavy metal contamination. *Br Med Bull* 68:167-82.

14. Zhang, X., T. Zhong, L. Liu, et al. 2015. Impact of soil heavy metal pollution on food safety in China. *PLoS ONE* 10(8):e0135182.

15. Mäder, P., A. Fliessbach, D. Dubois, et al. 2002. Soil fertility and biodiversity in organic farming. *Science* 296(5573):1694-97.

16. Bengtsson, J., J. Ahnström, and A.C. Weibull. 2005. The effects of organic agriculture on biodiversity and abundance: A meta-analysis. *J Appl Ecol* 42(2):261-69.

17. Ahlbom, I.C., E. Cardis, A. Green, et al. 2001. Review of the epidemiologic literature on EMF and health. *Environ Health Perspect* 109(Suppl 6):911-33.

18. International Agency for Research on Cancer. 2002. Non-ionizing radiation, Part I: Static and extremely low-frequency (ELF) electric and magnetic fields. *IARC Monographs on the Evaluation of Carcinogenic Risks to Humans*, Volume 80. Lyon: IARCPress.

19. Gifford, R. 2014. Environmental psychology matters. *Annu Rev Psychol* 65:541-79.

20. Oishi, S. 2014. Socioecological psychology. *Annu Rev Psychol* 65:581-609.

21. Cooper, R.F.D., C. Boyko, and R. Codinhoto. 2010. The effect of the physical environment on mental well-being. In Cooper C.L., J. Field, U. Goswami, et al., eds. *Mental Capital and Wellbeing.* West Sussex: Wiley-Blackwell, 967-1006.

22. Vischer, J.C. 2007. The effects of the physical environment on job performance: Towards a theoretical model of workspace stress. *Stress and Health* 23(3):175-84.

23. Woo, J.M., and T.T. Postolache. 2008. The impact of work environment on mood disorders and suicide: Evidence and implications. *Int J Disabil Hum Dev* 7(2):185-200.

24. Karasek, R., and T. Theorell. 1990. *Healthy Work: Stress, Productivity, and the Reconstruction of Working Life.* New York: Basic Books, 156.

25. Rich, M. 2002. Healthy hospital designs: Improving decor and layout can have impact on care; fewer fractures and infections. *The Wall Street Journal*, 27 November, B-1, B-4.

26. Devlin, A.S., and A.B. Arneill. 2003. Health care environments and patient outcomes: A review of the literature. *Environ Behav* 35(5):665-94.

27. Ulrich, R.S. 1991. Effects of interior design on wellness: Theory and recent scientific research. *J Health Care Inter Des* 3(1):97-109.

28. Frumkin, H. 2001. Beyond toxicity: Human health and the natural environment. *Am J Prev Med* 20(3):234-40.

29. Ryan, R.M., N. Weinstein, J. Bernstein, et al. 2010. Vitalizing effects of being outdoors and in nature. *J Environ Psychol* 30(2):159-68.

Chapter 6

1. Kaptchuk, T.J. 2000. *The Web That Has No Weaver.* 2nd ed. New York: McGraw-Hill, 47, 55-56.

2. Wild, C.P. 2005. Complementing the genome with an "exposome": The outstanding challenge of environmental exposure measurement in molecular epidemiology. *Cancer Epidemiol Biomarkers Prev* 14:1847-50.

3. Rappaport, S.M., and M.T. Smith. 2010. Environment and disease risks. *Science* 330(6003):460-61.

4. Alegría-Torres, J.A., A. Baccarelli, and V. Bollati. 2011. Epigenetics and lifestyle. *Epigenomics* 3(3):267-77.

5. Ornish, D., M.J.M. Magbanua, G. Weidner, et al. 2008. Changes in prostate gene expression in men undergoing an intensive nutrition and lifestyle intervention. *Proc Natl Acad Sci USA* 105(24):8369-74.

6. Ornish, D., L.W. Scherwitz, J.H. Billings, et al. 1998. Intensive lifestyle changes for reversal of coronary heart disease. *JAMA* 280(23):2001-07.

7. Fay, L.B., and J.B. German. 2008. Personalizing foods: Is genotype necessary? *Curr Opin Biotechnol* 19(2):121-28.

8. German, J.B., A.M. Zivkovic, D.C. Dallas, et al. 2011. Nutrigenomics and personalized diets: What will they mean for food? *Annu Rev Food Sci Technol* 2:97-123.

9. Minich, D.M., and J.S. Bland. 2013. Personalized lifestyle medicine: Relevance for nutrition and lifestyle recommendations. *Scientific World Journal* 2013.

Chapter 7

1. Anderson Jr, E.N. 1987. Why is humoral medicine so popular? *Soc Sci Med* 25(4):331-37.

2. Manderson, L. 1987. Hot-cold food and medical theories: Overview and introduction. *Soc Sci Med* 25(4):329-30.

3. Messer, E. 1981. Hot-cold classification: Theoretical and practical implications of a Mexican study. *Soc Sci Med Med Anthropol* 15B(2):133-45.

4. Jackson, W.A. 2001. A short guide to humoral medicine. *Trends Pharmacol Sci* 22(9):487-89.

5. Lad, V. 1984. *Ayurveda: The Science of Self-Healing.* Twin Lakes, WI: Lotus Press, 26.

6. Pool, R. 1987. Hot and cold as an explanatory model: The example of Bharuch district in Gujarat, India. *Soc Sci Med* 25(4):389-99.

7. Ni, L., X. Lin, and P. Rao. 2007. Validation of a mathematical model for determining the yin-yang nature of fruits. *Asia Pac J Clin Nutr* 16(Suppl 1):208-14.

8. Huang, C.J., and M.C. Wu. 2002. Differential effects of foods traditionally regarded as 'heating' and 'cooling' on prostaglandin E2 production by a macrophage cell line. *J Biomed Sci* 9(6):596-606.

9. Ou, B., D. Huang, M. Hampsch-Woodill, et al. 2003. When east meets west: The relationship between yin-yang and antioxidation-oxidation. *FASEB J* 17(2):127-29.

Chapter 8

Maciocia, G. 1995. *Tongue Diagnosis in Chinese Medicine.* 2nd ed. Seattle: Eastland Press.

1. Beinfield, H., and E. Korngold. 1991. *Between Heaven and Earth: A Guide to Chinese Medicine.* New York: Ballantine Books, 71-73.

Chapter 9

Beinfield, H., and E. Korngold. 1991. *Between Heaven and Earth: A Guide to Chinese Medicine.* New York: Ballantine Books.

Haas, E.M. 2003. *Staying Healthy With the Seasons.* 21st century ed. New York: Celestial Arts.

Kaptchuk, T.J. 2000. *The Web That Has No Weaver.* 2nd ed. New York: McGraw-Hill.

Pitchford, P. 2002. *Healing With Whole Foods: Asian Traditions and Modern Nutrition.* 3rd ed. Berkeley: North Atlantic Books.

Chapter 10

Haas, E.M. 2003. *Staying Healthy With the Seasons.* New York: Celestial Arts.

Kastner, J. 2004. *Chinese Nutrition Therapy.* Stuttgart, Germany: Thieme.

Leggett, D. 1999. *Recipes for Self-Healing.* Totnes, England: Meridian Press.

Leggett, D. 1994. *Helping Ourselves: A Guide to Traditional Chinese Food Energetics.* Totnes, England: Meridian Press.

Lind, M.B., and C. Hockman-Wert. 2009. *Simply in Season: A World Community Cookbook.* Harrisonburg, VA: Herald Press.

Lu, H.C. 1994. *Chinese Natural Cures: Traditional Methods for Remedies and Prevention.* New York: Black Dog and Leventhal Publishers.

Lu, H.C. 2000. *Chinese System of Foods for Health and Healing.* New York: Sterling Publishing.

Pitchford, P. 2002. *Healing With Whole Foods: Asian Traditions and Modern Nutrition.* 3rd ed. Berkeley: North Atlantic Books.

U.S. Department of Agriculture, Agricultural Research Service. 2010. USDA National Nutrient Database for Standard Reference, Release 23. Nutrient Data Laboratory Home Page. http://www.ars.usda.gov/ba/bhnrc/ndl

Walters, T. 2009. *Clean Food: A Seasonal Guide to Eating Close to the Source.* New York: Sterling Publishing.

Wood, R. 2010. *The New Whole Foods Encyclopedia.* New York: Penguin Books.

1. Amagase, H., B.L. Petesch, H. Matsuura, et al. 2001. Intake of garlic and its bioactive components. *J Nutr* 131(3):955S-62S.

2. Schäfer, G., and C.H. Kaschula. 2014. The immunomodulation and anti-inflammatory effects of garlic organosulfur compounds in cancer chemoprevention. *Anticancer Agents Med Chem* 14(2):233-40.

3. Wasser, S.P. 2002. Medicinal mushrooms as a source of antitumor and immunomodulating polysaccharides. *Appl Microbiol Biotechnol* 60(3):258-74.

4. Guaâdaoui, A., F. Bouhtit, and A. Hamal. 2015. The preventive approach of biocompounactives (1): A review in recent advances in common vegetables and legumes. *International Journal of Nutrition and Food Sciences* 4(1):89-102.

5. Kaur, C., and H.C. Kapoor. 2001. Antioxidants in fruits and vegetables – the millennium's health. *Int J Food Sci Tech* 36(7):703-25.

6. Kong, K.W., H.E. Khoo, K.N. Prasad, et al. 2010. Revealing the power of the natural red pigment lycopene. *Molecules* 15(2):959-87.

7. Mazza, G. 2007. Anthocyanins and heart health. *Ann Ist Super Sanità* 43(4):369-74.

8. Fraser, P.D., and P.M. Bramley. 2004. The biosynthesis and nutritional uses of carotenoids. *Prog Lipid Res* 43(3):228-65.

9. Krzyzanowska, J., A. Czubacka, and W. Oleszek. 2010. Dietary phytochemicals and human health. In Giardi, M.T., G. Rea, and B. Berra, eds. *Bio-Farms for Nutraceuticals: Functional Food and Safety Control by Biosensors.* New York: Springer, 74-98.

10. İnanç, A.L. 2011. Chlorophyll: Structural properties, health benefits and its occurrence in virgin olive oils. *Akademik Gida* 9(2):26-32.

11. Maiani, G., M.J.P. Castón, G. Catasta, et al. 2009. Carotenoids: Actual knowledge on food sources, intakes, stability and bioavailability and their protective role in humans. *Mol Nutr Food Res* 53(S2):S194-S218.

12. He, J., and M.M. Giusti. 2010. Anthocyanins: Natural colorants with health-promoting properties. *Annu Rev Food Sci Technol* 1:163-87.

13. Liu, R.H. 2003. Health benefits of fruit and

vegetables are from additive and synergistic combinations of phytochemicals. *Am J Clin Nutr* 78(3):517S-520S.

14. Borlinghaus, J., F. Albrecht, M.C.H. Gruhlke, et al. 2014. Allicin: Chemistry and biological properties. *Molecules* 19(8):12591-618.

15. Damalas, C.A., and I.G. Eleftherohorinos. 2011. Pesticide exposure, safety issues, and risk assessment indicators. *Int J Environ Res Public Health* 8(5):1402-19.

16. Gupta, S., and N. Abu-Ghannam. 2011. Bioactive potential and possible health effects of edible brown seaweeds. *Trends Food Sci Technol* 22(6):315-26.

17. Pitchford, P. 2002. *Healing With Whole Foods: Asian Traditions and Modern Nutrition.* 3rd ed. Berkeley: North Atlantic Books, 580-81.

18. Rajapakse, N., and S.K. Kim. 2011. Nutritional and digestive health benefits of seaweed. *Adv Food Nutr Res* 64:17-28.

19. Uzogara, S.G. 2000. The impact of genetic modification of human foods in the 21st century: A review. *Biotechnol Adv* 18(3):179-206.

20. Whitman, D.B. 2000. Genetically modified foods: Harmful or helpful? *Cambridge Scientific Abstracts Discovery Guides* 2000:1-13.

21. Benbrook, C.M. 2012. Impacts of genetically engineered crops on pesticide use in the U.S. – the first sixteen years. *Environmental Sciences Europe* 24(1):1-13.

22. Pitchford, P. 2002. *Healing With Whole Foods: Asian Traditions and Modern Nutrition.* 3rd ed. Berkeley: North Atlantic Books, 19-21.

23. Castellini, C., C. Mugnai, and A. Dal Bosco. 2002. Effect of organic production system on broiler carcass and meat quality. *Meat Sci* 60(3):219-25.

24. Lebret, B. 2008. Effects of feeding and rearing systems on growth, carcass composition and meat quality in pigs. *Animal* 2(10):1548-58.

25. Hansson, I., C. Hamilton, T. Ekman, et al. 2000. Carcass quality in certified organic production compared with conventional livestock production. *J Vet Med Series B* 47(2):111-20.

26. Daley, C.A., A. Abbott, P.S. Doyle, et al. 2010. A review of fatty acid profiles and antioxidant content in grass-fed and grain-fed beef. *Nutr J* 9:10.

27. Nuernberg, K., G. Nuernberg, K. Ender, et al. 2005. Effect of grass vs. concentrate feeding on the fatty acid profile of different fat depots in lambs. *Eur J Lipid Sci Technol* 107(10):737-45.

28. Hites, R.A., J.A. Foran, D.O. Carpenter, et al. 2004. Global assessment of organic contaminants in farmed salmon. *Science* 303(5655):226-29.

29. Valenzuela A., J. Sanhueza, and S. Nieto. 2003. Cholesterol oxidation: Health hazard and the role of antioxidants in prevention. *Biol Res* 36:291-302.

30. Staprans, I., X.M. Pan, J.H. Rapp, et al. 2005. The role of dietary oxidized cholesterol and oxidized fatty acids in the development of atherosclerosis. *Mol Nutr Food Res* 49:1075-82.

31. Siri-Tarino, P.W., Q. Sun, F.B. Hu, et al. 2010. Saturated fatty acids and risk of coronary heart disease: Modulation by replacement nutrients. *Curr Atheroscler Rep* 12(6):384-90.

32. Michas, G., R. Micha, and A. Zampelas. 2014. Dietary fats and cardiovascular disease: Putting together the pieces of a complicated puzzle. *Atherosclerosis* 234(2):320-28.

33. Siri-Tarino, P.W., Q. Sun, F.B. Hu, et al. 2010. Meta-analysis of prospective cohort studies evaluating the association of saturated fat with cardiovascular disease. *Am J Clin Nutr* 91(3):535-46.

34. Dehghan, M., A. Mente, X. Zhang, et al. 2017. Associations of fats and carbohydrate intake with cardiovascular disease and mortality in 18 countries from five continents (PURE): a prospective cohort study. *Lancet* 390(10107):2050-62.

35. Pitchford, P. 2002. *Healing With Whole Foods: Asian Traditions and Modern Nutrition*. 3rd ed. Berkeley: North Atlantic Books, 180-81.

36. Choe, E., and D.B. Min. 2006. Mechanisms and factors for edible oil oxidation. *Compr Rev Food Sci Food Saf* 5(4):169-86.

37. Malik, V.S., M.B. Schulze, and F.B. Hu. 2006. Intake of sugar-sweetened beverages and weight gain: A systematic review. *Am J Clin Nutr* 84:274-88.

38. Vartanian, L.R., M.B. Schwartz, and K.D. Brownell. 2007. Effects of soft drink consumption on nutrition and health: A systematic review and meta-analysis. *Am J Public Health* 97:667-75.

39. Fung, T.T., V. Malik, K.M. Rexrode, et al. 2009. Sweetened beverage consumption and risk of coronary heart disease in women. *Am J Clin Nutr* 89:1037-42.

Acknowledgments

We are grateful to our families, friends, patients, and all those who have assisted and supported us throughout the writing of this book. We would also like to thank the following people for helping us to realize our vision: our editor, Tom Pold, for his keen eye and guidance, Gary Tooth for his elegant book design, Narda Lebo for her beautiful illustrations, Beth Miller, and Stephen Callahan.

Index

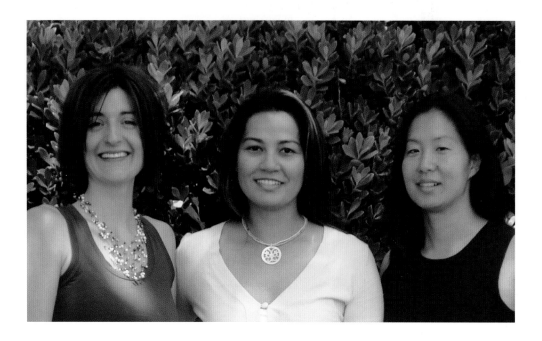

Brielle Kelly is a licensed acupuncturist in California and New York and is a nationally board certified Diplomate of Oriental Medicine (NCCAOM). She also has a certification in Applied Clinical Nutrition. Brielle has previously held professorships at Mercy College and the Swedish Institute in New York City. With over 15 years of clinical experience, she runs a successful acupuncture and holistic health care practice which specializes in the use of whole food nutritional therapies and traditional herbal remedies. For more information, please visit www.yinfinitewellness.com. Brielle lives with her wife, two sons, and dog in the San Francisco Bay Area.

Cherisse Godwin has a Bachelor of Social Work from the University of Hawaii and is a graduate of Tante Marie's Cooking School in San Francisco. She received a Healing with Whole Foods Certification from the Heartwood Institute in California, where she studied with renowned Traditional Chinese Medicine and nutrition author Paul Pitchford. Cherisse has worked in community outreach programs that promote disease prevention and healthy lifestyles. Her home is on the island of Kauai, where she lives with her husband and daughter.

Kristy Hsiao has a Bachelor of Science from Johns Hopkins University and is a graduate of the California Culinary Academy in San Francisco. She also received a Healing with Whole Foods Certification from the Heartwood Institute in California. Her professional experience includes work in the engineering, pharmaceutical, and food industries. As a second-generation Taiwanese American, Kristy is interested in reclaiming healing traditions and dietary therapies from her ancestry.

www.whatsyourseason.com